THIRD EDITION

DENTAL ASSISTING

Instruments & Materials Guide

Pat Norman
Donna Phinney
Judy Halstead

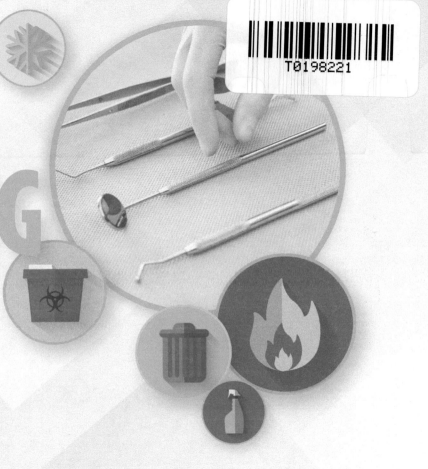

THIRD EDITION

DENTAL ASSISTING

Instruments & Materials Guide

Pat Norman
Donna Phinney
Judy Halstead

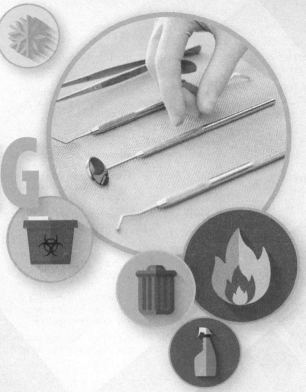

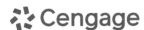 Cengage

Australia · Brazil · Canada · Mexico · Singapore · United Kingdom · United States

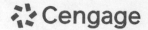

Dental Assisting Instruments & Materials Guide, Third Edition

Pat Norman, Donna Phinney, Judy Halstead

SVP, Higher Education & Skills Product: Erin Joyner

Product Director: Jason Fremder

Product Manager: Lauren Whalen

Product Assistant: Dallas Wilkes

Content Manager: Anubhav Kaushal, MPS Limited

Digital Delivery Lead: David O'Connor

Sr. Director, Marketing: Sean Chamberland

Marketing Manager: Courtney Cozzy

IP Analyst: Ashley Maynard

IP Project Manager: Kelli Besse

Production Service: MPS Limited

Sr. Art Director: Angela Sheehan

Cover Image Source: iStockPhoto.com/izusek

Interior image Source: GrooveZ/ShutterStock.com

For product information and technology assistance, contact us at **Cengage Customer & Sales Support, 1-800-354-9706** or **support.cengage.com**.
For permission to use material from this text or product, submit all requests online at **www.copyright.com**.

Library of Congress Control Number: 2021931702

ISBN: 978-0-357-45740-5

Cengage
5191 Natorp Boulevard
Mason, OH 45040
USA

Cengage is a leading provider of customized learning solutions. Our employees reside in nearly 40 different countries and serve digital learners in 165 countries around the world. Find your local representative at: **www.cengage.com**.

To learn more about Cengage platforms and services, register or access your online learning solution, or purchase materials for your course, visit **www.cengage.com**.

Printed in the United States of America

Print Number: 04   Print Year: 2024

CONTENTS

PREFACE

Dental instruments and materials are continually developing and changing as technology advances and clinical needs arise. Manufacturers of dental instruments provide many designs and sizes and are continually making improvements as new procedures and materials become available. Dentists select instruments and materials they feel the most confident and comfortable using when working with patients. Each procedure requires special instruments and materials to accomplish the task.

Many types of instruments and materials are used in the dental office. Examples include instruments and materials used in dental hygiene; diagnostic and restorative procedures; endodontic, oral maxillofacial surgery, implants, orthodontic, pedodontic, fixed and removable prosthodontic specialties; disinfection and sterilization of instruments and equipment; and laboratory settings. Having a comprehensive grasp of the instruments and materials used is beneficial for patient education and protection.

The dental assistant is responsible for
- keeping the instruments sterilized and in working condition
- ordering new instruments as needed
- keeping the instruments in sequence while assisting during procedures
- sterilizing and maintaining instruments
- knowing all the materials used in the dental office
- ordering, stocking, preparing, and mixing materials

This third edition of *Dental Assisting Instruments and Materials Guide* is designed to give dental assistants the basic knowledge necessary in relationship to each instrument and material presented. The instruments and materials are categorized in groupings that follow basic dental procedures in general and specialty dentistry. This allows students to easily study similar information. Students are able to view each instrument and learn its uses, parts, and other miscellaneous information. In addition, students will learn the use, composition, properties, Occupational Safety and Health Administration (OSHA) properties, mixing and setting times, and directions for each material associated within that section. There are too many different brands of each material to include in one text but we tried to include a variety of materials for dental assistants to gain an understanding of the basics so they can use this information and apply it to any brand name. The guide also covers sterilization equipment, solutions, and monitors.

Students will find this guide to be a helpful tool in their educational learning process in addition to their main textbook and clinic/laboratory experience.

New to This Edition
Updates have been made throughout the text to address changes in instruments and equipment.

Chapter 1
- Chapter renamed: Properties and Care of Dental Instruments
- Added information and images of precleaning, disinfecting, and sterilizing solutions

Chapter 2
- Updated images and information

Chapter 3
- Added coverage and images of the following: evacuator screens, air-water syringe, saliva ejectors, and water-line treatments
- Updated images and information

Chapter 4
- Updated images and information

Chapter 5
- Added numbers to clamps
- Updated images and information

Chapter 6
- Updated and added images and information

Chapter 7
- Updated images and information

Chapter 8
- Combined information about Black's numbering system

Chapter 9
- Added information and images on caries detectors/indicators solutions, desensitizers, relief gel, varnish, liners and low-strength bases, and core build-up materials
- Updated images

Chapter 10
- Added information and images on amalgam bonding agents, amalgam restorative materials, and best practices for handling amalgam and waste and its disposal
- Updated and added images

Chapter 11
- Added information on composite shade guides and composite polishers
- Updated and added images
- Added information and images on etching and bonding materials
- Added information and images on composite, compomer, and glass ionomer restorative materials

Chapter 12
- Added information and images on tooth slooth, glass bead sterilizers, and Bunsen burners
- Added information and images on sodium hypochlorite, formo cresol, root canal lubricant, and sealer
- Added information and images on temporary restoration materials
- Updated and added images

Chapter 13
- Added coverage of dry-socket materials

Chapter 14
- Combined content where appropriate

- Added information and images on alginate, alginate substitute, and impression material flavorings
- Added information and images on supplies needed: bowls, spatulas, and impression trays
- Added information and images on waxes and cement materials

Chapter 15
- Added information and images on preventive materials: pit and fissure sealants, prophy paste, and fluoride
- Added information and images on in-office and at-home whitening solutions
- Added information on tray setup for application of dental sealants

Chapter 16
- Added information and images on Florida periodontal probe system and periodontal dressing
- Updated and added images

Chapter 17
- Added information and images on bite registration materials and wax materials
- Added information and images on impression trays

- Added information and images on final impression materials
- Added information and images on temporary crown acrylic and materials
- Added information on temporary and permanent cementation materials

Chapter 18
- New chapter focusing on implant systems; content formerly combined with Chapter 16
- Added information and images on implant supplies and instruments

Chapter 19
- Updated images

Chapter 20
- Added information and images on plaster and stone
- Added information and images on pumice, laboratory waxes, thermoplastic, custom tray, and vacuum-forming materials

Chapter 21
- Added information and images of Scan X Digital

DESCRIPTION OF ICONS

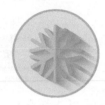 **Heat Sterilization**

 **Cold Sterilization**

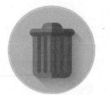 **Disposable**

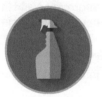 **Disinfect**

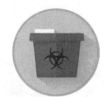 **Sharps Container**

ACCOMPANYING TEACHING AND LEARNING RESOURCES

Online Instructor Companion Website
An online Instructor's Manual accompanies this book. It contains information to assist instructors in designing the course, including a test bank powered by Cognero®, PowerPoint Lecture slides, and an Image gallery. Sign up or sign in at http://www.cengage.com to search for and access this product and its online resources.

PowerPoint Lecture® Slides
These vibrant Microsoft® PowerPoint lecture slides for each chapter assist you with your lecture by providing concept coverage using images, figures, and tables directly from the textbook!

Cengage Testing Powered by Cognero
Cengage Learning Testing Powered by Cognero is a flexible online system that allows you to author, edit, and manage test bank content from multiple Cengage solutions; create multiple test versions in an instant; and deliver tests from your learning management system, your classroom, or wherever you want.

ACKNOWLEDGMENTS

I want to thank those who encouraged and motivated me to update and develop this instrument and materials guide. Donna Phinney and Judy Halstead have been the most inspirational and motivational mentors I could have ever asked for. They encouraged and molded me through my education and career in dentistry. Thanks to my students for asking us to develop better ways to learn and remember instruments and materials that are used in dental procedures. Each year, students' quest for knowledge becomes more creative and inventive. A quick reference is necessary in the busy lives of students who must fit so many things into their schedules. My goal was a quick reference to meet their needs.

I would like to thank Cengage and its staff, including Senior Project Managers Anubhav Kaushal and Jenny Ziegler, and Product Manager Lauren Whalen, whose assistance and encouragement in this project are greatly appreciated.

Last, but never least, I would like to thank my husband, Jim, and my family, for their continued support throughout all of our endeavors.

REVIEWERS

Kelli Haskin, Genesis Career College
Julie Kupfer, Century College
Maria Martin, Southeastern Vocational Regional High School
Colleen Mee, Ross Medical Education Center
Donna Pruitt, Alamance Community College
Lori Scribner, ATA Career Education
Kim Turner, Vista College Fort Smith

CHAPTER 1

Properties and Care of Dental Instruments

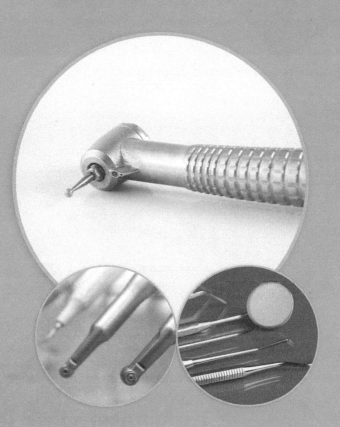

Basic Structural Parts and Working Ends of Dental Instruments

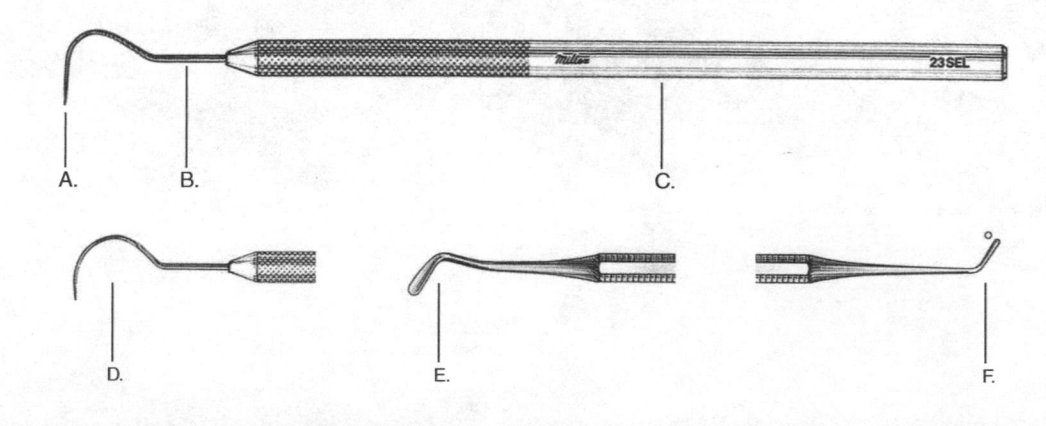

Use

Dental instruments are used to accomplish a variety of tasks. Each procedure requires special instruments for its unique tasks. Most instruments are constructed of stainless steel, high-tech plastic/resin, or anodized aluminum. The working end of an instrument performs the specific function of the instrument.

Properties

A. Working end
B. Shank
C. Handle

The working end may be a point, blade, or nib.

D. The point is sharp and is used to explore, detect, and reflect materials.
E. The blade may be flat or curved and may have a rounded or cutting edge.
F. The nib is a blunt end that may be serrated or smooth.

Notes

There are single- and double-ended instruments. On some double-ended instruments the primary working end is marked with an indented ring around the shank or the handle.

Ergonomically Designed Handles

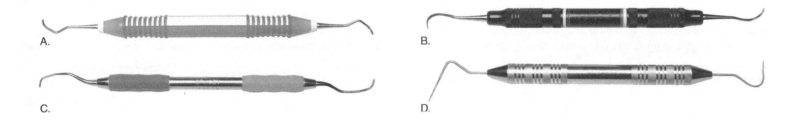

A.

B.

C.

D.

Use	The handle or shaft of an instrument is where the instrument is held by the operator. Some handles are ergonomically designed for easier handling and better grip.
Notes	• In traditional instruments, handles may be smooth, serrated, round, or hexagonal (six-sided). Some may have cone socket handles that allow the working ends to be replaced. • Ergonomic handles may be larger and designed with rests and grooves. • Some handles are covered with a soft, rubber-like material for more comfortable handling. • Handles are made of lightweight, sterilizable materials.

The Shank

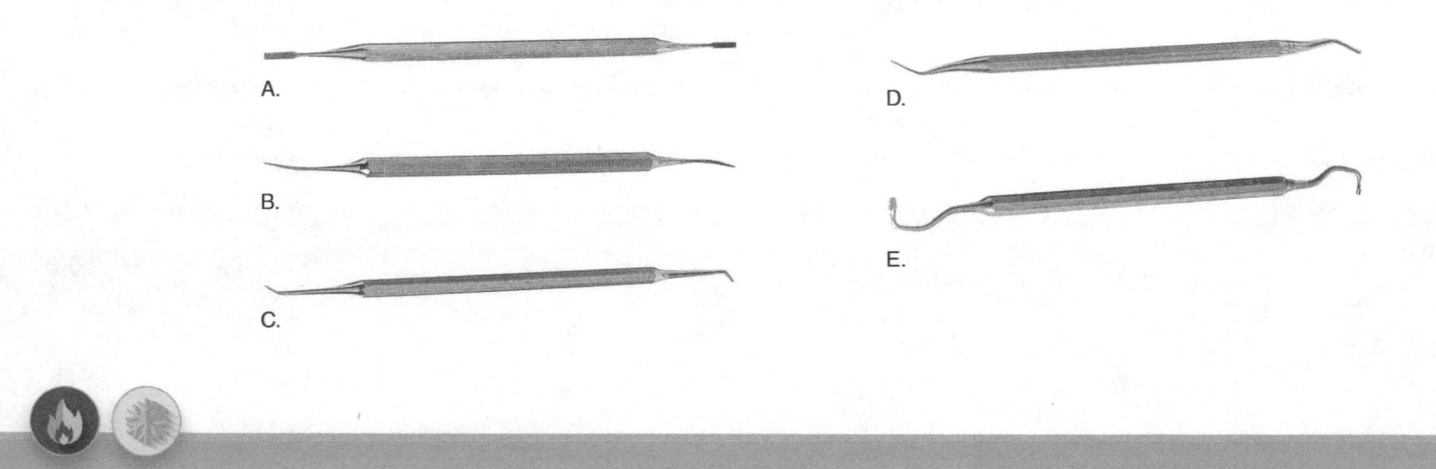

A.

B.

C.

D.

E.

Use   The shank connects the handle to the working end. It narrows or tapers from the handle to the working end. The shank may be angled to reach different areas of the mouth. Instruments that are used in the posterior regions of the mouth have more angles, whereas straighter or slightly curved instruments are used in the anterior regions.

Properties   **A.** Straight (no angles)
            B. Curved (slightly curved)
            C. Monangle (one angle)
            D. Binangle (two angles)
            E. Triple angle (three angles)

Color Coding

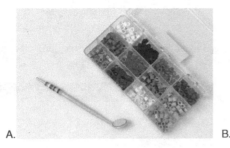

A.

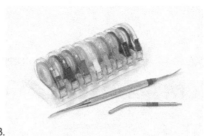

B.

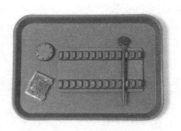

C.

Use	Color coding is a method used to easily identify instruments, tubs, and trays. Color coding may be used to indicate the sequence of a procedure, sets of instruments for specific procedures, treatment rooms where instruments are stored, individual operators, or any combination of these.
Properties	There are many types of materials used for color coding, including: **A.** Plastic rings. **B.** Tape. **C.** Color-coded tray, mouth mirror, bur block, tray mat, and plastic rings. (Color-coded tubs and various-size trays are also available.)
Notes	Materials used for color coding must be autoclavable and durable.

Dental Precleaners, Disinfectants, and Sterilants

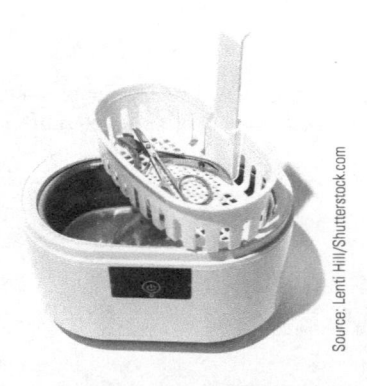

Source: Lenti Hill/Shutterstock.com

Use	• Used for cleaning and removing bioburden from instruments prior to disinfection and sterilization
Composition	• Proteolytic enzyme detergent
	• Concentrated formula
Properties	• Machine uses solution by cavitation.
	• Noncorrosive, nonammoniated, and nonsudsing solutions.
	• Solution available in different types.

Type I:	General purpose
	Dilution: 1 part solution to 10 parts water
Type III:	Plaster and stone remover: no dilution
Type IV:	Tarter and stain remover: no dilution
Type VI:	Temporary cement remover: no dilution

• Solution changed when cloudy.

Ultrasonic Machine and Cleaners

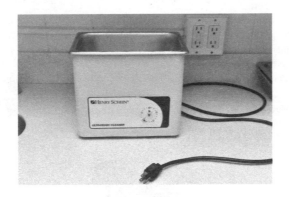

Precautions   Use appropriate personal protective equipment (PPE) and follow all Occupational Safety and Health (OSHA) guidelines.
1. Glasses
2. Mask
3. Heavy utility gloves

Directions

1. Dilute 1 part solution to 10 parts water into a clean ultrasonic cleaner.
2. Submerge the basket containing the contaminated instruments in the solution.
3. Place the lid on ultrasonic cleaner and set the timer for 2 to 10 minutes to remove debris.
4. Remove the lid and the basket of instruments and rinse thoroughly under warm water for 30 seconds.
5. Dispense instruments onto towel, blot dry, and separate instruments for cold/heat sterilization.

Banicide Plus®

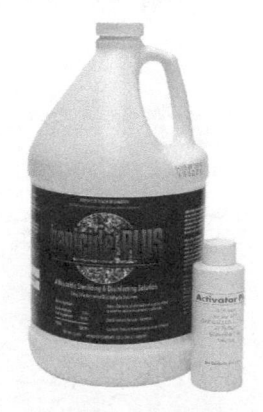

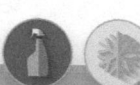

Use	• Used for cold sterilization and high-level disinfection
Composition	• Active ingredient: 3.4% glutaraldehyde
Properties	• Requires the addition of an activator prior to use. • Additional additives guard against corrosion. • Mint-scented. • Banicide may be used as a sterilant/high-level disinfectant for up to 28 days after initial use.

- Store at 24°C or 75.2°F.
- Can be deactivated with 850 g of glycine for disposal down drains.
- Sterilant: Submerge instruments for 10 hours.
- High-level disinfectant: Submerge instruments for at least 90 minutes.

Banicide Plus® *Continued*

Precautions Use appropriate PPE and follow all OSHA guidelines.
- Ingestion: It may cause irritation and possibly chemical burns of the mouth, throat, stomach, and esophagus.
- Eyes: Contact with the solution may cause damage to the eyes, including severe corneal injury, which may cause permanent impairment of vision. Vapors may cause stinging sensation in the eyes.
- Skin: Direct contact with the solution may cause skin irritation or aggravation of existing dermatitis. Skin may turn yellow or brown, which is harmless.
- Inhalation: Vapor is irritating to the respiratory tract.
- Ventilation and skin and eye protection should be used.

Directions

1. Open the screw lid on the gallon container and the activator.
2. Pour the activator into the plastic gallon container.
3. Place the lid back on the gallon container and move it to incorporate the activation into the entire solution.
4. Make a note of the date that the activator was placed in the container either on the bottle or somewhere close by. It is advisable to make such as note on any sterilizing or disinfecting tub/tray that is being used.
5. The solution is ready to use for 28 days.

Biocide G30™

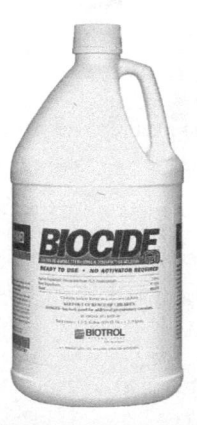

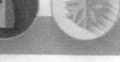
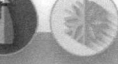

Use
- Used for cold sterilization and high-level disinfection
- Reusable for 30 days for sterilization and disinfection

Composition
- Active ingredient: 2.65% acidic glutaraldehyde

Properties
- Ready to use, no chemical activator required.
- Contains a rust inhibitor to protect instruments.
- Active for 30 days.
- Lemon-scented.
- Sterilant: Submerge instruments for 10 hours.
- High-level disinfectant: Submerge instruments for at least 45 minutes.

Precautions Use appropriate PPE and follow all OSHA guidelines.
- Ingestion: Contact with solution may cause irritation and possibly chemical burns.
- Eyes: Contact with solution may cause damage, including severe corneal injury, which could permanently impair vision. Vapors may cause a stinging sensation in the eyes.
- Skin: Direct contact with the solution may cause skin irritation or aggravation of existing dermatitis. Skin may turn yellow or brown, which is harmless.
- Inhalation: Vapor is irritating to the respiratory tract.
- Ventilation and skin and eye protection should be used.

Biocide G30™ *Continued*

Directions

1. The solution is ready to use.
2. Pour the solution into the disinfecting/sterilizing tub/tray directly from the gallon container.
3. Place a note on the container about when the solution was first used. Also make a note on the disinfecting/sterilizing tub/tray to indicate when the solution was first used.
4. Solution is active for 30 days.

Birex™ SE

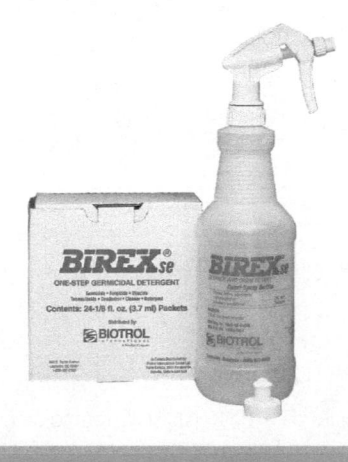

Use	• Broad-spectrum cleaner and antimicrobial, intermediate-level disinfectant for hard surfaces
Composition	• Phenylphenol • Phosphoric acid
Properties	• Complies with OSHA's BloodBorne Pathogen Standard and the CDC guidelines for intermediate-level disinfectants. • 14-day shelf life (after mixing). • Available in twenty-four 1/8-oz packets and spray bottle.

- Easy to store.
- 10-minute disinfecting contact time.
- Biodegradable.

Precautions Use appropriate PPE and follow all OSHA guidelines.
- Concentrate is corrosive to tissues.
- Dilution is slightly irritating to eyes.
- Concentrate is severely irritating to skin and eyes.
- It will cause an upset stomach.
- Chemical is listed as a carcinogen or potential carcinogen.

Birex™ SE   *Continued*

Directions

1. Fill water to the correct level in the quart spray bottle that comes with Birex.
2. Dispense one 1/8-oz packet into the water.
3. Label the spray bottle with the activation date.
4. Shake bottle slightly to evenly dispense the packet into the water.
5. It is ready to spray on hard surfaces for disinfecting in 10 minutes.

CaviWipes 1™

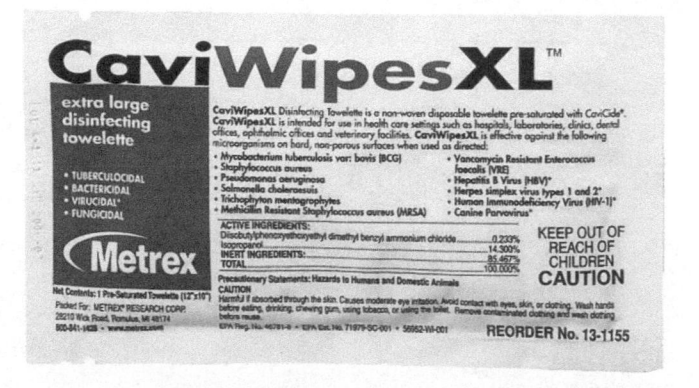

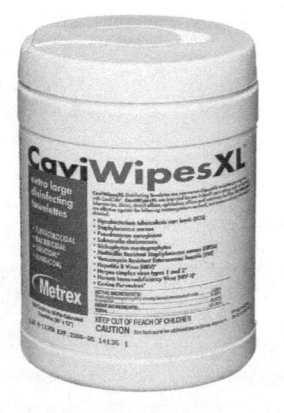

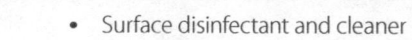

Use	• Surface disinfectant and cleaner
Composition	• Isopropanol
	• Ethylene glycol monobutyl ether
	• Diisobutyl phenoxy ethoxy ethyl dimethyl benzyl ammonium chloride
Properties	• Disposable towelettes presaturated with surface disinfectant.
	• Available in individually wrapped towelettes, XL (three times larger), or a dispensing canister.

- Nonwoven, nonabrasive towels.
- Recommended for all nonporous surfaces.
- A wall mount for the canister is available.
- 1- and 3-minute disinfectant available.

Precautions Use appropriate PPE and follow all OSHA guidelines.
- Skin: Not considered an irritant.
- Eyes: Contact with eyes can cause reversible damage.
- Inhalation: May cause mild irritation.

CaviWipes 1™ *Continued*

Directions

1. Pop-up center-hinged plastic lid.
2. Towelettes can be dispensed as a single sheet by tearing at the perforated line or by taking as many as needed before tearing at the perforated line.
3. Use one towelette to preclean the surface of debris, then dispose of the towelette.
4. Use a second towelette to wipe nonporous surfaces to disinfect; leave surface wet for 1 to 3 minutes depending on surface contact disinfectant used.

Cetylcide II

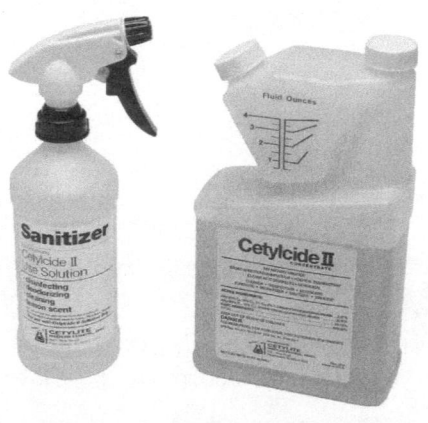

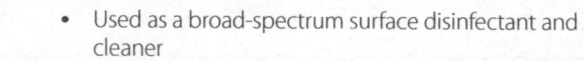

Use
- Used as a broad-spectrum surface disinfectant and cleaner

Composition
- Dual quaternary ammonium compound
- Sodium carbonate
- Tergitol NP-10
- Ethylenediaminetetraacetic acid

Properties
- Environmental Protection Agency (EPA)–registered broad-spectrum disinfectant.
- Complies with OSHA's BloodBorne Pathogen Standard.
- Environmentally safe/biodegradable.
- Lemon-scented.
- Tip and pour bottle for easy mixing.
- Each quart yields 16 gallons of solution.
- Biodegradable detergent with cleaning properties.
- No alcohol, bleach, iodophor, phenol, or glutaraldehyde.

Cetylcide II *Continued*

Precautions Use appropriate PPE and follow all OSHA guidelines.
- Eye: Corrosive and irritant; prolonged contact may cause corneal burns.
- Skin contact: Corrosive and irritant.
- Ingestion: May be fatal. Burning pain, swelling in digestive tract, paralysis, circulatory shock may occur.
- Inhalation: Will cause irritation of mucous membranes, coughing, and shortness of breath.
- Systemic and other effects: None reported.

Directions

1. Fill measuring device with 1/2 oz of concentrate.
2. Dispense concentrate into 1-quart spray bottle that comes with the solution or obtained separately.
3. Fill the quart bottle with water.
4. One-step cleaning and disinfecting.
5. 10-minute disinfecting contact time.

Coecide™ XL and Coecide™ XL Plus

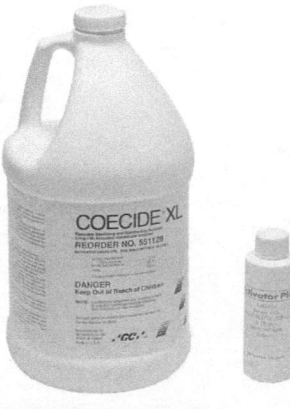

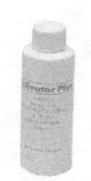

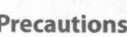

Use	• Used for sterilization, high-level disinfection, and intermediate-level disinfection
Composition	• Coecide™ XL: 2.5% alkaline glutaraldehyde • Coecide™ XL Plus: 3.4% alkaline glutaraldehyde
Properties	• Corrosion inhibitor. • Activator included. • EPA-registered for use and reuse up to 28 days after activation. • Can activate 1 quart at a time for economy.

• Sterilization: 10 hours at 25°C.
• High-level disinfection: 90 minutes at 25°C.

Precautions Use appropriate PPE and follow all OSHA guidelines.
• Acute and chronic: Avoid skin contact. Repeated contact with skin may cause sensitization in some people, resulting in allergic contact dermatitis. Moderate to severe irritation to skin, eyes, and mucous membranes. Low to mild irritation by inhalation. Toxic if ingested.
• Ventilation and skin and eye protection should be used.

Coecide™ XL and Coecide™ XL Plus *Continued*

Directions

1. Open the container top on both the activator and the solution.
2. Pour the activator into the solution.
3. Place the top on the solution and mix slightly to incorporate the activator thoroughly. Dispense into disinfecting tub/tray.
4. Write on the bottle the date of activation and/or on the disinfecting tub/tray to note the active duration of 28 days at 25°C.

MetriCide 28

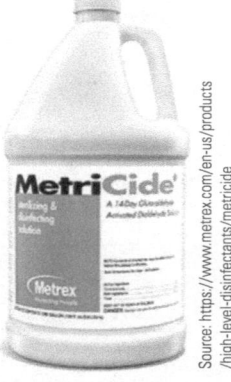

Source: https://www.metrex.com/en-us/products/high-level-disinfectants/metricide

Use	• High-level disinfectant or sterilant on immersible instruments
Composition	• 2.5% buffered glutaraldehyde
Properties	• Attains an alkaline pH of between 7.5 and 8.5. • Active up to 28 days at 25°C. • Sterilization: 10 hours at 25°C. • Disinfection: 90 minutes at 25°C.
Precautions	Use appropriate PPE and follow all OSHA guidelines.

• Skin: Mild to moderate irritation.
• Eye: Direct contact can cause irritation.
• Ingestion: Toxic.
• Inhalation: Low or mild irritation.

Directions

1. No dilution.

2. Place solution in the sterilizing/disinfecting tub/tray.

3. Immerse instruments in the solution.

4. Write the date of use on the disinfecting tray to note the active duration of 28 days at 25°C.

Sporox II

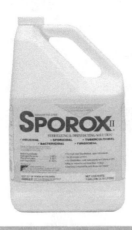

Use	• Sterilizing and high-level disinfecting solution
Composition	• Active ingredient: hydrogen peroxide 7.5%
Properties	• Ready to use; no mixing or activation required.
	• No noxious odors.
	• Oxidizes away dental debris and contaminants.
	• High-level disinfecting: 30 minutes at 20°C.
	• Sterilization: 6 hours at 20°C.
	• May be reused for up to 21 days.
Precautions	Use appropriate PPE and follow all OSHA guidelines.
	• Corrosive to eyes.

• May be harmful or fatal if swallowed.
• Do not get in eyes, on skin, or on clothing.
• Use safety glasses and gloves.

Directions

1. Place the solution in sterilizing/disinfecting tub/tray. No activation is required.
2. Immerse instruments in the solution.
3. Sterilization: 10 hours at 20°C.
4. Disinfection: 90 minutes at 20°C.
5. Write the date of use on the disinfecting/sterilizing tray to note the active duration of 21 days.

Procedure: Precleaning, Disinfecting, and Sterilizing Basic Dental Instruments

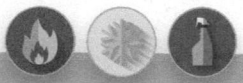

This procedure is performed by the dental assistant in the sterilization area. See Chapter 6 for cleaning, lubricating, and sterilizing handpieces and Chapter 7 for sterilization of burs.

Equipment and Supplies
- Ultrasonic unit ready with solution
- Disinfecting solution in spray bottle mixed and ready
- 4 × 4 and 2 × 2 gauze

Procedure: Precleaning, Disinfecting, and Sterilizing Basic Dental Instruments *Continued*

Directions

1. Review the Material Safety Data Sheet (MSDS) for all solutions.
2. Wear appropriate PPE.
3. Wash hands and pull on utility gloves.
4. Remove all disposable supplies and dispose of correctly in biohazard bag, sharps container, or nonregulated garbage can.
5. Submerge instruments in the ultrasonic solution for 2 to 10 minutes to removed biofilm.
6. While ultrasonic unit is running, use a surface disinfectant following manufacturer directions to disinfect tray, mats, material bottles, pens/pencils, and anything that cannot be placed in heat sterilization. All surfaces need to be sprayed and cleaned first, then wiped to remove debris. The surfaces are then sprayed a second time and the solution is left on surfaces for the time designated time by the manufacturer.
7. Once ultrasonic cleaning is complete, remove basket and rinse all instruments under warm water for 30 seconds.
8. Dispense instruments onto towel on the decontaminated area and pat dry.
9. Divide instruments for cold and heat sterilization as appropriate.
   a. Place heat-sterilized instruments into the autoclave.
   b. Place items that cannot be heat-sterilized into the cold sterile solution.
10. After the time has elapsed for spray disinfectant area, dry tray, mat, and any miscellaneous items used in procedure.
11. Disinfect all areas touched (control pads, counters, lids, etc.).
12. Remove glasses and mask, wash utility gloves, then remove utility gloves and wash hands.
13. Do not break aseptic technique.

CHAPTER 2
Disposables and Barriers

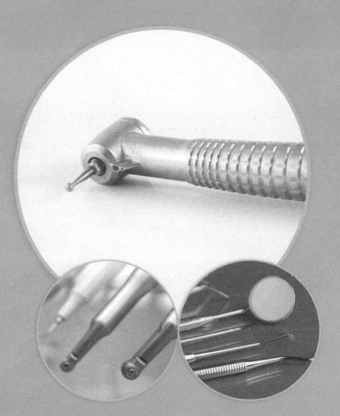

Micro Applicator and Brushes

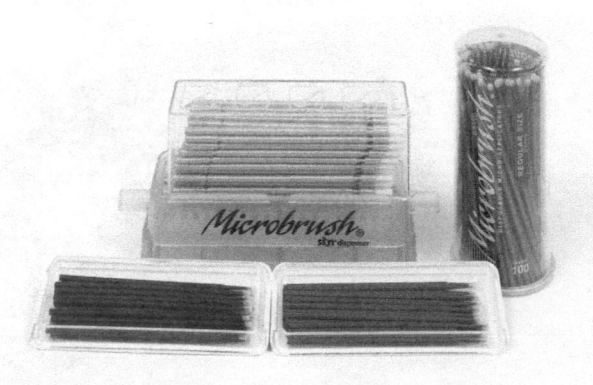

Use
- To place etchants
- To apply bonding agents
- To apply primer
- To apply sealants
- To apply varnishes
- To apply hemostatic solutions
- To get into those hard-to-reach areas

Properties Plastic handles with micro ball end of nonabsorbent fiber or bristled tip brushes.

Notes
- Instruments normally come with bendable neck to allow easy placement and precise application.
- Micro applicators are available in regular, fine, superfine, and ultrafine.
- Micro brush tips are available in fine or regular.
- Micro applicators and brushes are available in a variety of styles, sizes, and colors.
- Both micro applicators and brushes are disposable.

Cotton Rolls and Cotton Pellets

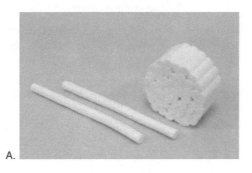

A.

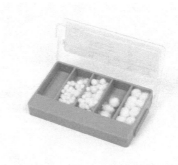

B.

Use

A. Cotton rolls are used in all procedures:
- to dry an area,
- for isolation.
- to provide a rest for the evacuation tip.
- to apply topical anesthetic.
- To retract tissues.

B. Cotton pellets are used to:
- dry tissues and tooth structures.
- place dental materials, such as cavity varnish.

Properties Cotton rolls are made of super absorbent and nonlinting cotton. They are either smooth or braided with silky yarn. Cotton pellets are small balls of absorbent cotton. Both cotton rolls and cotton pellets come in several sizes.

Notes
- Some cotton rolls are designed not to adhere to mucous membranes or sensitive tissues.
- Cotton rolls are available in different lengths and widths, both sterile and nonsterile.
- Cotton roll dispensers are available.
- Cotton pellets come in different sizes.
- Cotton pellet containers designed for easy dispensing are available.

Cotton-Tipped Applicators

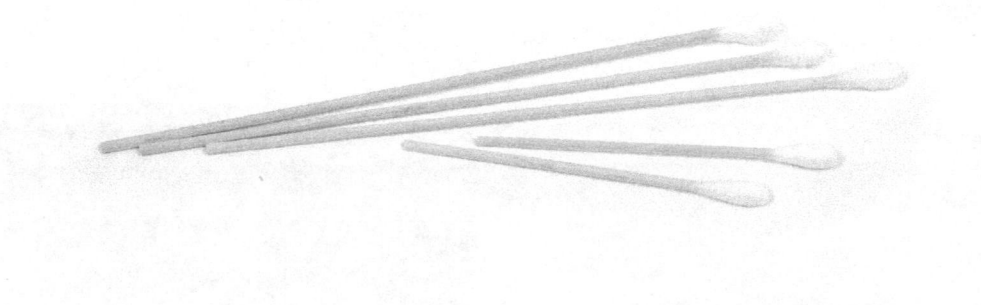

Use
- To dry and remove debris from the oral cavity and the tooth
- To apply lip lubricant
- To apply topical anesthetic or medication

Properties Wood handles with tightly wrapped cotton tips.

Notes
- Cotton-tipped applicators are available in 3-inch and 6-inch lengths.
- Some are sealed in autoclavable bags of 100 tips.
- These are disposable.

Gauze Sponges

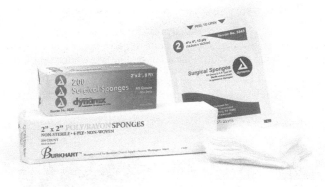

Use Gauze sponges have many functions, including their use in:
- Absorbing moisture.
- Retracting tissues such as the tongue, cheeks, and lips.
- Receiving debris or teeth/tooth fragments.
- Keeping instruments clean during a procedure.
- Applying pressure to a bleeding area.
- Disinfecting equipment, instruments, and the procedure area.

Properties Gauze sponges are folded pure virgin white cotton gauze; some are filled with 100 percent cotton fiber filling.

Notes
- Gauze sponges are available in various sizes (e.g., 2 × 2, 3 × 3, 4 × 4, and 5 × 5), and they come filled and unfilled.
- Nonwoven sponges, which are made of a rayon/polyester blend, are also available. These sponges are softer, very absorbent, and are less adhesive to the wound. The unfilled sponges come in 4, 8, and 12 ply (layers).
- Both sterile and nonsterile gauze sponges are available. They are usually purchased by the case but also can be purchased in individual presterilized packets of two cotton-filled sponges.

Face Masks and Shields Used in Dentistry

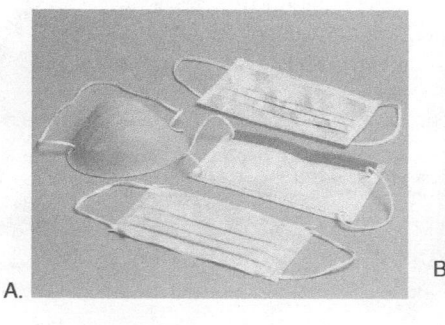

A.

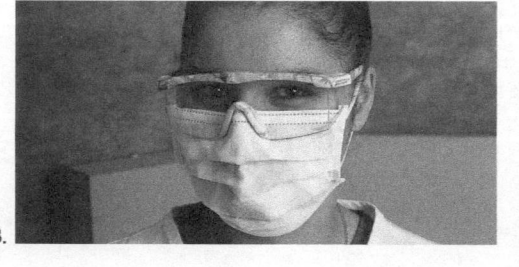

B.

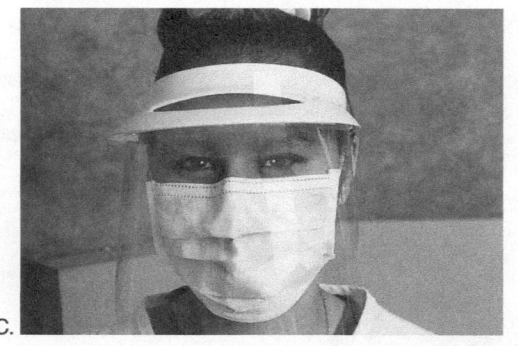

C.

Use   Face masks and shields are part of infection control techniques to prevent the spread of disease by protecting the dentist and dental auxiliary personnel from exposure to blood, debris, and dust while performing skills/tasks. Masks and shields also prevent cross-contamination between the dental team members and the patient.

Properties   One-piece masks are made of soft white, 3-ply, fluid-resistant, nonwoven fabric made from polypropylene. There are inner and outer layers designed to resist moisture and to prevent irritation for sensitive skin. These masks are secured in place with elastic loops that fit around the ears or with ties that tie in the back of the head. Other masks are molded and are constructed of several layers of fluid-resistant material. Most masks have a flexible aluminum nosepiece that secures the mask around the nose to prevent safety glasses from fogging.

Face Masks and Shields Used in Dentistry *Continued*

Disposable face shields are clear, distortion free, and fog free, and wrap around the face for protection. They are held in place by a soft or hard plastic headband.

A. Face masks in a variety of types, colors, and designs.

B. Face mask in place with eyewear.

C. Face mask in place with disposable face shield.

Notes
- Face masks should be worn with a disposable face shield or eyewear.
- Face masks are disposable.
- Face shields are disposable.

Protective Eyewear

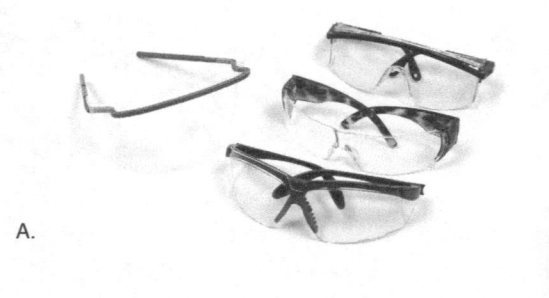

A.

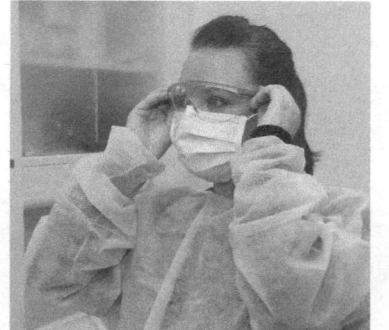

B.

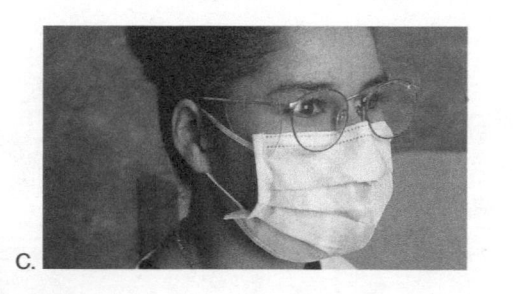

C.

Use Protective eyewear protects the eyes of the dentist, assistant, and patient from blood, saliva, and debris during dental treatment. Eyewear also offers protection from infectious diseases and aerosol droplets that may be transferred during treatment.

Properties Eye protection used in dentistry consists of eyeglass frames and lenses, which are usually made of lightweight plastic material.
  A. Examples of protective eyewear
  B. Eyewear on dental assistant
  C. Eyewear on dental assistant

Notes • Eyewear comes in many styles and colors and is often adjustable. All styles

- Anti-fog products are available to minimize fogging. Eyewear can be run under warm water to reduce fogging.
- If glasses are worn, side shields (Figure C) or goggles can be worn over them to ensure protection.
- The lenses of some eyewear are amber, gray, or dark; such eyewear is worn when the curing light is used during a procedure.
- Preassembled disposable eye shields are available.
- Eyewear needs to fit properly and be comfortable so that it can be worn for long periods of time.

Protective Gowns

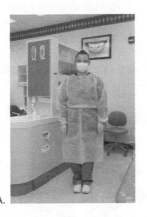
A.

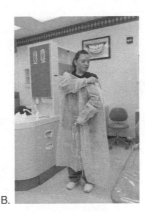
B.

Use   Gowns are used to cover clothing and protect from saliva, blood, debris, and fluids during dental treatment and sterilization procedures.

Properties   Disposable gowns are made with polyethylene or polypropylene; have long sleeves, often with elastic or knit cuffs; and are constructed to fit closely around the neck. The length can be jacket length, at the knee, or longer.
A. Example of disposable protective gown that is knee length.
B. Example of a dental assistant placing a protective gown.

Notes
- Gowns should be impervious to most liquids and aerosols.
- Gowns can be disposable or made from fabric for continued use.
- Both types are available in many colors and styles.
- Gowns should be changed daily or when contamination occurs.
- Gowns should be removed prior to leaving the dental office.

Examination Gloves

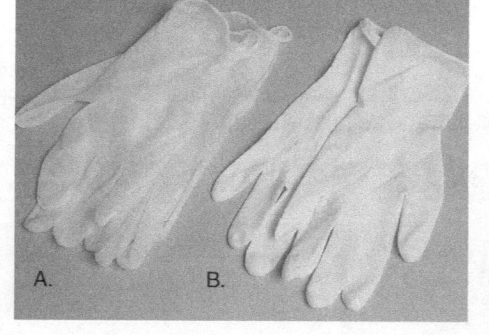

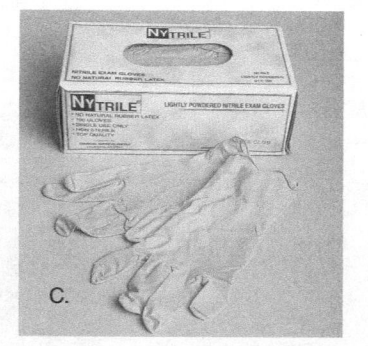

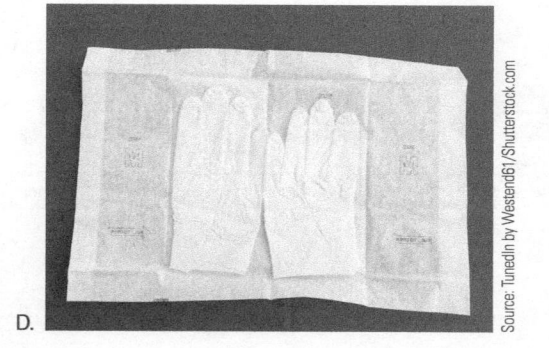

Source: Tunedln by Westend61/Shutterstock.com

Use Gloves are used as a barrier against microorganisms. Gloves are worn to protect dental team members from contact with saliva, blood, and debris.

Properties Examination gloves are made of several types of materials, including latex, nitrile, and vinyl. Gloves fit either the right or left hand and are powder free. They come in a variety of sizes, from extra small through extra large.
  A. Vinyl gloves
  B. Latex examination gloves
  C. Colored nitrile examination gloves
  D. Surgical gloves

Notes
- Some gloves are scented, and some offer more tactile sensitivity and a nonslip grip on the fingertips.
- Nitrile and vinyl gloves are designed for dental assistants and for use with patients with latex sensitivity or allergies.
- Gloves are available in nonsterile (worn for most dental treatment) and sterile (for surgical treatment) types.
- Gloves are worn over the cuffs of the protective gown.
- Gloves are purchased in boxes of 100.
- If gloves are penetrated or torn, or if the user leaves the area, the gloves should be removed, hands washed, and new gloves placed before treatment continues.

Overgloves and Utility Gloves

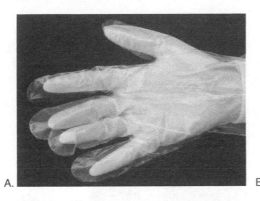

A.

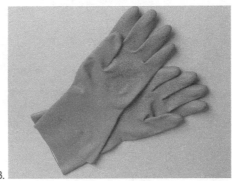

B.

Use   Overgloves are used to prevent cross-contamination. They are worn over examination gloves or alone when something outside the treatment area needs to be handled. An example would be holding a patient chart or if the assistant needs to retrieve an instrument from another area.

Utility gloves are used when disinfecting the dental unit and in the sterilizing area when cleaning and preparing instruments and trays for sterilization.

Properties A. Overgloves are clear polyethylene gloves that are sometimes textured. They are nonsterile.

B. Utility gloves come in a variety of colors and sizes to fit the left and right hands. They are one-piece, heavy-duty vinyl/nitrile gloves that can be sterilized.

Notes
- Overgloves come in a box or bag of 100 or more. They are often referred to as food-handler gloves. They are available in numerous sizes.
- The fingers of utility gloves are textured to prevent slippage. They are puncture- and chemical-resistant. Each individual should have his or her own gloves. They need to be used not only when handling contaminated instruments, but also when performing housekeeping tasks involving contact with blood or other potentially infectious materials (OPIM). They should be washed thoroughly after each use.

Mouth Props

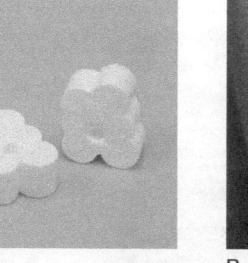
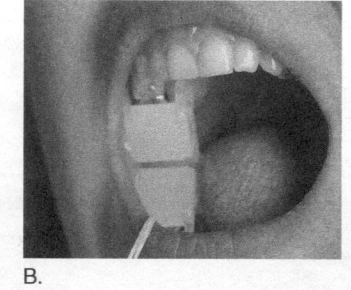
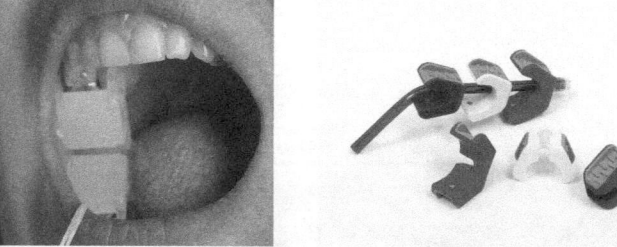

A.

B.

C.

D.

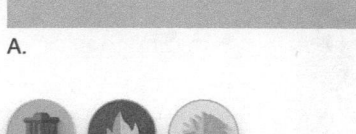

Use Props are used to assist the patient in keeping his or her mouth open during treatment.

Properties Mouth props are one-piece, wedge-shaped structures designed to fit the oral cavity. They may be made of rubber, plastic, or Styrofoam.

A. Styrofoam disposable mouth prop

B. Mouth prop in patient's mouth with ligature attached

C. Variety of sizes and colors of mouth props

D. Rubber bite block (prop)

Notes
- Mouth props are placed in the posterior space between the maxillary and mandibular teeth.
- They are available as disposable or autoclavable items.
- They come in a variety of colors and sizes, from pediatric to adult.
- They are used often for sedated patients.
- For patient safety and to prevent choking, a ligature should be tied to the mouth prop.

Cotton Roll Holders and Dry Angles/Dry Aids

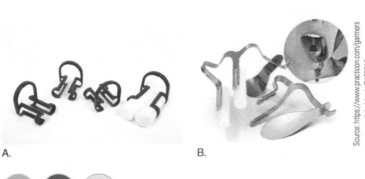

A.

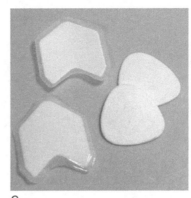

B.

Source: https://www.practicon.com/garmers-cotton-roll-holder/p/7125010

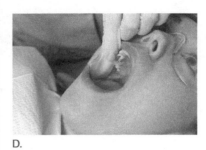

C.

D.

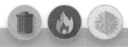

Use

Cotton roll holders are used to hold cotton rolls on buccal and lingual surfaces of the teeth in a specific area on the mandibular arch. They are also used to isolate, retract, and hold cotton rolls to keep an area dry.

Dry angles/dry aids are used to keep the mouth dry by covering the Stensen's (parotid) duct to restrict the flow of saliva. They absorb saliva and keep the working area dry. They also protect the cheek during dental treatment.

The backing on some dry angles reflects light to improve visibility.

Properties A. A cotton roll holder is a one-piece plastic device with two clamps sized to hold a cotton roll connected with a flexible bow.

B. Garmer cotton roll holders are smooth polished steel that keep cotton rolls in place; a sliding chin strap keeps the holder in place.

C. Dry angles/dry aids are thin absorbent wafers/pads. They are angular in shape, with one side made of absorbent cotton and the other side consisting of moisture-proof backing. Some have a silver backing that reflects light into the oral cavity.

D. Dry Angles in a patient mouth

Cotton Roll Holders and Dry Angles/Dry Aids *Continued*

Notes
- Cotton roll holders may be disposable or Garmer clamps made of stainless steel can be sterilized. They are available in different sizes and colors.
- Dry angles restrict the flow of saliva from the parotid gland for up to 15 minutes. They are considered a cotton roll substitute.
- Dry angles are ideal for bonding procedures, sealant application, placement of restorations, and cementation.

Patient Bibs and Bib Holders

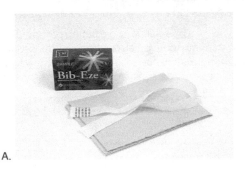

A.

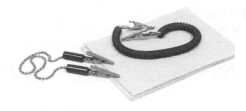

B.

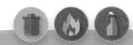

Use
- Bibs cover the patient to protect against moisture and debris. Bib clips hold the bib in place.

Properties Patient bibs are two- or three-ply tissue with poly backing. Bib holders have two clips connected by a tube, strip, chain, or coiled expandable plastic.
- **A.** Patient disposable bibs and disposable bib holders
- **B.** Disposable bib with bib clips

Notes
- Patient bibs come in a variety of sizes and contours, and are disposable.
- They may be purchased in many colors and printed designs with different features.
- Some bibs come with adhesive tabs so that bib clips are not required to secure the bib on the patient.
- Bib clips can be disposable, disinfectable, and/or autoclavable.

Tray Covers

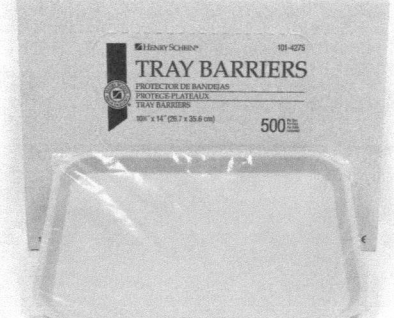

A.

B.

Use
Tray covers are used to cover the trays that are used to hold dental instruments, supplies, and materials used for a specific procedure; they protect the tray from moisture/liquid that may be produced during a procedure.

Properties Made from heavyweight paper or a polyethylene-backed paper
A. Plastic tray barriers: A plastic envelope that the tray is inserted into
B. Paper tray covers: Low absorbency tray covering to place instruments onto

Notes
- Tray covers come in many sizes to cover all sizes of trays.
- Tray covers come in many colors and several designs.
- Some offices use tray covers on the counter or cart without a tray.
- Tray covers impede the flow of moisture and protect the surface.
- Plastic tray barriers are available for increased aseptic technique.

Traps, Screens, and Filters

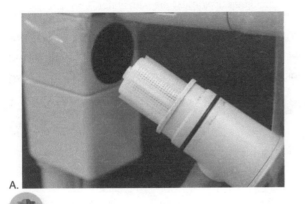

A.

5507	5506	5505	5508-S	5503	5502	5501
(2 3/4")	(2 3/4")	(3 3/4")	(Universal)	(1 7/8")	(2 15/16")	(2 1/8")

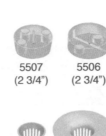

6400-C	6200-C	5500-SC	5512	5511	5509	5504	5500
B. (Universal)	(Universal)	(Universal)	(2 3/4")	(1 15/16")	(1 1/2")	(1")	(1 1/4")

Use	• Traps, screens, and filters are used to catch debris from the salvia ejector and high-volume evacuation (HVE) systems. • They keep evacuation systems from becoming clogged with debris, which would reduce efficiency during a procedure.
Properties	• Traps, screens, and filters are usually one-piece plastic devices designed to adapt to the different types of dental equipment. • They are ordered by unit type and system used.

A. High-volume disposable trap. Shown is the disposable trap removed from the dental unit for replacement.

B. Variety of high-volume disposable traps. The image shows multiple traps available; their use depends on the practices dental unit.

Notes	• Traps, screens, and filters come in many shapes, sizes, and designs. • Traps, screens, and filters are disposable in biohazard containers.

Fluoride Trays

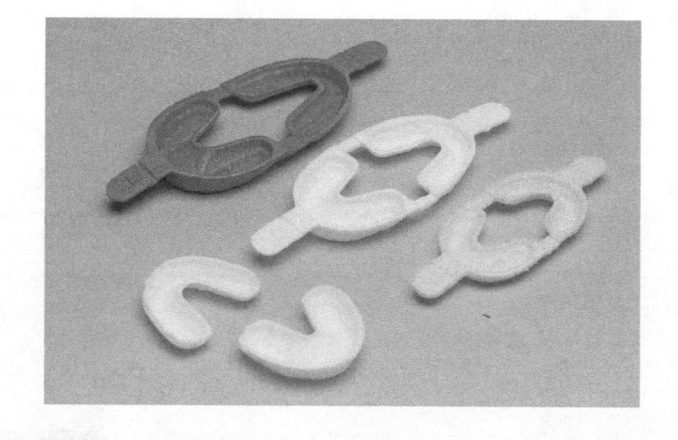

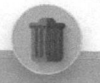

Use   Fluoride trays are used to hold fluoride gel/solution in the mouth around the teeth.

Properties Dual-arch trays, fold-over trays, or single-arch applicator trays are normally made from closed-cell foam.

Notes
- Trays are available in multiple colors and sizes.
- They are disposable.
- Fluoride trays are available in single-arch, double-fold-over, and dual-arch trays with a saliva ejector feature.
- Some folding-design trays have locking handles that allow for easy placement and removal.
- They are often sold in amounts of 50 or 100.

Surface Barriers

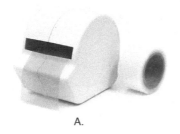

A.

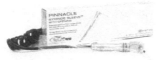

B. 1

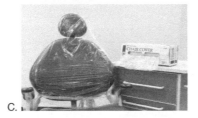

C.

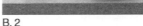

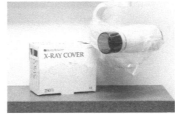

B. 2

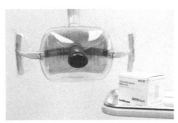

B. 3

Use Improve infection control, prevent cross-contamination, protect surfaces, give the patient confidence in the infection control techniques used by the dentist.

Properties • Perforated control film with adhesive backing.
• Come in 4 × 6- and 2½1/2 × 6-inch sizes.
• Available in colors, clear, or designs.
• Most often used with dispenser.
A. Sleeves/sheaths: Medical-grade plastic that is available in many sizes and shapes to cover most equipment in dental treatment rooms
B.1 Syringe sleeve
B.2 X-ray cover
B.3 Covers for light handles

C. Chair cover: Medical-grade plastic that is available in half- and full-chair cover designed to fit a variety of dental chairs.

Notes • These barriers are disposable and are designed for easy placement and removal.
• There are barriers to cover everything in the dental treatment room, from the dental chair to the handpieces, dental light, curing light, impression gun, air-water syringe, high-volume evacuator (HVE) handle, saliva ejector, computer keyboards, instruments and trays, x-ray tube heads, controls, and sensors.
• Surface barriers are designed to be easy to place and remove for efficient room turn-around.

CHAPTER 3

Basic Instruments, Evacuation, and Air-Water Syringe

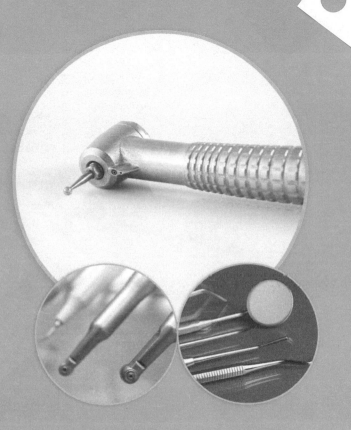

Basic Examination Instruments

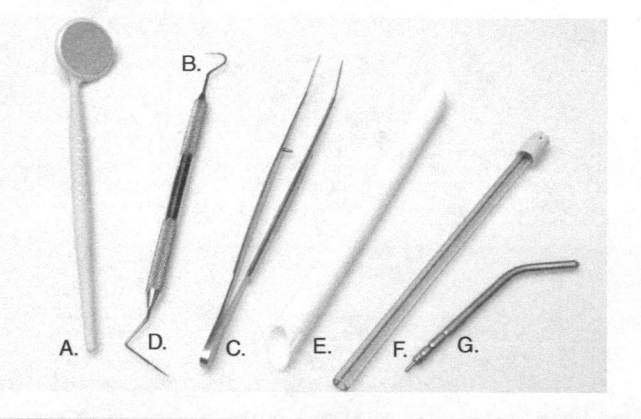

Use The basic tray setup includes instruments that are used for the examination of the oral cavity and the dentition. They can be used alone for the initial examination and are found on all procedure tray setups. The primary instruments on the basic tray setup are the mouth mirror, explorer, cotton pliers, and periodontal probe; these are sterilized after each use. These instruments are used with the evacuator, saliva ejector, and air-water syringe, which can be disposable or sterilizable.

Properties The basic tray setup includes:
- **A.** Mouth mirror
- **B.** Explorer
- **C.** Cotton pliers/forceps
- **D.** Periodontal probe
- **E.** Evacuator tip
- **F.** Saliva ejector
- **G.** Three-way syringe tip (also called air-water syringe tip)

Mouth Mirror

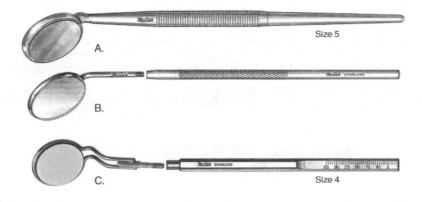

A.

Size 5

B.

C.

Size 4

Use
- To provide indirect vision in the oral cavity
- To reflect light into the mouth to illuminate an area being examined
- To retract oral tissues such as the lips, tongue, and cheeks
- To reflect light (transillumination) through the tooth surface to detect fractures
- To protect tissues from the handpiece or bur

Properties A. Single-ended instrument made of plastic or metal
B. and **C.** Metal straight handle with option of removable replacement head

Notes
- Mirrors are available in different sizes and types.
- Common sizes of mirrors are #4 and #5.
- Front-surface mirrors are more accurate and give a clear view.
- Concave-surface mirrors magnify the image.
- Flat-surface mirrors are used in the disposable models.
- Plane- or regular-surface mirrors reflect from the back of the glass and give a "ghost-like" image.

Explorer

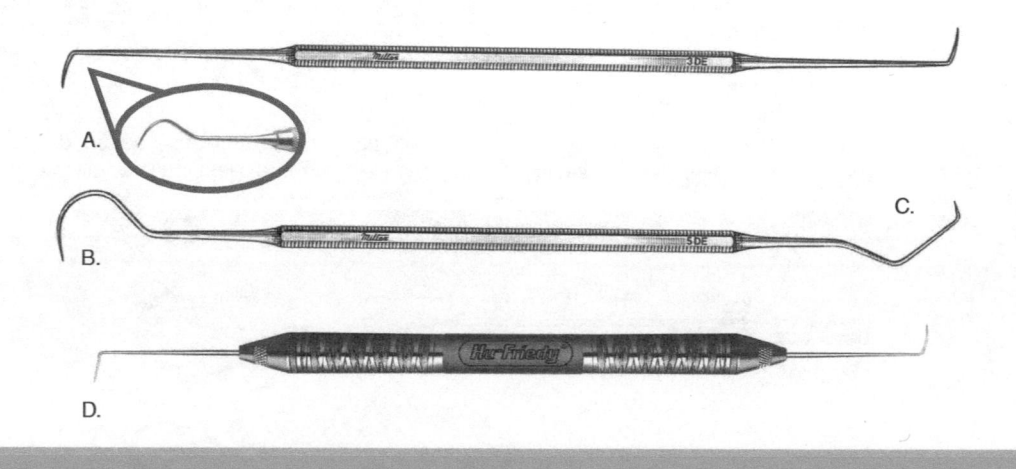

A.

B.

C.

D.

Use
- To examine the tooth structure for any defects or areas of decay
- To examine restorations and check for faulty margins or fractures
- To remove excess materials from around the margins of restorations or from bases and liners during cavity preparation

Properties **A.** Pigtail
B. Shepherd's hook
C. Orban, also called #17
D. Right angle

Notes
- Explorers can be single- or double-ended.
- The end is characterized by a thin, sharp point of flexible steel.
- Explorers come in a variety of angles and with several different ends.

Cotton Forceps (Pliers)

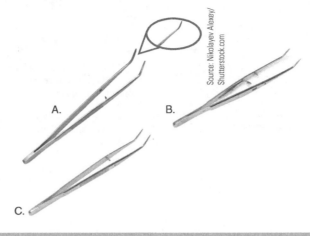

Source: Nikolayev Alexey/
Shutterstock.com

A.

B.

C.

Use	To place and remove items from the oral cavity, such as cotton rolls, cotton pellets, wedges, and large pieces of debris
Properties	**A.** The ends can be smooth or serrated on the beaks. **B.** Handles can be locking. **C.** Handles can be nonlocking.
Notes	• Cotton forceps (pliers) are shaped like large tweezers. • The ends can be smooth or serrated (A) on the beaks. • May have either locking (B) or nonlocking handles (C). • The tips may be angled or straight.

Expro

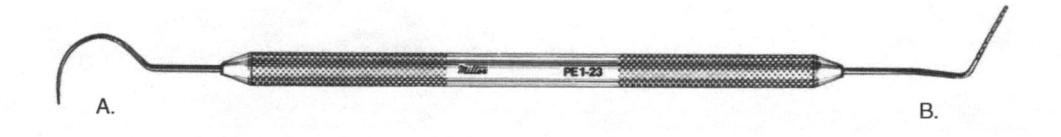

A.

B.

Use
- The Expro is a combination instrument that has an explorer on one end and a periodontal probe on the other end.
- Use of this instrument cuts down on the number of instruments needed on the tray.

Properties A. Explorer end
B. Periodontal probe end

Evacuator Tips, Handle, and Screens

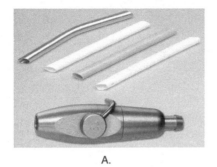

A.

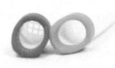

B.

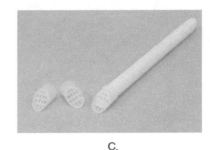

C.

Use	• To remove fluids and debris from the oral cavity • To retract soft tissues • To prevent discomfort to soft tissue • Screens prevent crowns, inlays, veneers, excess materials, etc. from being lost into the evacuation system. • Evacuation system cleaners are used after each patient, at the end of the day, and at the end of the week to keep the evacuation system clean and odor free and to prevent buildup of debris from blood, salvia, tissue, and dental materials, such as fluoride, inside the lines. • Evacuation system cleaners can be tablets, solutions, packets, or systems that are usually mixed and then suctioned into the

tubing. Some systems require the solution to sit for a few minutes, and others require repeated flushing.

Properties
A. Various evacuators with dental unit attachment
B. Soft tipped evacuator
C. Screens for evacuator tip

Parts
• Evacuator tips
• Evacuator handle
• Plastic sleeve with a beveled screen that sits over the end of the evacuator tip

Evacuator Tips, Handle, and Screens *Continued*

Misc.
- Placed into the evacuator handle that is connected to the high-volume evacuation system.
- Made from metal or plastic.
- Tips can be rubber coated for patient comfort.
- Straight or curved.
- Tips normally beveled.
- The screens can be used on all standard plastic and metal evacuator tips.
- Low cost.
- Can be sterilizable or disposable.
- Screens are purchased in bags of 100.

Saliva Ejector, Safe-Flo Saliva Ejector Valve

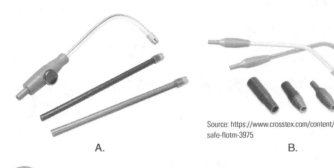

A.

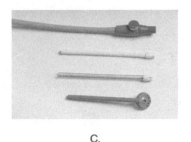

Source: https://www.crosstex.com/content/
safe-flotm-3975

B.

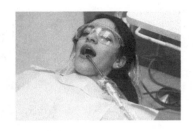

C.

D.

Use	• A low-volume (low-velocity) evacuation system used to remove fluids from the oral cavity.
	• One-way valve to prevent back-flow.
Properties	• Flexible, plastic tube about one-third in diameter of the size of the high-volume evacuation tip
	• Bendable with a guard cover on the end that is placed into the patient's mouth
	• Disposable valves that fit into hosing and used with any brand of saliva ejector
	A. Saliva ejectors inserted into dental unit
	B. Safe-flo saliva ejector

C. Variety of saliva ejectors
D. Saliva ejector placed in patient mouth

Notes
• Disposable
• Available in multiple colors
• Used primarily on mandibular arch
• Commonly used during coronal polish, sealant, and fluoride procedures
• Used during preventive treatment when the operator does not have an assistant
• Some are designed with a soft smooth tip to prevent patient discomfort
• One-way valve closes preventing cross-contamination

Three-Way Syringe Tip/Air-Water Syringe Tip

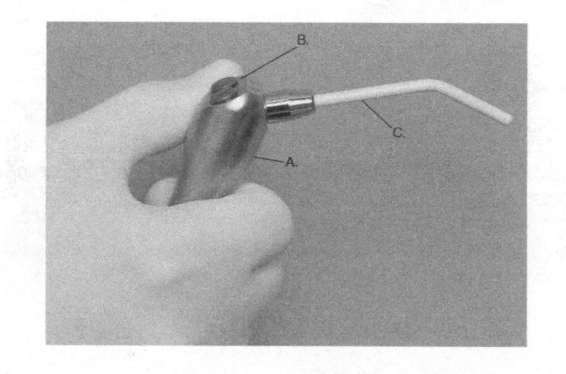

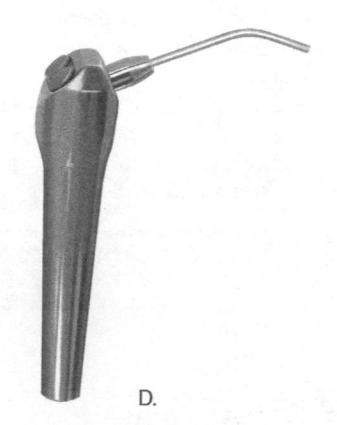

Use	• Emits water, air, or a combination of the two in a spray
	• Directs the air, water, or spray
	• Used for retraction of the tongue, cheeks, lips, and tissues of the oral cavity

Properties A. Handle
　　　　　　B. Controls
　　　　　　C. Disposable tip
　　　　　　D. 3-way syringe tips

Isolite System

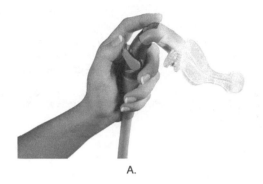

A.

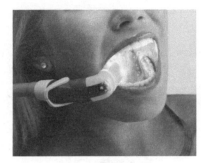

B.

Notes
- Allows water or air or spray to dispense
- Plastic or metal
- Disposable or able to be sterilized

Use
- Provides isolation, retraction, evacuation, and a light source in one piece of equipment. It also provides a mouth prop for the patient.

Parts
- Titanium control head, power/vacuum hose, and a one-time-use mouthpiece.
- The control head contains a light emitter, a dual-channel vacuum, and controls for both.

- The system is connected to the dental unit vacuum system and an electrical source.
- **A.** Isolite insert
- **B.** Isolite placed in patient mouth

Misc.
- The mouthpiece is available in different sizes.
- The mouthpiece is disposable.
- The light setting can be controlled for light-sensitive material.
- The mouthpiece isolates an entire quadrant and can be used on both the maxillary and mandibular arches.

Self-Contained Water Unit and Water Line Treatments

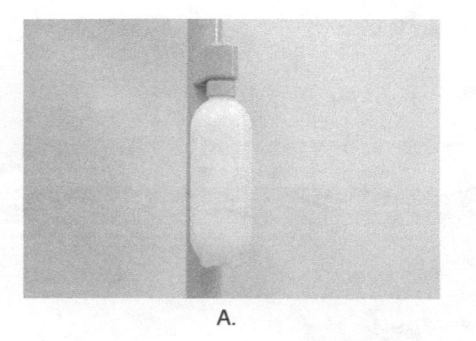

A.

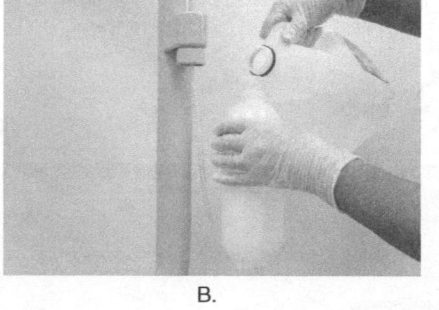

B.

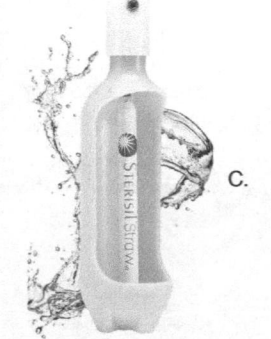

C.

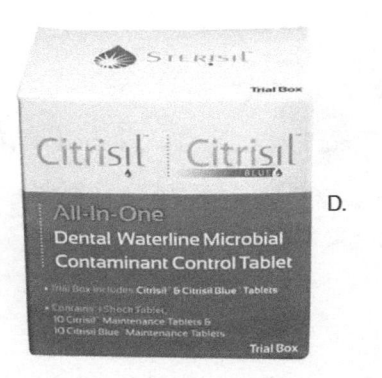

D.

Source: https://www.sterisil
.com/sterisil-straw-v2

Use
- A reservoir that houses high-quality water to be used by dental handpieces and air-water syringes. High-quality water is water that has been treated and has the biofilm (bacteria) removed.
- Water line treatment aids in the control and prevention of water contamination.

Properties A. Plastic bottles that attach to the dental unit
   B. Designed with a cap and a plastic tube where the plastic bottle attaches
   C. Sterisil straw
   D. Citrisil water tablets

Notes
- The water bottle is filled when empty, and water line tablets are added prior to each filling to prevent odor and foul taste due to bacteria.
- Or a straw is inserted into the dental unit and changed yearly, eliminating the need to empty the water bottle and purging and drying lines.
- The Centers for Disease Control and Prevention (CDC) requires ongoing monitoring of water lines.

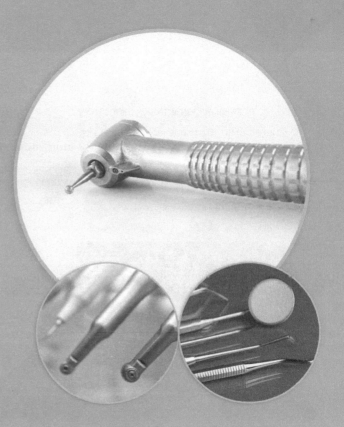

CHAPTER 4

Topical and Local Anesthetic and Nitrous Oxide Sedation

Topical Anesthetics

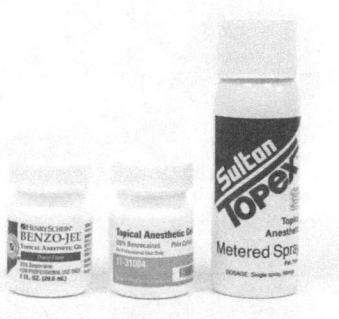

A.

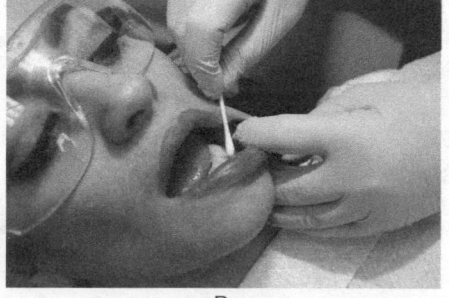

B.

Use Topical anesthetics are placed on the surface of the oral mucosa to desensitize the tissue for a brief period of time. They are used prior to placement of local anesthetic, during subgingival scaling, during root planing, when seating crowns, in dental dam placement, when placing matrix bands, when taking radiographs, for suppressing the gag reflex, and sometimes for periodontal probing. Topical anesthetic comes in gels, ointments, liquids, metered sprays, patches, and single doses.

Composition A. Ointments and metered spray
B. Placing topical anesthetic on a patient

Misc. Most topical anesthetics are flavored.

Local Anesthetic—Aspirating Syringe

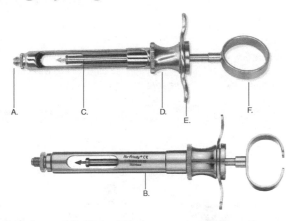

| **Use** | • To administer local anesthetic to a specific area. The American Dental Association (ADA) recommends the aspirating syringe. The harpoon is securely placed in the rubber stopper, which then allows the operator to aspirate.
• Aspirating when administering anesthesia ensures that the clinician has not introduced the needle into a blood vessel. |

Composition
A. Threaded end (needle adapter)
B. Syringe barrel
C. Piston rod with harpoon

D. Finger grip
E. Finger bar
F. Thumb ring

Notes
• Local anesthetic syringes are autoclavable.
• An anesthetic syringe without a harpoon is known as a nonaspirating syringe.
• Many anesthetic syringes must have the piston rod with harpoon retracted to allow insertion of the cartridge.

Local Anesthetic Needle

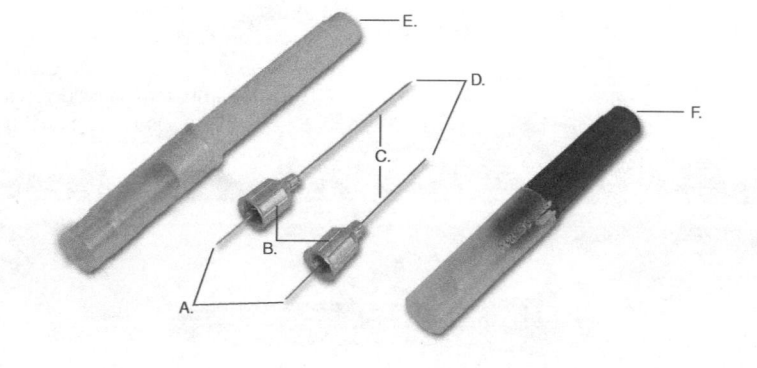

Use
- To penetrate the tissues
- To direct the local anesthetic solution from the carpule (anesthetic cartridge) into the surrounding tissues

Composition
A. Syringe end
B. Hub
C. Shank
D. Bevel
E. Long needle: Used for administration of nerve block injections
F. Short needle: Used for administration of infiltration and field block injections

Notes
- Needles come in different gauges or diameters. The most common are 25, 27, and 30 gauges.
- With anesthetic needles, the smaller the gauge of the needle, the larger the diameter of the needle.

Local Anesthetic Cartridge

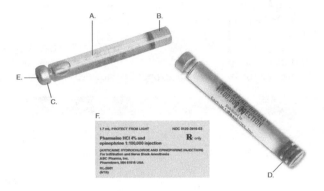

Use   The anesthetic cartridge, also called the carpule, is a glass cylinder that contains the anesthetic solution.

Composition **A.** Glass cartridge (carpule).
B. Rubber stopper or plunger: Where the harpoon of syringe inserts.
C. Aluminum cap.
D. Color coding of local anesthetic (required by the ADA).
E. Diaphragm: Where the needle inserts.
F. Mylar plastic label: Prevents breakage and provides identification information, including type of anesthetic, percentage of anesthetic, with or without epinephrine, strength of epinephrine, and expiration date.

Notes
- Local anesthetics follow the ADA color-coding band, which indicates types of anesthetic and vasoconstrictor combinations.
- Cartridges should be carefully examined for expired shelf-life date, large bubbles, extruded plungers, corrosion, or rust. All of these are reasons for cartridges to be discarded.
- The rubber stopper or plunger is slightly indented.
- The higher the percentage of epinephrine (vasoconstrictor), the longer the anesthetic lasts.

Recapping Devices and Needle Stick Protection

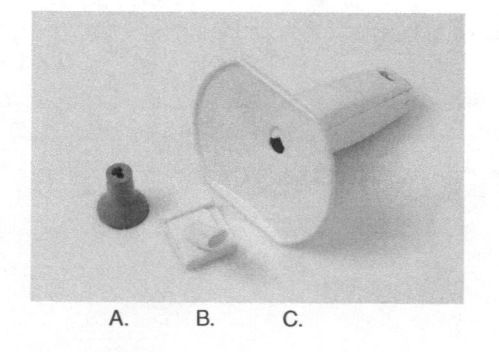
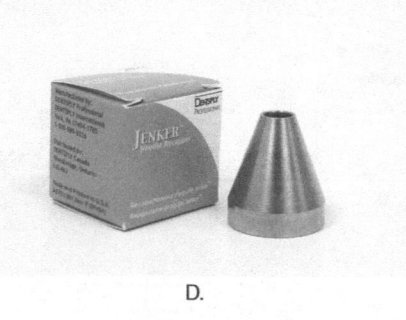
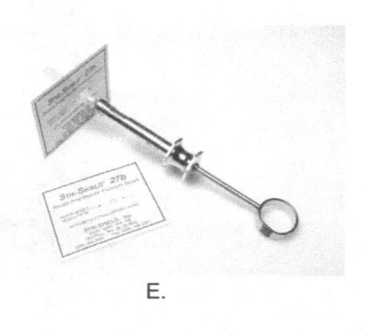

A.   B.   C.   D.   E.

Use

- Recapping devices are used to hold the needle cap; this allows the operator to safely recap the needle after delivery of anesthetic. Recapping devices help to prevent needlesticks.
- Needlestick guards prevent needlestick injury when capping and recapping the needle. They protect the dental assistant, dentist, and dental hygienist when recapping the needle.

Composition
A. Rubber recapping device
B. Needle capper
C. Handheld recapping device
D. The Jenker Needle Stick Protector
E. The needlestick guard is a square of cardboard material with a hole in the middle for the needle cap. The needle guard shown on a needle cap and syringe.

Recapping Devices and Needle Stick Protection *Continued*

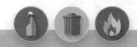

Notes

- The needle is slid into the protective guard using one hand or by placing the needle of the syringe in a mechanical recapping device.
- Most recapping devices can be sterilized.
- The needlestick guard is placed after the needle is placed on the syringe.
- The needle can be capped and recapped with one hand when using the needle guard.
- At no time should fingers or the thumb be in the front toward the syringe of the needle guard.
- The needle guard also acts as a prop to hold the syringe when it is not in use.
- Needle guards are available in boxes/packs of 100 or 500.

Anesthetic Tray Setup

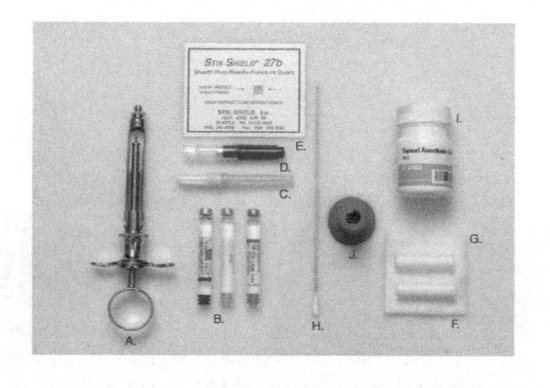

Use   Instruments and materials needed to place topical and local anesthetic are assembled on the treatment tray. Usually the anesthetic tray setup is part of the procedure tray.

Composition
A. Aspirating syringe
B. Selection of local anesthetic cartridges
C. Long needle
D. Short needle
E. Needlestick shield

F. Cotton rolls
G. 2 × 2 gauze sponge
H. Cotton-tip applicator
I. Topical anesthetic
J. Recapping device

Local Anesthetic—Computer-Controlled Delivery System (The Wand)

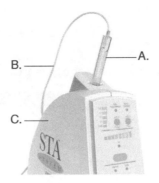

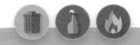

Use
This system is used to administer single-tooth, palatal, mandibular, and all other injections. The system's microprocessor delivers a controlled pressure and volume of anesthetic solution at a rate that is below the pain threshold.

Composition
A. Standard anesthetic cartridge
B. Plastic microtubing
C. Microprocessing unit

Notes
- It is used with a pen-like grasp that allows for flexibility in administration.
- The auxiliary can prepare the wand/single-tooth administration prior to treatment, similar to the anesthetic syringe.
- The computer manages the flow of the anesthetic while the operator focuses on needle placement.
- It improves ergonomics for the operator while increasing patient comfort.

Local Anesthetic—Periodontal Ligament Injection Syringe

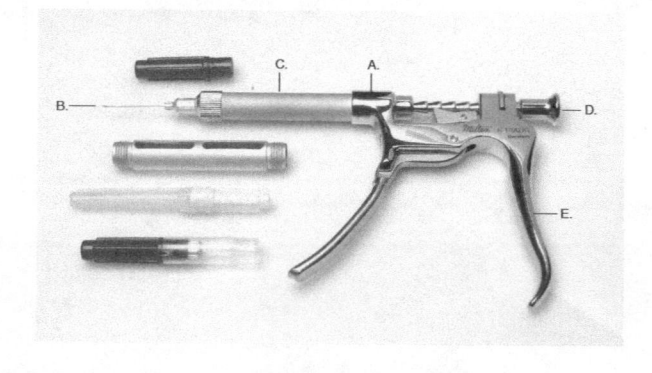

Use   Delivers a precise amount of anesthesia to one or two teeth in a quadrant and is sometimes used as an adjunct to another injection where the patient is only partially anesthetized

Composition **A.** Pressure syringe
        B. Needle end
        C. Barrel
        D. Plunger
        E. Handle

Nitrous Oxide Sedation Equipment

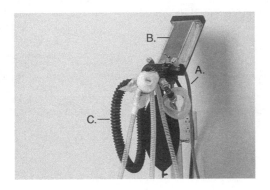

Use	• To provide relaxation
	• To relieve apprehension for patients during dental treatment
Composition	**A.** Nitrous oxide (blue tank) and oxygen (green or white tank) gases are used together to allow a safe method of sedation.
	B. The nitrous oxide unit has controls and gauges to administer the proper amount of nitrogen and oxygen.
	C. Each unit has a scavenger system to carry away exhaled and additional gas.
Notes	• Hoses connect to a tank of nitrous oxide and a tank of oxygen located in the dental cabinetry or storage area
	• Breathing tubes (hoses) connect the nitrous oxide and oxygen tanks to the nasal hoods for administration.

Nitrous Oxide Sedation Nasal Hoods

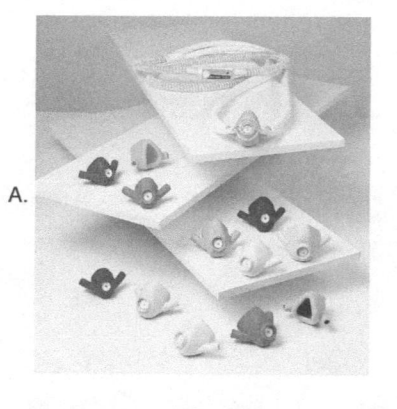

A.

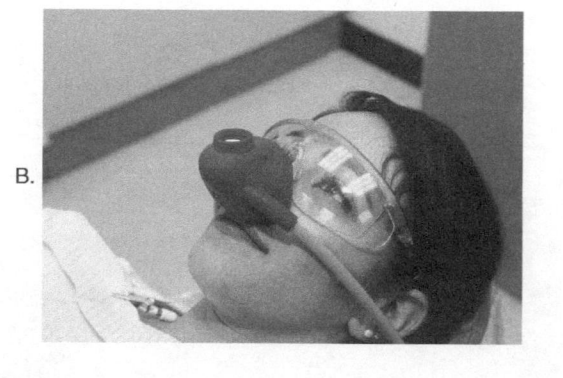

B.

Use　　　　Placed over the patient's nose so that the gases flow through to the patient

Composition • Rubber nose covers come in a variety of colors.
　　　　　　 • They are attached to a scavenging circuit.
　　　　　　 • Some are scented for patient comfort.
　　　　　　 • They attach to the breathing tubes that come from the nitrous oxide tank, which is blue, and the oxygen tank, which is green or white.

　　　　　　 A. Variety of color-coded nasal hoods/nosepieces
　　　　　　 B. Patient with nasal hood/nosepiece in place

CHAPTER 5
Dental Dam

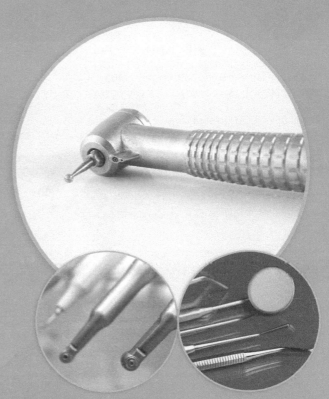

Dental Dam

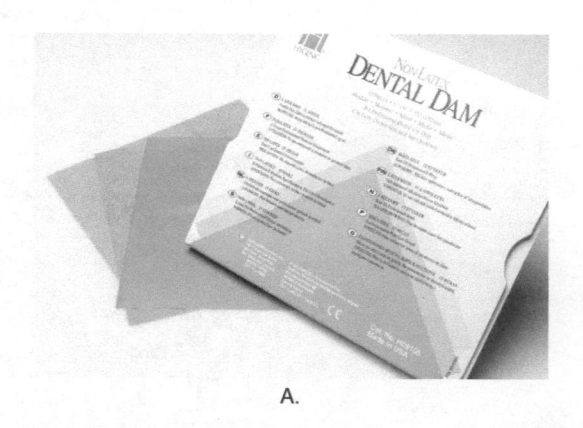

A.

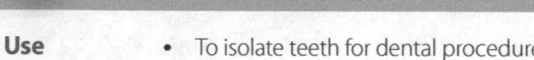

Use
- To isolate teeth for dental procedures
- To keep the area clean and dry while performing dental procedures

Composition
- Made from either latex or latex-free material.
- Comes in sizes 4 × 4 inches, 5 × 5 inches, or 6 × 6 inches.
- **A.** Dental Dam Material.

Notes
- The dental dam is often referred to as the rubber dam.
- Available in a wide range of colors, including green, blue, and pastels.
- Colors allow for increased visibility and contrast.
- Scented and flavored dams also are available.
- Dams are available in a variety of thicknesses: thin (light), medium, and heavy.

Dental Dam Stamp and Template

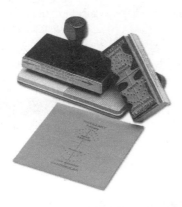

A.

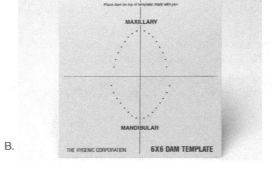

B.

Use
- The stamp is used to mark where the holes should be punched for correct dental dam placement.
- The template is used as a guide for marking the correct position for punching holes for dental dam placement.

Composition
- The stamp has 32 dots located on a punch and is used with a stamp pad to mark the rubber dam material.
- The template is made of durable plastic and has holes where an ink pen can be used to mark the correct position for punching.

A. Dental Dam Stamp.
B. Dental Dam Template.

Notes
The operator should examine the oral cavity before punching the dental dam to adjust positioning for the specific patient's dentition.

Dental Dam Punch

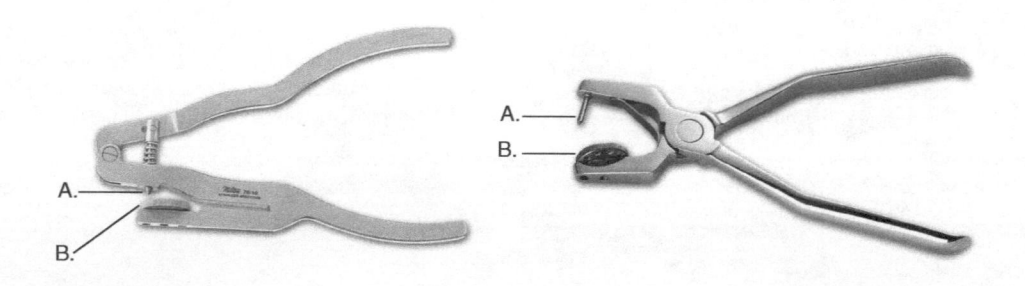

Use To punch holes in dental dam for each identified tooth the dentist wants isolated

Composition **A.** A stylus, which is a sharp projection to punch through the dental dam.

B. A punch table or plate, which is a rotating disc containing several hole sizes:
- No. 1 hole size (smallest hole): Used for lower incisors
- No. 2 hole size: Used for upper incisors
- No. 3 hole size: Used for premolars and cuspids
- No. 4 hole size: Used for molars
- No. 5 hole size (largest hole): Used for molars and the anchor tooth

Notes
- The operator should examine the oral cavity before punching the dental dam to adjust positioning for the specific patient's dentition.
- The space between the holes is approximately 3 to 3.5 mm.

Dental Dam Forceps

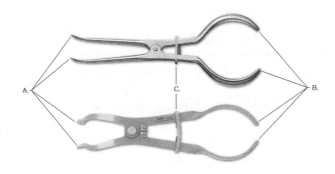

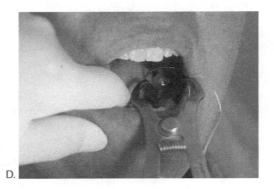

Use To place and remove the dental dam clamp

Composition **A.** Two beaks that fit into the holes of the jaws of the clamp.
B. Handle (where the pressure is applied to open the beaks).
C. Lock (sliding bar) that keeps the beaks of the forceps open to secure the clamp in position until it is placed on the anchor tooth. The sliding bar can be released once the clamp is placed, and then the beaks of the forceps will come together.
D. Clamp Placement.

Notes The forceps open with a spring motion.

Dental Dam Clamp

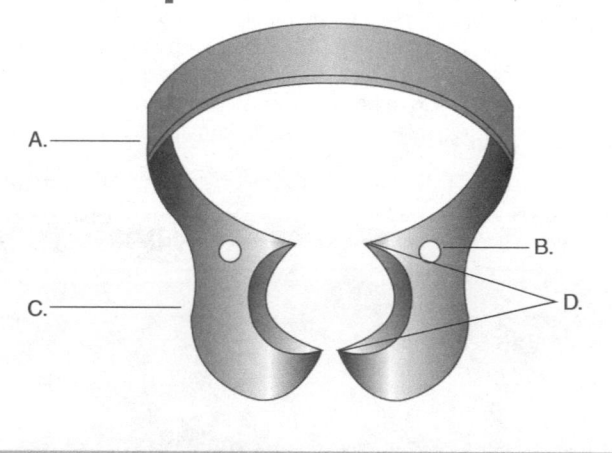

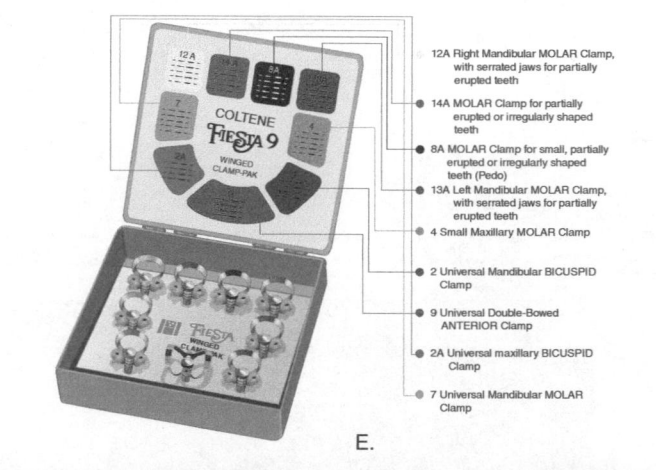

12A Right Mandibular MOLAR Clamp, with serrated jaws for partially erupted teeth

14A MOLAR Clamp for partially erupted or irregularly shaped teeth

8A MOLAR Clamp for small, partially erupted or irregularly shaped teeth (Pedo)

13A Left Mandibular MOLAR Clamp, with serrated jaws for partially erupted teeth

4 Small Maxillary MOLAR Clamp

2 Universal Mandibular BICUSPID Clamp

9 Universal Double-Bowed ANTERIOR Clamp

2A Universal maxillary BICUSPID Clamp

7 Universal Mandibular MOLAR Clamp

Use	To stabilize and secure the dental dam material in place
Composition	**A.** Bow (connects the jaws of the clamps and is positioned distal to the tooth being worked on).
	B. Forceps hole (utilized by the forceps to place the clamp).
	C. Jaw (rounded part of the clamp that fits tightly to the lingual and buccal/facial surfaces of the tooth).
	D. Jaw points (four points on the jaws of the clamp that are located at different widths and angles that fit to secure the clamp on the tooth near the cementoenamel junction).
	E. Clamp Kit.

Notes

- The tooth to be clamped must be evaluated before the clamp selection is made.
- The width of the tooth must be about the same as the width medial/distal between the points of the jaws of the clamp.
- Ensure that the clamp fits tightly.
- Ligatures of dental floss should be tied to the bow as a safety measure in case the clamp dislodges from the tooth.
- Clamps that have the letter A following the number have jaws that bend sharply downward toward the gingiva.
- Clamps without the letter A have jaws that are on a flat plane.

Anterior or Cervical Clamp

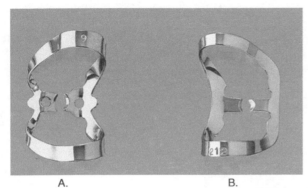

A.   B.

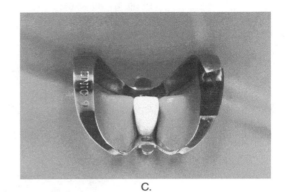

C.

Use   To stabilize and secure the dental dam material in place on an anterior tooth

Composition   Double bowed
    A. Winged.
    B. Wingless.
    C. Clamp placed for single tooth isolation.

Notes
- Clamp numbers are 00, 1A, 9, and 212.
- Clamps are sterilized.
- Dental floss ligatures are placed on clamps for rescue of a dislodged clamp.
- Used for restorations and endodontic treatment on the anterior teeth.

Premolar Clamp

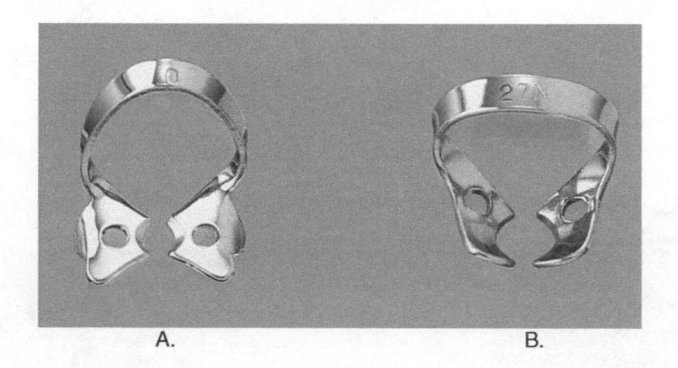

A.   B.

Use   To stabilize and secure the dental dam material in place on a premolar

Composition   **A.** Winged
                 B. Wingless

Notes
- The clamp used is determined by tooth size and shape.
- Variety of styles and sizes available.
- Clamp numbers are 0, 1, 2A, 2, 27N, and 29.
- Dental floss ligatures are placed on clamps for rescue of a dislodged clamp.
- Clamps are sterilized.

Universal Maxillary Clamp

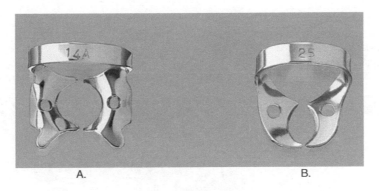

A.   B.

Use   To stabilize and secure the dental dam material in place on a maxillary molar

Composition   **A.** Winged
B. Wingless

Notes
- These clamps can be used on right or left maxillary molars.
- A variety of styles and sizes are available.
- Clamp numbers are 4, 5, 8, 8A, 14, 14A, 25, 26N, 30, 31, 201, and 205.
- Dental floss ligatures are placed on clamps for rescue of a dislodged clamp.
- Clamps are sterilized.

Universal Mandibular Clamp

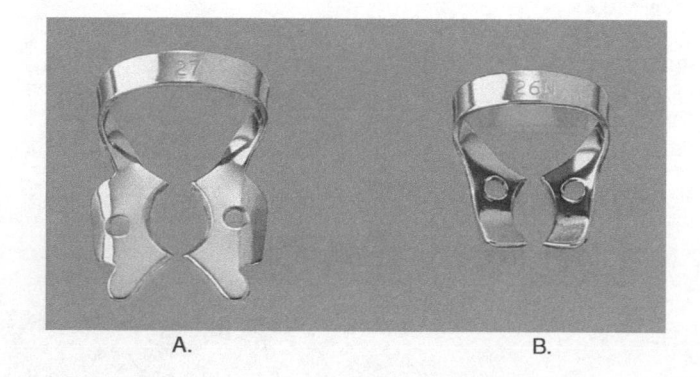

A. B.

Use   To stabilize and secure the dental dam material in place on a mandibular molar

Composition **A.** Winged
                B. Wingless

Notes
- Can be used on right or left mandibular molars.
- A variety of styles and sizes are available.
- Clamp numbers are W3, 3, 7A, 7, 12A, 13A, 26, 27 and 28.
- Dental floss ligatures are placed on clamps for rescue of a dislodged clamp.
- Clamps are sterilized.

Dental Dam Frames

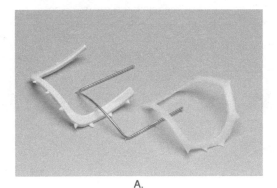

A.

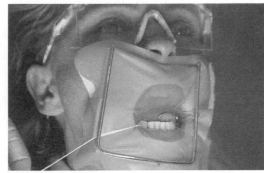

B.

Use   Used to stretch and secure the dental dam in place across the patient's face

Composition
- U- or oval-shaped frames made from metal or plastic.
- Small projections around the borders to secure the dental dam.
- **A.** Frames.
- **B.** Frame placement.

Notes
- Plastic frames are radiolucent.
- The U-shaped frame is common and is known as the (metal) Young frame or (plastic) U-frame.
- Frames can be placed over or under the dental dam material according to the dentist's preference.
- Frames are sterilized.
- The oval-shaped frame is known as the Ostby frame.

Dental Dam Napkin

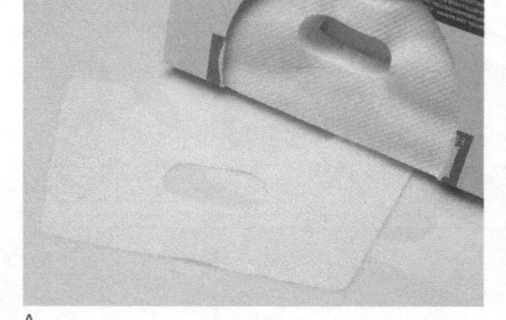

A.

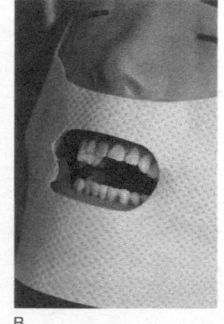

B.

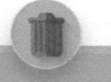

Use   For patient comfort and to absorb saliva, water, and
perspiration

Composition   **A.** Precut dental dam napkin.
     B. Dental dam napkin with correct placement shown.
     • Made of soft, absorbent fabric
     • Precut
     • Designed to prevent the dam material from touching
the face by covering the area around the mouth and the
cheeks

Notes   • Dental dam napkins are available in several sizes.
     • They are disposable.

Quick and Instant Dental Dam

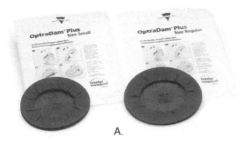

A.

Source: https://www.ivoclarvivadent.us /explore/OptraDam

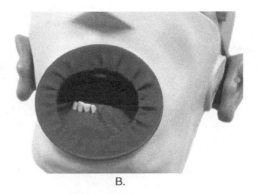

B.

Use	For quick and easy placement of the dental dam for full-quadrant or single-use isolation
Composition	**A.** Latex preframed dental dams **B.** Dental dam placement

Notes
- Instant dental dams are available in several styles.
- They are compact and comfortable for the patient.
- They allow for easy placement by the operator.
- They are disposable.

Dental Dam Tray Setup

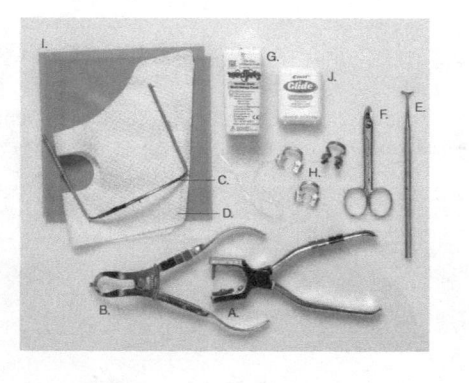

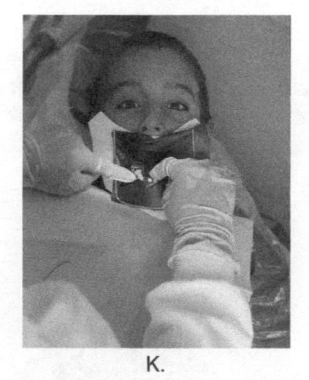

K.

Composition

A. Dental dam punch
B. Dental dam forceps
C. Dental dam frame
D. Dental dam napkin
E. Tucking instrument (T-ball burnisher)
F. Crown and bridge scissors
G. Widgets ligature (a stretchable cord placed like dental floss to hold the dental dam in place)

H. Clamps
I. Stamped dental dam
J. Dental floss (for inverting the dental dam material)
K. Dental Dam Placement.

CHAPTER 6
Dental Unit and Handpieces

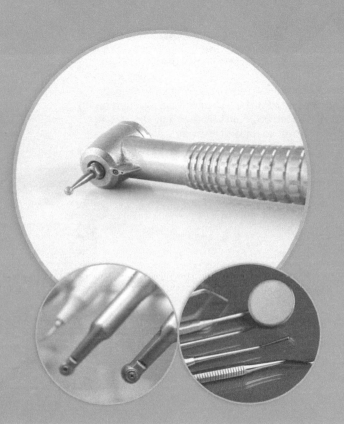

The Dental Delivery System

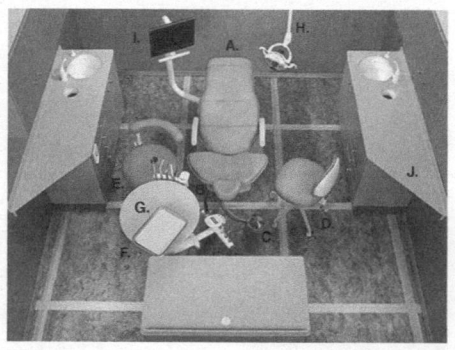

Use   Comprehensive unit for delivering patient dental care.

Composition **A.** Ergonomically designed patient chair that provides comfort and support during treatment.

B. Patient chair adjustments (not pictured).

C. Rheostat to control handpieces.

D. Ergonomically designed chair for operator with lumbar support.

E. Ergonomically designed chair for assistant with extended arm.

F. Rear delivery system with air-water syringe, high-volume evacuator (HVE), and saliva ejector on assistant's side and handpieces and air-water syringe on operator's side.

G. Tray table for placement of tray setups and auxiliary items.

H. Operating light attached to the dental unit or mounted on the ceiling.

I. Computer screen for digital radiographs and patient information.

J. Cabinetry with sinks and countertops.

The Dental Delivery System *Continued*

Notes
- Units are available in many sizes, designs, colors, and features to meet practice needs.
- The photo shown is of a rear delivery system; units are available with front and side delivery.
- Operator and assistant chairs need to be adjustable and have stable bases.
- Units are designed to allow for easy cleaning and disinfecting.

The Dental Unit

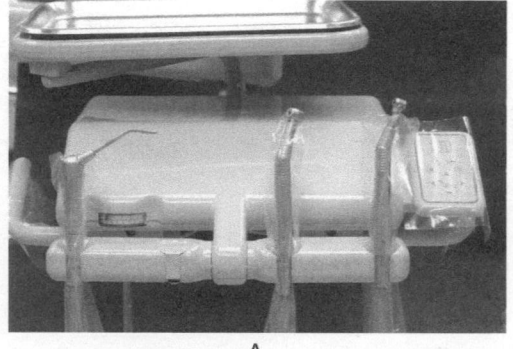
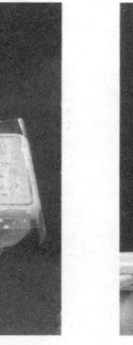
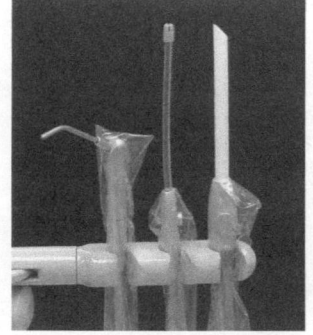
A.

B.
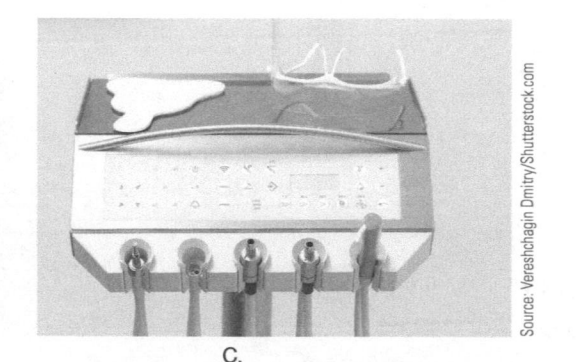
C.

Use Provides placement of the air-water syringe, dental handpieces, HVE, saliva ejector, ultrasonic scaling unit, curing light, and other options used by the operator and the dental assistant. Units are available in front, rear, and side delivery systems.

Composition **A.** Unit shown with handpieces and air-water syringe used by the operator.

B. Unit shown with air-water syringe, saliva ejector, and HVE used by the assistant.

C. Unit shown without attachments prior to seating a patient.

Notes
- Units have a self-contained water bottle, a vacuum system, and electrical connections, including fiber optics.
- Units can be designed according to the operator's preference; for example, curing lights may be attached.
- Barriers are often placed over hard-to-clean areas.

The Parts of the Dental Handpiece

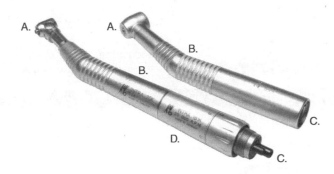

Use

Many dental handpieces are available for various procedures, both in the oral cavity and in the laboratory. Handpieces are used to remove dental decay, prepare the cavity for filling, polish the teeth, and polish and finish restorations and dental appliances.

Composition

A. Working end (head) where rotary instruments and attachments are held.

B. Shank-handle portion of the handpiece.

C. The connection end of the handpiece attaches to the power source here.

D. Forward and reverse controls on the low-speed handpiece.

Notes

- Shown on the left is the low-speed handpiece with a prophy attachment; on the right is a high-speed handpiece.
- All handpieces and attachments can be cleaned, lubricated, and sterilized; the manufacturer's directions should be followed.

High-Speed Handpiece

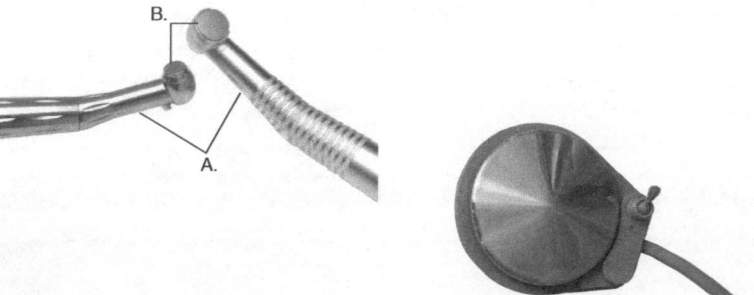

Use   The high-speed handpiece is used with a bur to rapidly cut teeth, as well as to smooth surfaces and finish restorations.

Composition **A.** High-speed handpiece.
B. Button/release lever to allow for bur placement and removal.
C. Rheostat (foot control of handpiece speed and on/off water switch).

Notes
- High-speed handpieces operate at 400,000 revolutions per minute (rpm) or higher.
- The high-speed handpiece produces frictional heat and needs a coolant such as air, water, or an air-water spray.
- The high-speed handpiece does not hold any attachments but does hold burs and other rotary instruments.

High-Speed Handpiece *Continued*

- The power source for the handpiece comes from compressed air. The rheostat is used to activate and control the speed of the handpiece. Also, on the rheostat there is a switch to turn the water to the handpiece on or off.
- The burs are held in place by a small metal cylinder called a chuck. To tighten or loosen the chuck, a button/release lever on the back of the head of the handpiece is used.
- To insert a bur into the high-speed handpiece, push the button on the back of the handpiece head, insert the bur, and release. Pull on the bur to ensure that it is fully engaged into the chuck of the handpiece.
- Handpieces are kept in sterilization bags until ready for use.
- High-speed handpieces are to be cleaned, lubricated, and sterilized per the manufacturer's directions.

Fiber-Optic High-Speed Handpiece

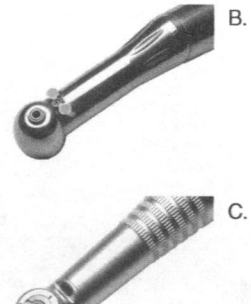

B.

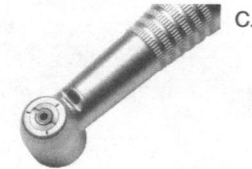

C.

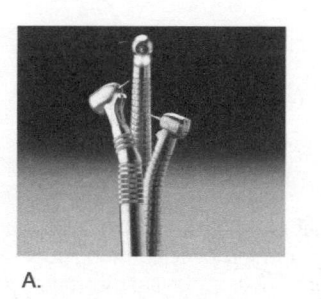

A.

Use
The fiber-optic system greatly improves the visibility of the treatment area by illuminating the area for the dentist.

Composition
Small illuminated area on the handpiece head that provides light during tooth preparation.
A. High Speed Handpieces.
B. High Speed Handpiece with two fiber optic lights.
C. High Speed Handpiece with water openings on the head.

Notes
- The fiber-optic light is carried along optical bundles in the tubing of the handpiece.
- The light source for the fiber-optic light is placed in the head of the tubing, where the fiber-optic handpiece attaches. This tubing attachment can be used only with the fiber-optic handpiece.
- Fiber-optic handpieces should be attached only to the fiber-optic tubing on the dental unit.
- High-speed handpieces are to be cleaned, lubricated, and sterilized per the manufacturer's directions.

Low-Speed Handpiece

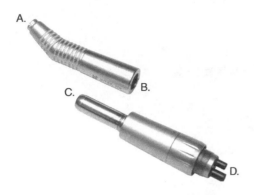

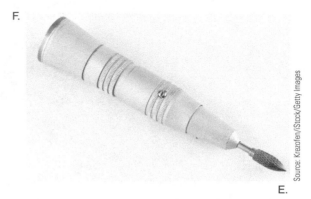

Source: Krezofen/Stcck/Getty Images

Use   The low-speed handpiece is used in both the dental treatment room and the laboratory. In the dental unit, the low-speed handpiece is used to polish teeth and restorations, remove soft carious material, and define cavity margins and walls. In the laboratory, the low-speed handpiece is used to trim, smooth, and polish removable dental appliances, such as dentures and partials.

Composition   **A.** Working end of the low-speed handpiece attachment.
            B. End for connecting to low-speed motor.
            C. Low-speed motor that attaches to the connecting end of attachments.

D. Low-speed motor that attaches to dental unit and compressed air.
E. Low-speed handpiece with nose cone, vulcanite bur with long shank placed in nose cone
F. Low-speed motor that attaches to dental unit and compressed air.

Notes

- Low-speed handpieces operate at or under 30,000 revolutions per minute (rpm).
- The low- or slow-speed handpieces are referred to as the straight handpieces because the shank and head are in a straight line.

Low-Speed Handpiece *Continued*

- Low-speed handpieces are used with or without attachments. The attachments are either a contra angle or a prophy angle. These attachments are used in the mouth.
- Low-speed handpieces can also be used without attachments. Long-shanked burs are inserted into the working end of the nose cone and used in the dental laboratory.
- Low-speed handpieces and attachments can operate in forward or reverse rotations.
- Low-speed handpieces are to be cleaned, lubricated, and sterilized per the manufacturer's directions.

Low-Speed Handpiece with Contra-Angle Attachment

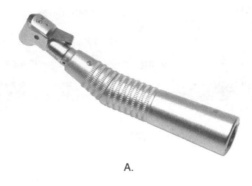

A.

Use
- To hold burs, discs, stones, rubber cups, and brushes for intraoral and extraoral procedures
- To remove soft decay
- To polish amalgams
- To make or finish composite restorations
- To adjust crowns and bridges
- To adjust partials and dentures
- To adjust temporary restorations

Composition Contra-angle latch attachment on a low-speed handpiece.
A. Contra Angle with latch.

Notes   This attachment uses latch-type burs, discs, stones, rubber cups, and brushes.

Low-Speed Handpiece with Prophy-Angle Attachment

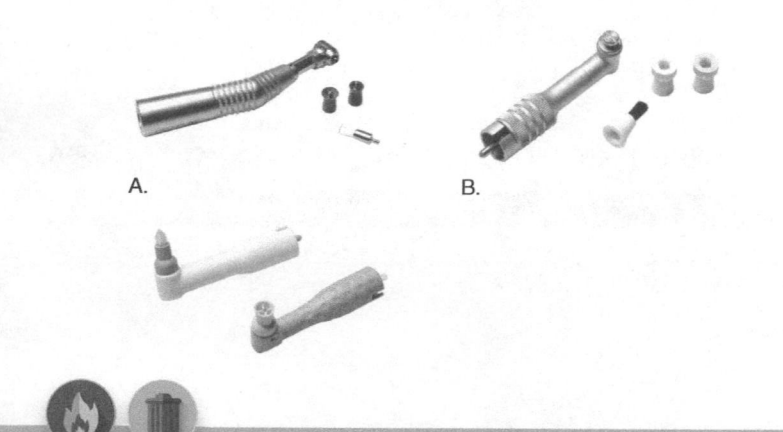

A.

B.

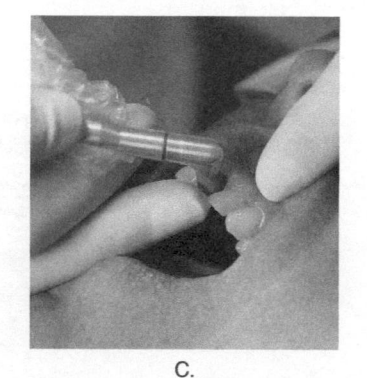

C.

Use To polish the teeth with rubber cups or brushes

Composition A. Screw-type prophy-angle attachment with screw-type cup and brush.
B. Snap-on type prophy-angle attachment with snap-on-type cup and brush.
C. Prophy-angle attachment with a cup in use.

Notes
- Some low-speed handpieces are designed to be lightweight to reduce hand and finger fatigue.
- There are also disposable prophy-angle attachments with cups and brushes to attach to low-speed handpieces.
- These handpieces are to be cleaned, lubricated, and sterilized per the manufacturer's directions.

Equipment to Clean and Lubricate the Handpieces

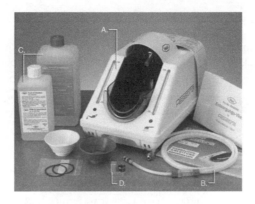

Use To clean and lubricate both high- and low-speed handpieces

Composition **A.** Assistina machine
B. Connecting hoses
C. Solutions
D. High-speed adapter

Notes
- These units must be connected to compressed air.
- They have attachments so that both the high- and low-speed handpieces can be run in the same unit.
- Handpieces must be wiped off after the cycle is complete, and then they are ready to be sterilized.
- Several models are available, including the Assistina and the QUATRROcare. The manufacturer's directions should be followed.

Electric Handpiece

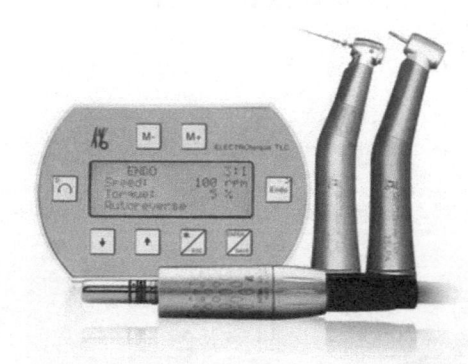

Use

The electric handpiece is used for cavity preparation; endodontic procedures; contouring and trimming provisional crowns and bridges; and adjusting crowns, bridges, and permanent restorations.

Composition
- Control unit
- Motor and hose
- High-speed attachment with fiber optics
- Low-speed attachment
- Endodontic attachment
- Straight attachment

Notes
- Electric handpieces are an alternative to air-driven handpieces.
- Electric handpieces run from 27,000 to 200,000 rpm.
- Electric handpieces are quiet, vibration free, and efficient.
- Electric handpieces are to be cleaned, lubricated, and sterilized per the manufacturer's directions.

Laboratory Handpiece

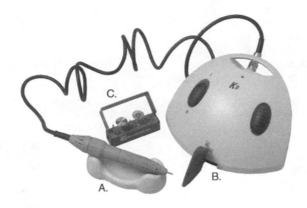

Use
- To trim and contour provisional crowns, bridges, and custom trays
- To adjust and polish partials and dentures

Composition
A. Handpiece with holder
B. Foot control
C. Selection of burs, stones, and discs

Notes
- Laboratory handpieces are used for multiple purposes in the dental office.
- Laboratory handpieces can be used in the reverse or forward direction. The manufacturer's directions should be followed.

Air Abrasion

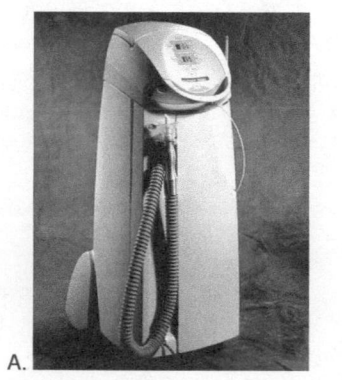

A.

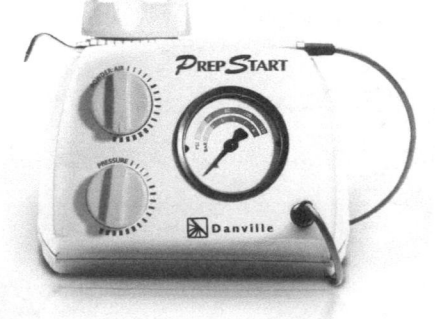

B.

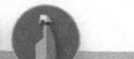

Use
- To clean fissures for sealants
- To prepare tooth and remove decay in small cavities (example: Class I)
- To clean restorations
- To make special repairs in restorations
- To roughen the inside of restorations before bonding

Composition
- Base unit
- Control panel
- Foot switch
- Air-pressure gradient
- Handpiece
- Abrasive flow control
- External suction device
- **A.** Floor model
- **B.** Table unit

Air Abrasion *Continued*

Notes
- Each unit requires an air pressure source and an abrasive.
- Air abrasion units come in a variety of models, including floor models and countertop units.
- When using air abrasion units, minimal anesthetic is required.
- Abrasive particles are different sizes and made of various materials such as aluminum oxide.
- Abrasive particles must be evacuated while his unit is used, and eye protection must be worn.

Laser Handpiece

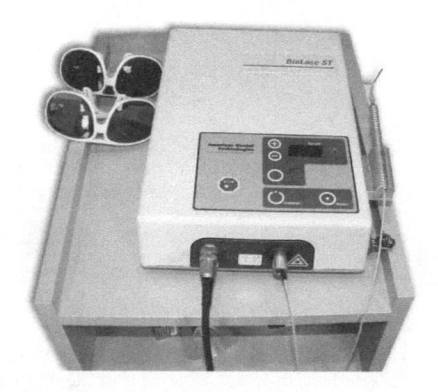

Use
The laser handpiece is used to cut and remove soft tissue, to control bleeding, and to biopsy tissue. Dental lasers are also used to cure some dental materials, in cavity preparation and caries removal, in diagnostic transillumination for detection of caries microfractures, in endodontic therapy, in pulpotomy treatment, to whiten teeth, and to treat lesions such as cold sores.

Composition
Dental laser unit with handpiece attachment and safety glasses.

Notes
- The dental laser is a medical device that generates a precise beam of concentrated light energy.
- With technology constantly improving, there are many types of dental lasers.

Surgical Unit with Light for Implant Systems

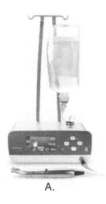

A.

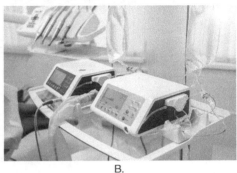

B.

Source: Terelyuk/Shutterstock.com

Use	Precise surgical placement of implants, extractions, and oral surgery procedures.
Composition	• Motor and tubing • Speed control • Surgical unit with memory chip • Irrigation–hygienic unit • Contra angle with light **A.** Free Standing Implant Unit. **B.** Implant Unit in Operatory.
Notes	• Sterile water is utilized with the handpiece for cooling. • Surgical handpieces come with a light. • Surgical handpieces are electrical and run at a lower speed (used for implants) of 10 to 50 rpm to a maximum speed of 40,000 rpm. • Unit displays actual speed, direction, and torque.

CHAPTER 7
Burs, Stones, and Discs

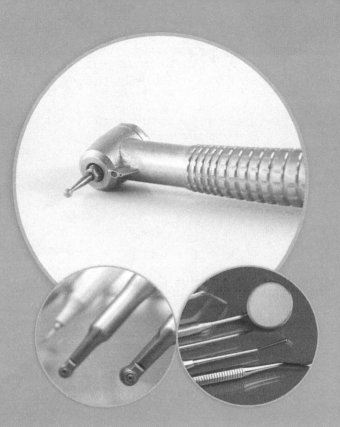

Burs

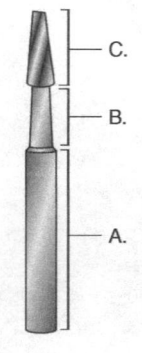

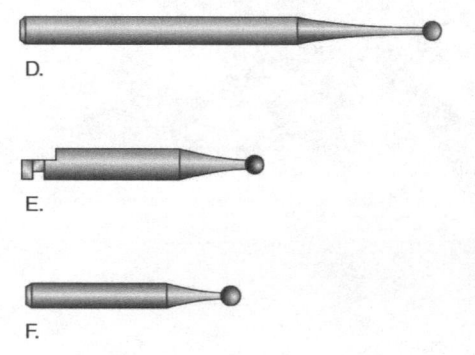

Use
Burs are part of a group of instruments referred to as rotary instruments that cut or polish tooth structure. They are used with high- or low-speed handpieces. Burs are used in numerous laboratory functions.

Composition
A. The shank is the part that is inserted into the handpiece.
B. The neck is the tapered connection of the shank to the head.
C. The head is the working end of the bur.
D. Straight Shank.
E. Latch-type Shank.
F. Friction Grip Shank.

Notes
- The straight shank, or long shank, functions with the straight, low-speed handpiece.
- The latch-type shank has a notch that fits into the contra-angle/right-angle handpiece and latches securely in place.
- The friction-grip shank functions with the high-speed handpiece.
- Burs are purchased individually in packages or several in one package.

Round Bur

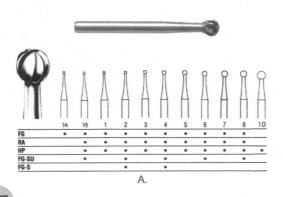

	¼	½	1	2	3	4	5	6	7	8	10
FG	•	•	•	•	•	•	•	•	•	•	
RA		•	•	•	•	•	•	•	•	•	•
HP		•	•	•	•	•	•	•	•	•	•
FG-SU		•		•		•		•		•	
FG-S				•		•					

A.

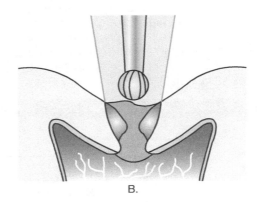

B.

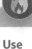

Use
- To open the cavity and remove carious tooth structure
- To open the tooth for endodontic treatment

Composition Bladed cutting bur with a shank (friction grip, latch, or straight) and a round cutting head.
A. Round Burs.
B. Round Bur Opening a Cavity Preparation.

Notes
- Available in a range of sizes: 1/4, 1/2, 1, 2, 3, 4, 5, 7, 8, and 10.
- The smallest is 1/4, and 10 is the largest.

Burs are sterilized and reused until dull, and then they are disposed of in the sharps container.

Inverted Cone Bur

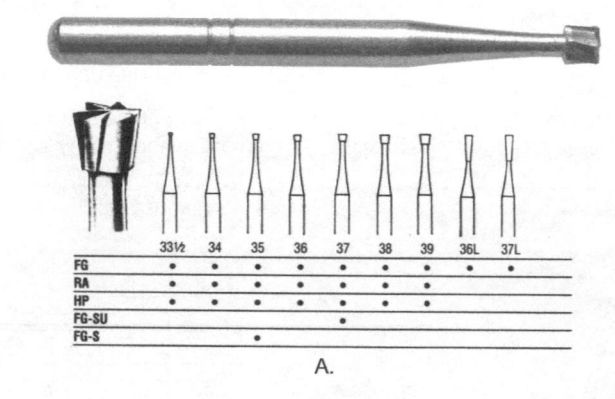

	33½	34	35	36	37	38	39	36L	37L
FG	•	•	•	•	•	•	•	•	•
RA	•	•	•	•	•	•	•		
HP	•	•	•	•	•	•	•		
FG-SU					•				
FG-S			•						

A.

Use
- Removes caries
- Makes undercuts in the preparation for retention

Composition Bladed cutting bur with a shank (friction grip, latch, or straight) and a short tapered cutting head.
A. Inverted Cone.

Notes
- Available in a range of sizes: 33 1/2: 34, 35, 36, 37, 38, 39, 36L, and 37L.
- The smallest is 33½, and 39 is the largest; 36L and 37L have a longer head.
- *L* indicates long head on the bur.
- *S* indicates short head on the bur.
- Burs are sterilized and reused until dull, and then they are disposed of in the sharps container.

Plain Fissure Straight Bur and Plain Fissure Cross-Cut Bur

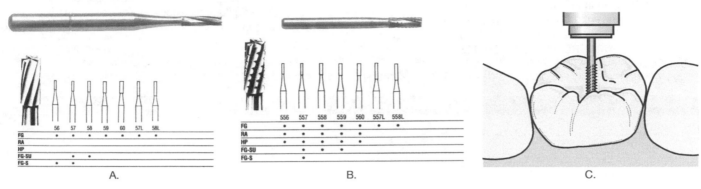

	56	57	58	59	60	57L	58L
FG	•	•	•	•	•	•	•
RA							
HP							
FG-SU			•	•			
FG-S	•	•					

A.

	556	557	558	559	560	557L	558L
FG	•	•	•	•	•	•	•
RA	•	•	•	•	•		
HP	•	•	•	•	•		
FG-SU		•	•	•			
FG-S			•				

B.

C.

Use
- Forms the cavity walls of the preparation
- Places retention grooves in walls of cavity preparation

Composition This is a bladed cutting bur with a shank (friction grip, latch, or straight) and a long straight cutting head. The cross-cut bur has horizontal cuts.
- **A.** Straight Fissure.
- **B.** Straight Fissure Cross-cut.
- **C.** Fissure use in Cavity Preparation.

Notes
- Head has parallel sides (cross-cut with horizontal cutting edges).
- Available in a range of sizes: 56, 57, 58, 59, 57L, and 58L (straight) and 556, 557, 558, 559, 557L, and 558L (cross-cut).
- *L* indicates long head on the bur.
- *S* indicates short head on the bur.
- Burs are sterilized and reused until dull, and then they are disposed of in the sharps container.

Tapered Fissure Straight Bur and Tapered Fissure Cross-Cut Bur

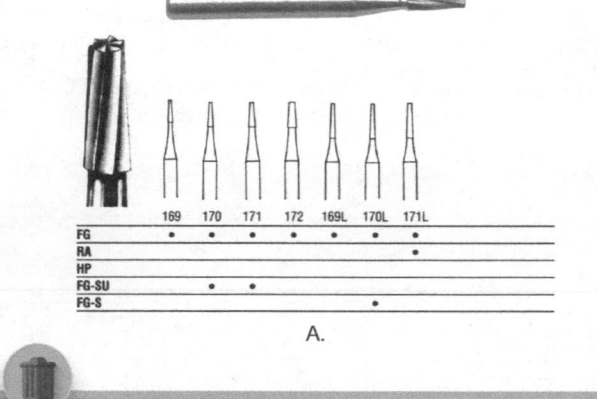

	169	170	171	172	169L	170L	171L
FG	•	•	•	•	•	•	
RA							•
HP							
FG-SU		•	•				
FG-S							•

A.

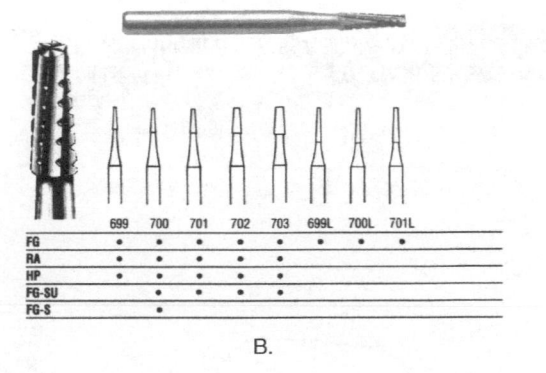

	699	700	701	702	703	699L	700L	701L
FG	•	•	•	•	•	•	•	•
RA	•	•	•	•	•			
HP	•	•	•	•	•			
FG-SU	•	•	•	•	•			
FG-S	•							

B.

Use
- Forms divergent walls (angles) of the cavity preparation
- Places retention grooves in the walls of the cavity preparation

Composition This is a bladed cutting bur with a shank (friction grip, latch, or straight) and a long-tapered cutting head.
  A. Tapered Fissure.
  B. Tapered Fissure Cross-cut.

Notes
- These are available in a range of sizes: 169, 170, 171, 172, 169L, 170L, and 171L (straight) and 699, 700, 701, 702, 703, 699L, 700L, and 701L (cross-cut)
- *L* indicates long head on the bur.
- *S* indicates short head on the bur.
- The head of the cross-cut bur is tapered and has horizontal cutting edges.
- Burs are sterilized and reused until dull, and then they are disposed of in the sharps container.

End-Cutting Bur

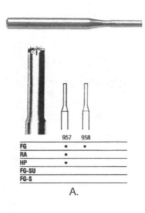

A.

Use   Forms the shoulder for crown preparations

Composition This is a cutting bur with a shank (friction grip, latch, or straight); bladed only on the end of a cylinder head.
A. End Cutting.

Notes
- These are available in sizes 957 and 958.
- Burs are sterilized and reused until dull, and then they are disposed of in the sharps container.

Wheel

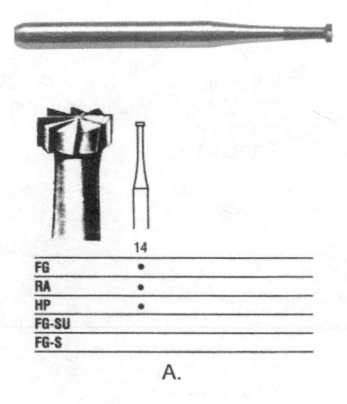

	14
FG	•
RA	•
HP	•
FG-SU	
FG-S	

A.

Use Forms retention in preparations, often used in Class V preparations

Composition A bladed cutting bur with a shank (friction grip, latch, or straight) and wheel-shaped short head.
A. Wheel.

Notes
- The head has cutting edges on the top and the sides.
- It comes in size 14.
- Burs are sterilized and reused until dull, and then they are disposed of in the sharps container.

Pear Bur

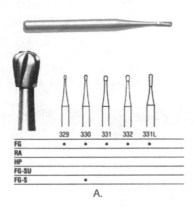

	329	330	331	332	331L
FG	•	•	•	•	•
RA					
HP					
FG-SU					
FG-S		•			

A.

Use
- Opens and extends the cavity preparation
- Removes dental decay

Composition This is a bladed cutting bur with a shank (friction grip, latch, or straight) and a pear-shaped head.
A. Pear.

Notes
- The head of the bur is shaped like a pear, with the largest part away from the neck of the bur.
- The bur has cutting edges on all sides of the head.
- The common sizes are 329, 330, 331, 332, and 331L.
- *L* indicates long head on the bur.
- *S* indicates short head on the bur.
- Burs are sterilized and reused until dull, and then they are disposed of in the sharps container.

Diamond Bur Flat-End Taper and Flat-End Cylinder

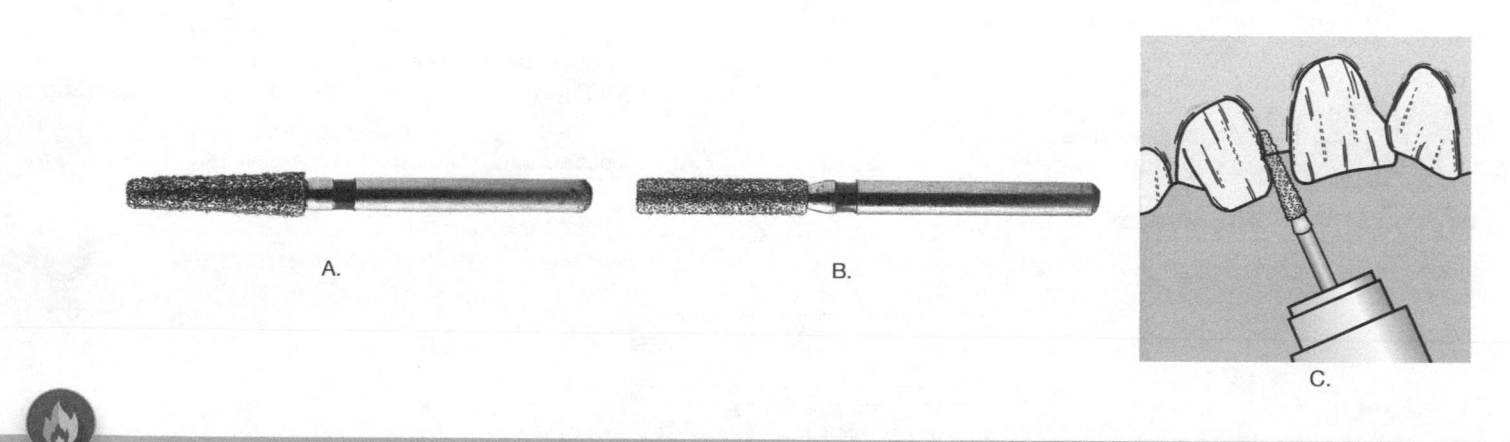

A.

B.

C.

Use
- Rapid reduction of tooth for crown preparation when a square shoulder is needed (taper) or when parallel wall and flat preparation floor is needed (cylinder)
- Rapid reduction of tooth for crown preparation

Composition The head of the diamond bur is embedded with diamond particles through an electroplating or a bonding process.
- **A.** Tapered Diamond.
- **B.** Cylinder Diamond.
- **C.** Diamond use in Preparation.

Notes
- This is available in a variety of shapes, sizes, and grits.
- Super-fine is used to finish restorations.
- Grit is designated by the color band on the shank of the diamond bur or by the letter after the name of the diamond bur. Grit ranges include super-fine to super-coarse.
- Burs are sterilized and reused until dull, and then they are disposed of in the sharps container.

Diamond Bur Flame and Diamond Bur Wheel

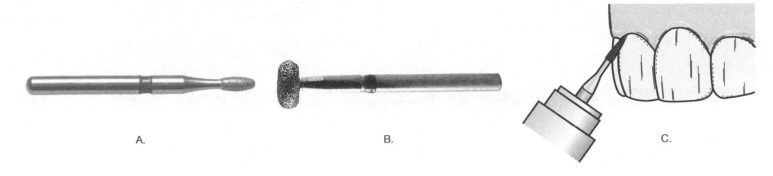

A.

B.

C.

Use
- Rapid reduction of tooth for crown preparation when a beveled subgingival margin is needed (flame).
- Rapid reduction of the incisal edge during crown preparation (wheel).
- Rapid reduction of the lingual aspect of the anterior teeth during crown preparation (wheel)
- Contouring anatomy into composite restorations.

Composition The head of the diamond bur is embedded with diamond particles through an electroplating or bonding process.
- **A.** Flame Diamond.
- **B.** Wheel Diamond.
- **C.** Diamond use in Smoothing a Restoration.

Notes
- This comes in a variety of shapes, sizes, and grits. Grit ranges include super-fine to super-coarse.
- The flame shape can be short, as shown, or long and tapered.
- Super-fine grits are used to finish restorations.
- The wheel is sometimes called a donut shape.
- Burs are sterilized and reused until dull, and then they are disposed of in the sharps container.

Diamond Turbo or Speed Cut and Diamond Composite Finishing Bur

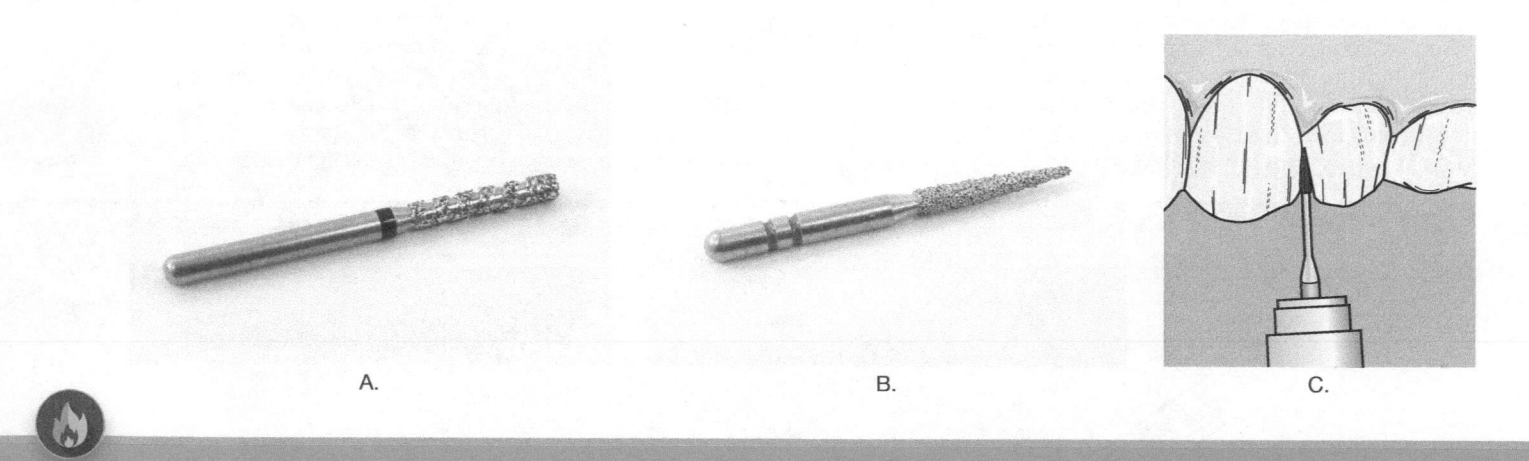

A.

B.

C.

Use	• Rapid cutting and gross reduction of the tooth structure
	• Used to finish composite restorations
	• Used to finish glass ionomer and porcelain restorations
Composition	• Cross-cuts or spiral cuts on head of diamond bur; head is embedded with diamond particles through an electroplating or bonding process.
	A. Turbo Diamond
	B. Composite Diamond
	C. Diamond use in Smoothing a Restoration

Notes
- These are available in a variety of shapes with cross-cuts or spiral cuts in the diamond head.
- Diamonds are designed with diamond-free cooling zones that absorb normal heat production.
- Burs are sterilized and reused until dull, and then they are disposed of in the sharps container.
- Grits from ultra-fine to extra-coarse are available.
- A super-fine grit is used to finish restorations.
- They are available in long and short shanks.

Finishing Bur

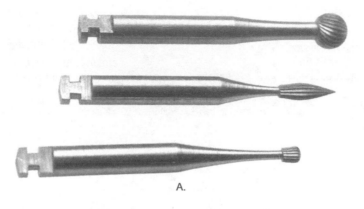

A.

Use	• To smooth, trim, and finish metal restorations • To smooth, trim, and finish natural-tooth-colored material restorations
Composition	Up to 30 or more blades for ultra-fine finishing **A.** Variety of Shapes of Finishing Burs.

Notes
- Finish burs come in a variety of shapes and sizes.
- They are identified by the manufacturer's number.
- They are available in latch (as shown) and friction grip.
- Burs are sterilized and reused until dull, and then they are disposed of in the sharps container.

Surgical Bur

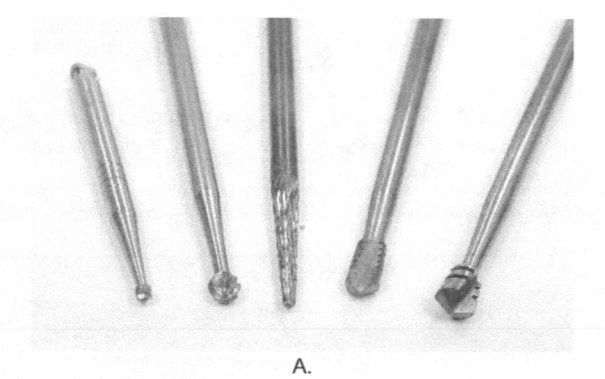

A.

Use   Used in low-speed handpiece straight nose cone to reduce and contour the alveolar bone and tooth structure

Composition
- Extra-long shanked bur available in many shapes.
- The head is designed to cut tooth or bone structure.
- **A.** Variety of Shapes of Surgical Burs.

Notes
- Heads come in various sizes and shapes.
- Long shanks.
- Burs are sterilized and reused until dull, and then they are disposed of in the sharps container.

Laboratory Burs

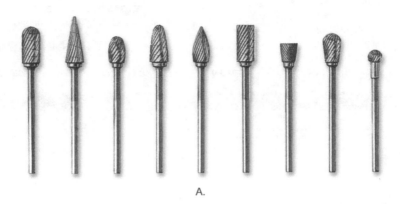

A.

Laboratory burs are sometimes referred to as vulcanite burs.

Use
- To make adjustments on acrylic materials, such as partials, dentures, and custom trays
- Used on plaster, stone, and metal materials

Composition
- Long shanks insert into straight nose cone low-speed handpieces.
- Large working ends.

A. Variety of Shapes of Laboratory Burs.

Notes
- A variety of sizes and shapes are available.
- They are available in titanium-nitrate-coated carbide.
- Titanium-nitrate-coated burs are faster, cooler, and longer-lasting.

Mandrel Snap-On and Mandrel Screw-On

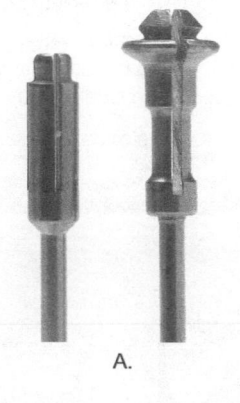

A.

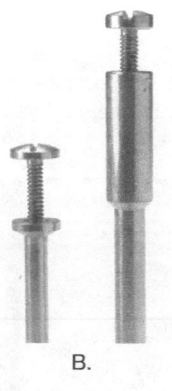

B.

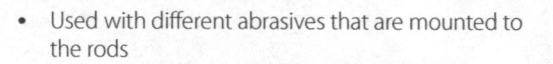

Use
- Used with different abrasives that are mounted to the rods
- Used to hold the discs that finish and polish

Composition Rods of various lengths that are used in low-speed handpieces with snap-on or screw-on attachments.
A. Snap-On Mandrel.
B. Screw-On Mandrel.

Notes
- Short-shanked snap-on or screw-on mandrels are used with a contra-angle slow-speed handpiece.
- A long shank is used with a straight slow-speed handpiece.
- These are available in friction grip.
- These can be sterilized, or they are available in disposable types.

Sandpaper Discs

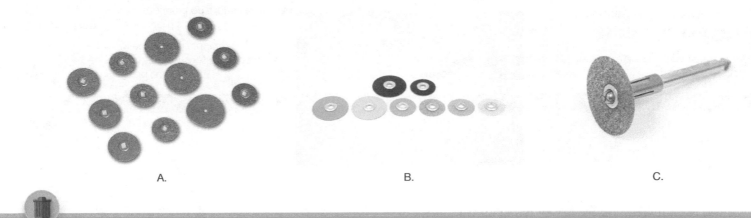

A.

B.

C.

Use
- To polish, smooth, and adjust restorative materials
- To polish, smooth, and adjust dental appliances

Composition
- Circular discs
- Abrasive texture on one or both sides
- Mounted to mandrel for use
- **A.** Sandpaper discs
- **B.** Soft sandpaper discs in various sizes and grits
- **C.** Snap on garnet disc attached to mandrel

Notes
- Sandpaper discs can be rigid or flexible.
- They are available in a variety of sizes and grits.
- Colors on discs represent grit abrasiveness.
- When using discs, begin with more abrasive material then move to less abrasive materials.
- When ordering, the size, grit, abrasiveness, and type of mandrel must be specified.

Diamond Disc

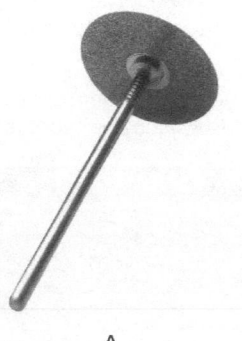

A.

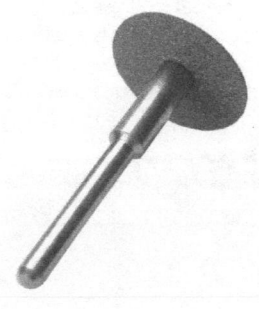

B.

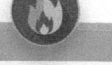

Use
- Rapid cutting
- Polishing composite restorations
- Interproximal reduction

Composition Circular steel discs
- **A.** Disc mounted on a long shank mandrel for use in a Slow Speed Straight Nose Cone.
- **B.** Disc mounted on a friction grip mandrel for use in a High Speed Handpiece.

Notes
- These are available in solid or patterned discs.
- These steel discs have diamond particles or chips bonded to both sides.
- Discs are sterilized and reused until dull, and then they are disposed of in the sharps container.

Carborundum Discs

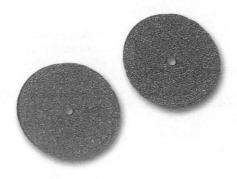

Use
- Used primarily in the dental laboratory to cut and finish gold restorations
- Used for trimming acrylic provisional restorations

Composition
- Circular, thin, and brittle discs that break easily
- Carborundum on both sides
- Mounted to a mandrel

Notes
- These are called separating discs.
- Discs are disposable.
- Carborundum discs are also known as Joe Dandy discs.

Rubber Points and Polishing Points

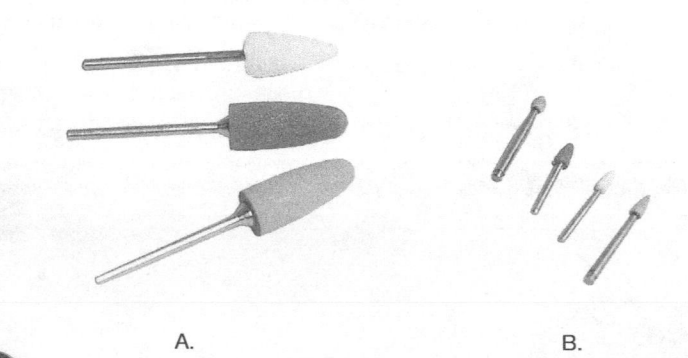

A.

B.

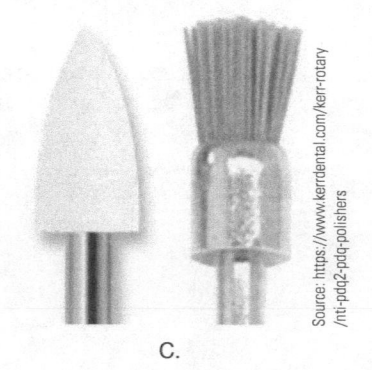

C.

Source: https://www.kerrdental.com/kerr-rotary/nti-pdq2-pdq-polishers

Use To polish restorations

Composition
- Rubber-tipped head impregnated with abrasive material
- Can be made out of many types of materials and shapes
- Latch-type or friction-grip shanks
- **A.** Long shank polishing point for use in a Slow Speed Straight Nose Cone.
- **B.** Variety of polishing points for use in a Slow Speed Contra Angle or a Friction Grip High Speed Handpiece.
- **C.** Polishing point and brush.

Notes
- White points are for polishing.
- Green points (greenies) are not as abrasive as brown points.
- Brown points (brownies) are more abrasive than green points.
- Occlubrush polishers are for finishing restorations.
- Many shapes and materials of polishers are available.

Bur Blocks

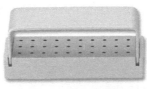

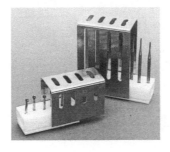

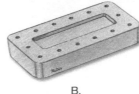

A.

B.

Use	On dental tray setups
Composition	Holding device for burs
	A. Burs placed in Bur Blocks.
	B. Bur Blocks.

Notes

- Bur blocks come in a variety of shapes and sizes from different manufacturers.
- Most bur blocks can be sterilized.
- They hold both friction-grip and latch-type burs.
- Some are magnetic to hold burs in place.

CHAPTER 8
Hand-Cutting Instruments

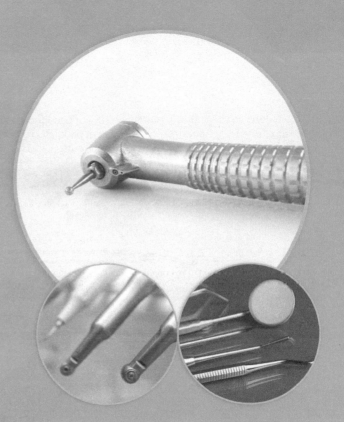

Three-Number and Four-Number Instruments

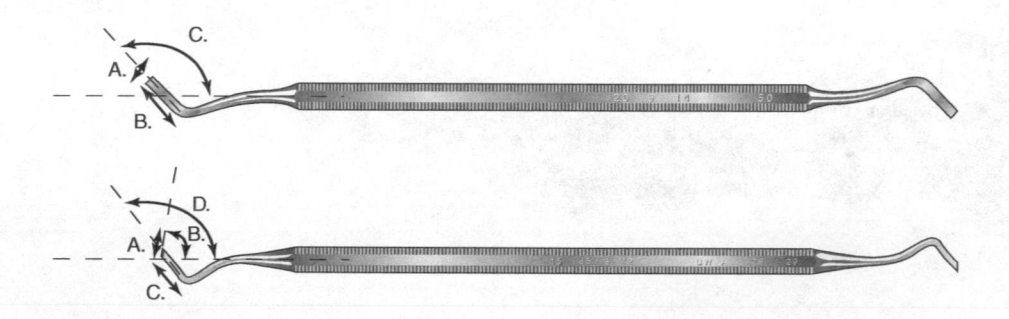

Black's formula was developed by G. V. Black to standardize the exact size and angulation of an instrument. Black's formula for three-number hand-cutting instruments includes the length and width of the blade and the angle at which the blade is positioned to the handle. The formula for four-number hand-cutting instruments includes the length and width of the blade, the angle at which the blade is positioned to the handle, and the angle of the cutting edge of the blade to the handle. Many cutting instruments have been replaced with rotary instruments (burs).

Straight Chisel

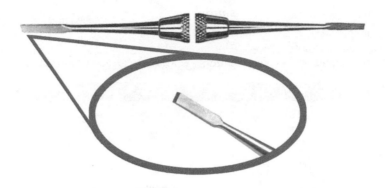

Use	• To shape and plane enamel and dentin walls of the cavity preparation • Used in a pushing action • Used in Class II or IV cavity preparations • Used with a mallet to remove crowns	**Composition**	• Straight-shanked instrument with bevel on one side of the cutting edge • Single- or double-ended
		Notes	• Straight chisels need to be sharpened. • This is a three-number instrument.

Wedelstaedt Chisel

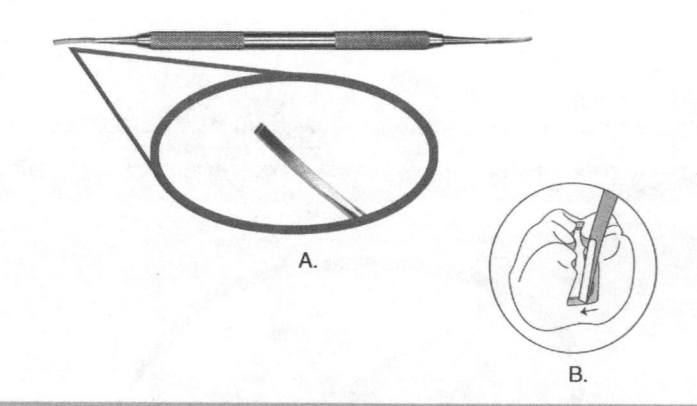

A.

B.

Use
- To shape and plane enamel and dentin walls of the cavity preparation
- Used in a pushing action
- Used for Classes III and IV cavity preparations

A. Wedelstaedt Chisel.
B. Wedelstaedt Chisel placement inside of a Cavity Preparation.

Composition
- Slightly curved blade on a shanked instrument with bevel on one side of the cutting edge
- Single- or double-ended

Notes This is a three-number instrument.

Binangle Chisel

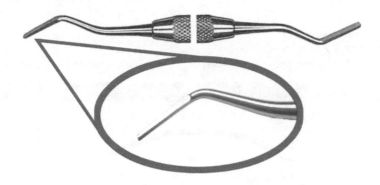

Use	• To shape and plane enamel and dentin walls of the cavity preparation • Used in a pushing action • Used in a Class II cavity preparation
Composition	Two angles in the shank of the instrument
Notes	• This is usually a double-ended instrument. • This is a three-number instrument.

Hatchets

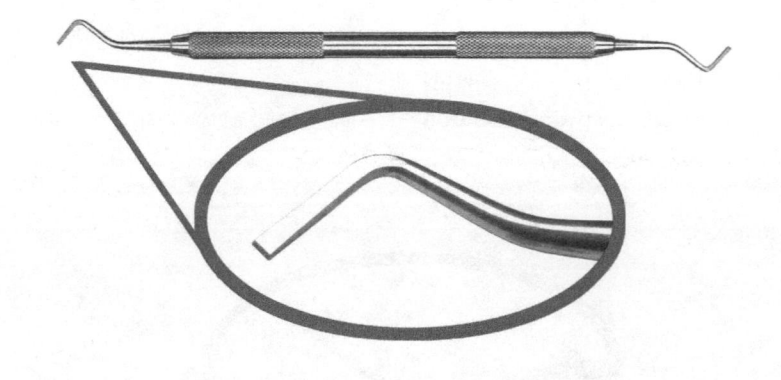

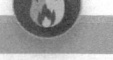

Use
- To refine the cavity walls and to obtain retention in the cavity preparation
- Used in a downward motion

Composition
- Paired left and right with the bevel on one side of the blade on one end of the instrument and on the reverse side of the blade on the other end.

Notes
- Hatchets are usually double-ended instruments.
- They are sometimes referred to as enamel hatchets.
- This is a three-number instrument.

Hoes

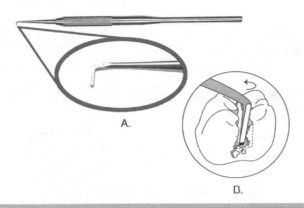

A.

B.

Use	• To smooth and shape the floor of the cavity preparation • Used in a pulling motion
Composition	A shank and head shaped similarly to a garden hoe with straight and angled shanks. **A.** Hoe. **B.** Hoe placement inside of Cavity Preparation.
Notes	• The cutting edge of the blade is nearly perpendicular to the shank/handle. • This is a three-number instrument. • Hoes are normally single-ended.

Gingival Margin Trimmers

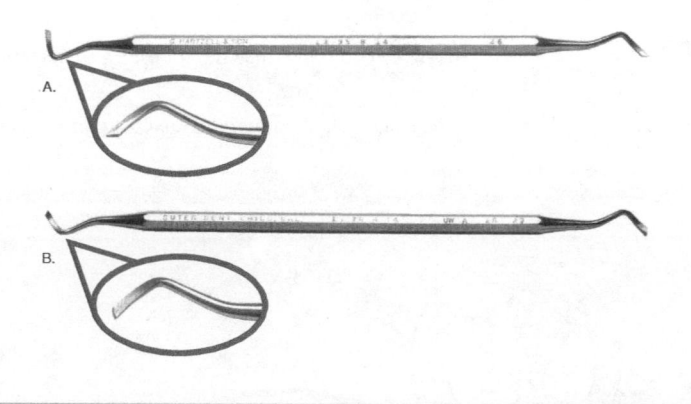

A.

B.

Use

To bevel the gingival margin wall of the cavity preparation

Composition • A pair of instruments with binangled shanks used to smooth the mesial and distal cervical margins of the cavity preparation.
  • The blade is curved rather than straight. One end curves to the right; the other curves to the left.
  • The cutting edge is slanted.
A. Distal gingival margin trimmer (GMT)
  • Close-up of the working end of the distal GMT
B. Mesial gingival margin trimmer
  • Close-up of the working end of the mesial GMT

Notes

  • A pair of GMTs is used during cavity preparation because one instrument is used for the distal surfaces (A) and another for the mesial surface (B).
  • This is a four-number instrument. If the second number of the four-number formula is 90 or above, it is used on the distal surface of the cavity preparation. If it is 85 or below, it is used on the mesial surface.

Angle Formers

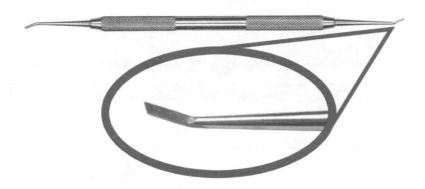

Use	To form and define point angles and to sharpen line angles in a cavity preparation
Composition	This is a double-ended instrument in which the cutting edge is slanted and ends in a point. The slanted cutting edge is beveled differently on each end of the instrument to allow access to the mesial and distal surfaces of the cavity preparation.
Notes	• Angle formers are four-number instruments. • These are usually double-ended instruments.

Excavators—Spoon and Blade Excavators

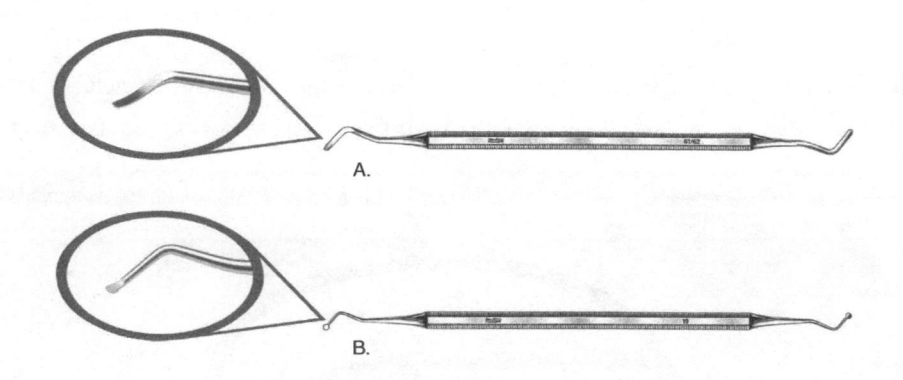

A.

B.

Use
- To remove carious materials and debris from the teeth
- To assist in the tucking/inverting of the dental dam around the teeth
- To remove temporary crowns and bridges during fabrication
- To remove excess temporary cement from around temporary restorations

Composition
- A bladed instrument with a binangled shank that is rounded at the working end of the blade.
- **A.** Blade excavator
- **B.** Spoon excavator

Notes
- Excavator ends are spoon-shaped with cutting edges.
- These instruments can be single- or double-ended.
- The ends vary in size.
- This is the most commonly used cutting instrument.

CHAPTER 9

Diagnostic Aids, Matrices, Instruments and Materials used for Cements, Bases, Liners, and Buildup

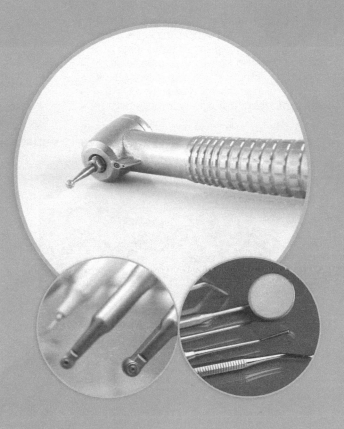

Intraoral Camera

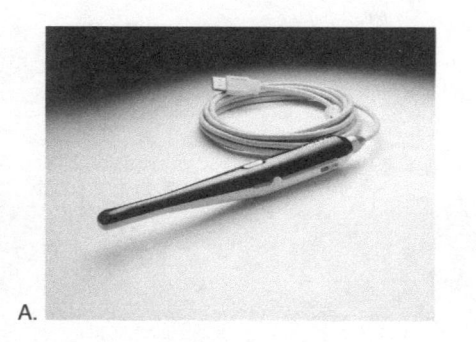

A.

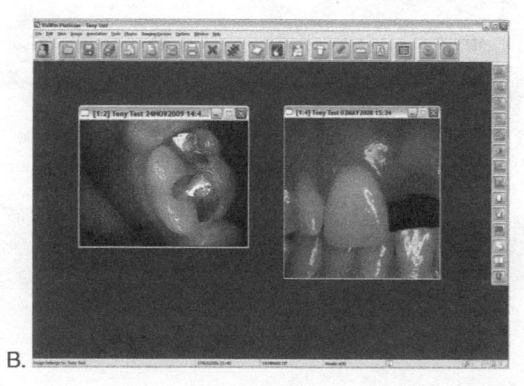

B.

Use
- Allows patients to see areas and conditions inside their mouths while the dentist is discussing them
- To take photos that can be saved in patients' electronic records or printed for their paper records
- Used for marketing, patient presentation, and helping the patient understand needed treatment
- Aids in insurance claims

Composition
- Handheld wand with camera that takes intraoral pictures and is attached to the dental unit and computer terminal or is wireless

Properties
A. Intraoral Camera image
B. Images on computer screen

Notes
- The intraoral camera allows the office to be paperless.
- It may be attached to the dental unit, a mobile unit or is available wireless
- It can be used by the dentist or auxiliary personnel.
- Barriers are used on the wand.
- The systems are designed to obtain different views of the tooth/teeth for better diagnosis.

Caries Detectors/Indicators

Caries detectors or caries indicators are special machines or dyes used to detect caries by distinguishing between good, sound, hard dentin and dentin that is infected with bacteria and is softened.

Cavity Detection/DIAGNOdent

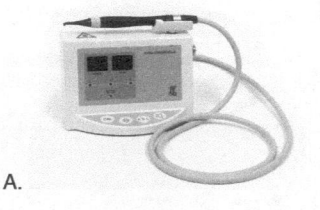

A.

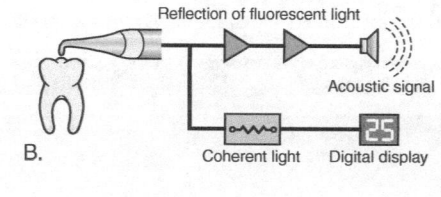

Reflection of fluorescent light

Acoustic signal

B.

Coherent light   Digital display

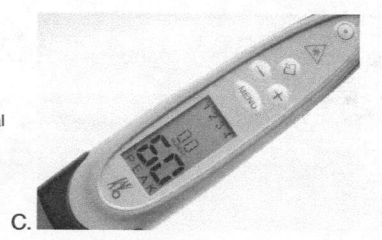

C.

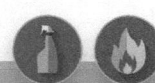

Use
- To detect carious material in the tooth
- To ensure that the tooth is free of caries prior to sealant placement
- To quantify caries progression

Composition
- Battery-operated microprocessor-controlled display unit with handpiece and tips or handheld pen unit with tips for easier handling and greater mobility
  - **A.** KaVo DIAGNOdent unit
  - **B.** How caries detection works
  - **C.** Close-up of the handheld pen unit

Notes
- Tips must be sterilized.
- Lasers may also emit audio signals.
- A decayed tooth structure and bacteria fluoresce (give off light) when exposed to specific wavelengths of light. Thus, a healthy tooth exhibits little or no fluorescence, whereas a tooth with decay fluoresces according to the extent of decay.

Caries Detector

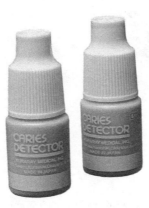

Use	• Identification of carious dentin
	• Aids in the removal of the carious dentin layer for a conservative preparation
	• Minimizes removal of remineralizable, healthy dentin, thus protecting the pulp
Composition	• Propane-1,2-diol with D&C red 30 dye
Properties	• Supplied in small bottles.
	• Comes in red dyes.
	• Must be rinsed off after a reaction time of 10 seconds.

• Do not use after expiration date.
• Do not store at temperatures above 77°F (25°C).
• Avoid exposure to sunlight.

Precautions
• Eye and skin irritation is possible.
• Product should not be ingested.
• Product is flammable. Keep away from open flame.
• Avoid cross-contamination.

Mixing and Setting Time No mixing is required. Apply for 10 seconds.

Caries Detector *Continued*

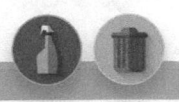

Directions

1. Place a couple of drops in a dappen dish.
2. Use a small applicator tip to dip into the dye.
3. Place the dye in the cavity preparation and let it set for about 10 seconds.
4. Rinse the dye off of the cavity preparation.
5. Use burs and spoon excavators to remove the stained dentin.
6. This process is repeated until no caries remain.

Caries Indicator

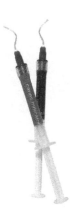

Use
- Identification of carious dentin
- To preserve maximum amount of inner dentin while infected dentin is removed
- Assists in locating fractures, root canal orifices, and calcified canals

Composition
- VistaRed: glycol based with 1% acid red 52 solution
- VistaGreen: propylene glycol with FD&C green

Properties
- Supplied in unit dose packages and prefilled syringes.
- Must be rinsed off after reaction time of 10 seconds.
- Do not use after expiration date.

- Do not store at temperatures above 77°F (25°C).
- Avoid exposure to sunlight.

Precautions
- Eye and skin irritation possible.
- Product should not be ingested. If ingested, may cause nausea and vomiting.
- Product is flammable. Keep away from open flame.
- Avoid cross-contamination.

Mixing and Setting Time No mixing is required. Apply for 10 seconds.

Caries Indicator *Continued*

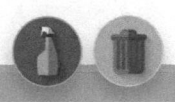

Directions

1. Dispense dye into the cavity prep using the disposable tip.
2. Place the dye in the cavity preparation and let it set for about 10 seconds.
3. Rinse the dye off of the cavity preparation.
4. Use burs and spoon excavators to remove the stained dentin.
5. This process is repeated until no caries remain.

Desensitizers

Desensitizers are agents used to reduce or eliminate the sensitivity of the teeth. Sensitivity may be caused by abrasions that expose dentin; caries; abfraction associated with bruxism; leaking restoration, scaling, and root planing; and some restorative materials.

There are several categories of desensitizing agents, including toothpastes, fluoride gel/varnish, inorganic salts, and resin agents.

Relief Gel

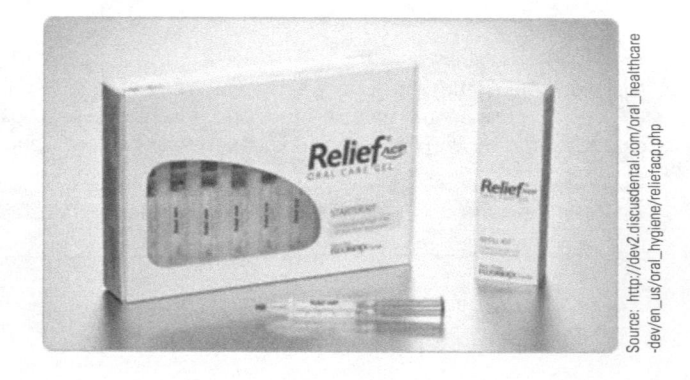

Source: http://dev2.discusdental.com/oral_healthcare-dev/en_us/oral_hygiene/reliefacp.php

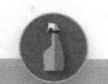

Use	• Reduces sensitivity associated with thermal changes, tooth whitening, acid penetration, sweets, and/or direct contact • Assists in preventing tooth decay by aiding in rebuilding enamel • Improves luster of teeth
Composition	Potassium nitrate 5% and fluoride 0.240%
Properties	• Comes in a mint-flavored gel • Also comes in a syringe for easy application

Precautions
- Eye and skin irritation is possible.
- Product should not be ingested.

Mixing and Setting Time No mixing is required.

Directions
Patient may apply directly into whitening tray or apply with a soft toothbrush.

Gluma Desensitizer

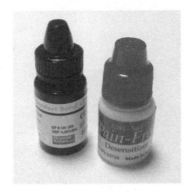

Use
- Prevents dentinal hypersensitivity
- Treats cervical sensitivity
- Prevents postoperative sensitivity
- Applied under all restorations, under resin-bonded veneers, inlays, onlays, and crowns
- Applied after root planing or periodontal treatment

Composition
- 5% glutaraldehyde
- 35% HEMA-hydroxyethyl, methacrylate, pentanedial
- Water

Properties
- Refrigerate if not used for a long time.
- Place pulp protection before placing GLUMA if cavity preparation is close to pulp.
- Drying the tooth before placement is not necessary; tooth can be moist.

Precautions
- Eye and skin irritation is possible; if contact occurs, rinse immediately.
- Product should not be ingested.
- Product is flammable. Keep away from open flame.
- Avoid cross-contamination.

Gluma Desensitizer *Continued*

**Mixing and
Setting Times** No mixing is required. Apply for 30 seconds.

Directions

1. Use a small sterile cotton pellet, applicator tip, or single-dose applicator.
2. Apply material to the dentin of the tooth using a gentle but firm rubbing motion for 30 seconds.
3. Dry thoroughly but do not rinse.

D/Sense® Crystal

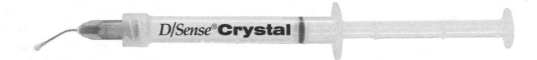

Use
- Desensitizer and cavity liner
- Prevention of cervical erosion and gingival recession
- Applied under crowns and bridges when standard cement is used
- Applied to exposed dentin, such as around the margins of a temporary crown
- Applied under restorations

Composition
- Solution of potassium binoxalate and nitric acid in water
- Free of HEMA, glutaraldehyde, and other toxic chemicals

Properties
- One-step, dual-action material.
- Fast-acting.
- Long-lasting results.
- Reacts with the dentin to precipitate microcrystals of calcium oxalate and potassium nitrate.
- Occludes dentinal tubules with calcium oxalate and potassium nitrate.
- Time saving and less waste.
- Gentle on soft tissues.

D/Sense® Crystal *Continued*

Precautions
- Eye and skin irritation is possible; if contact occurs, rinse immediately.
- If ingested, give a solution of sodium bicarbonate or liquid antacid medication.

Mixing and Setting Times No mixing is required. Setting (drying) time is 30 seconds using a gentle air spray or 2 minutes without the air spray.

Directions

1. Remove the cap from the syringe and securely attach a SofNeedle foam tip or dispense a few drops of liquid from the syringe into a dappen dish and use a small applicator.

2. To improve the comfort of the patient, warm the syringe to body temperature.

3. Check the flow of the material from the syringe on a paper pad and then pass the syringe to the dentist for placement.

4. The material is rubbed until the dentin is saturated for about 20 seconds.

5. After the material is placed, gently use the air-water syringe and air-dry for 30 seconds or let airdry the preparation for 2 minutes. The material has a frosty white precipitate.

6. Repeat if needed.

Tofflemire Matrix

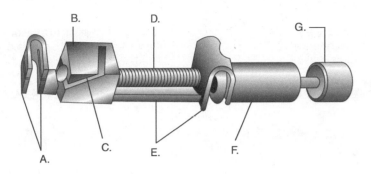

Use
- To hold the matrix band that establishes the normal contour of the prepared tooth while the tooth is being filled with the restorative material
- Class II cavity preparations

Composition **A.** Guide channels: The slots in the end of the retainer that hold the matrix band; slots direct the band to the right or left of the retainer.

B. Vise (locking): Holds the ends of the matrix band in place in the diagonal slots.

C. Diagonal slot: Where the matrix band is placed; slides up and down on the spindle.

D. Spindle: A screw-like rod used to secure the band in the vise.

E. Frame: The main body of the retainer.

F. Inner knob (adjusting knob): Used to adjust the size (circumference) of the matrix band loop by moving the vise along the frame of the retainer.

G. Outer knob (locking knob): Used to tighten and loosen the spindle against the band in the vise.

Matrix Bands

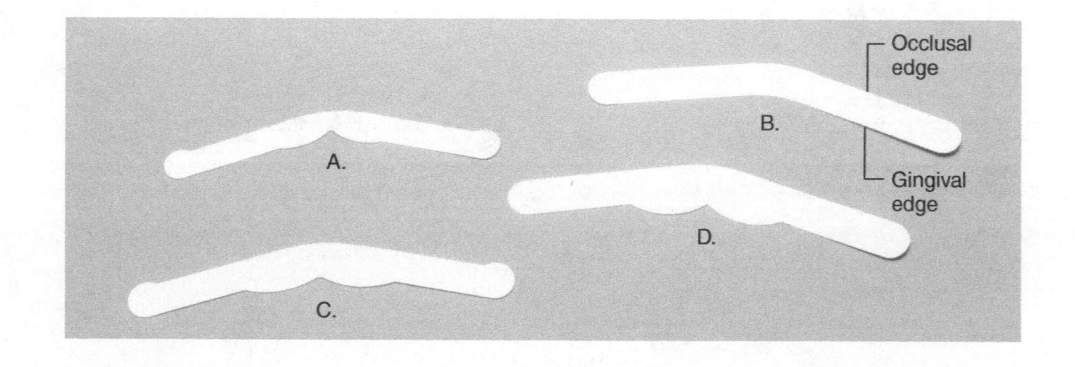

Use
- Form the missing surface or wall and reestablish the normal contour of the prepared tooth while the tooth is being filled with the restorative material
- Class II preparations.

Composition
- **A.** Pediatric band used for primary teeth
- **B.** Universal band
- **C.** Premolar band
- **D.** Molar band

Notes
- Matrix bands are made of stainless steel.
- Matrix bands are normally the same length.
- Matrix bands differ in the shape of one edge and in their widths.
- The size of the cavity prep indicates which band is used.

Auto-Matrix Kit

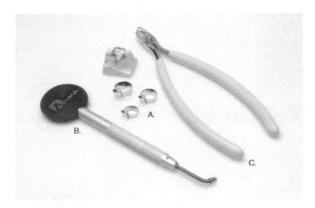

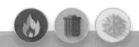

Use
- Forms the missing surface or wall and reestablishes the normal contour of the prepared tooth while the tooth is being filled with the restorative material
- Class II preparations

Composition
A. Matrix and coil: Used to loop the tooth and replace the missing surface or tooth wall
B. Tightening device and rotation handle: Used to tighten the matrix around the tooth; fits into the coil and tightens as the handle is rotated
C. Removal pliers: Used to clip the end of the autolock loop

Notes
- The stainless-steel bands are conical shaped and come in four sizes.
- The matrix and coil (bands) are circles with autolock loops that lock the matrices on the teeth.
- There is no retainer to obstruct the operator's access or vision.

Cure-Thru Clear Cervical Matrices

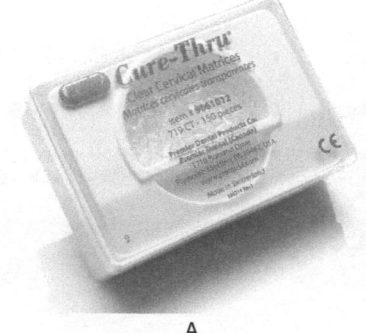

A.

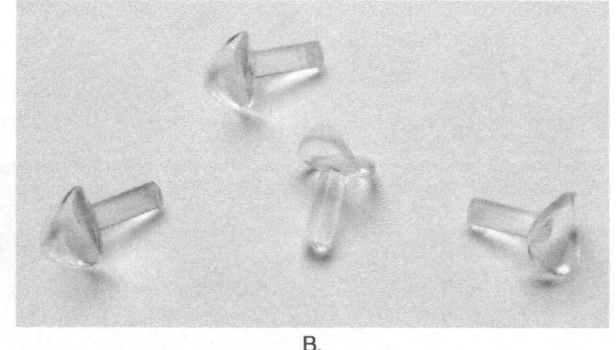

B.

Use To compress and contour restorative material into cervical area as it is light cured

Composition **A.** A plastic tab attached to a contoured matrix that fits the cervical area of the tooth.

B. Some cervical matrices come with a positioning instrument instead of a tab.

Notes • Matrices are available in an assorted box of 250.

• Box contains (50) anterior/premolar and molar matrices.

• Box contains (35) matrices in other shapes.

• A positioning instrument, which is also clear, is included.

• Product is flexible to fit the exact contour of the tooth.

• Matrix allows for excellent marginal integrity.

• Material can be cured directly through this matrix.

• For a composite interproximal matrix, a plastic strip matrix is used.

Plastic Strip Matrix and Clip

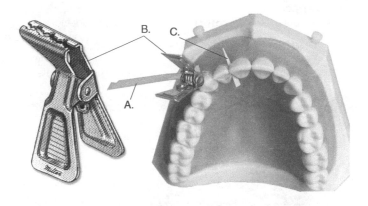

Use		• Provide anatomical contour and proximal contact relation to the tooth	

Use
- Provide anatomical contour and proximal contact relation to the tooth
- Prevent excess material at the gingival margin
- Confine the restorative material under pressure while the material is being cured
- Protect the restorative material from losing or gaining moisture during the setting time
- Allow the polymerizing light to reach the composite restorative material

Composition
- **A.** Strip matrix
- **B.** Clip retainer
- **C.** Wedge

Notes
- Plastic strip matrix is used with composite, glass ionomer, or compomer restorative materials on anterior teeth.
- Product is made of nylon, acetate, celluloid, or resin.
- It is approximately 3 inches long and 3/8 inches wide

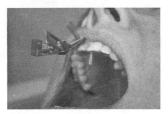

Sectional Matrix System

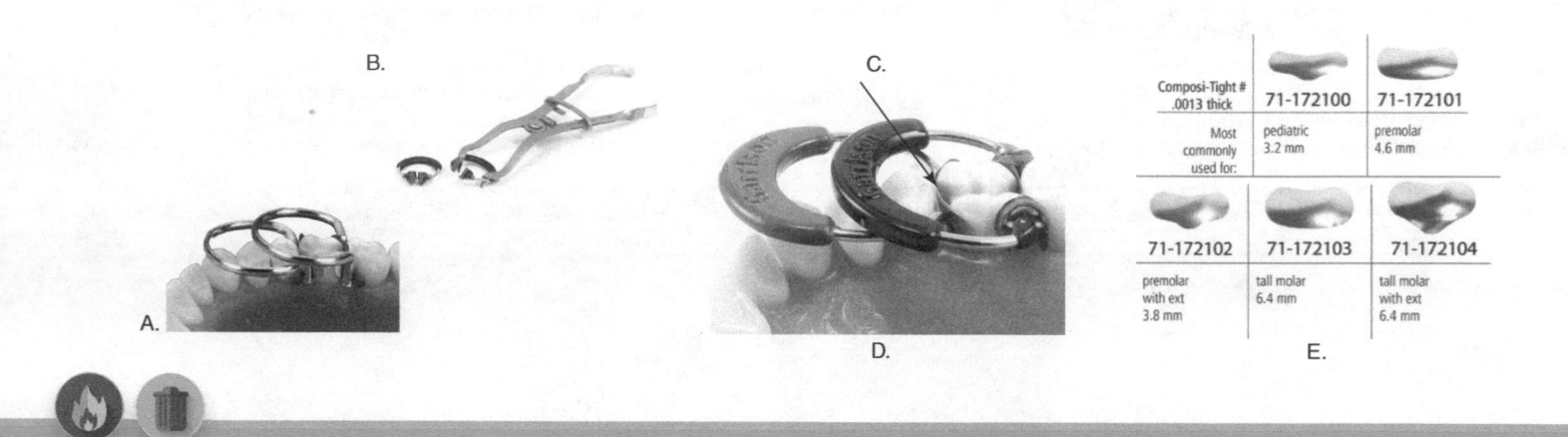

B.

C.

A.

D.

E.

Composi-Tight # .0013 thick	71-172100	71-172101
Most commonly used for:	pediatric 3.2 mm	premolar 4.6 mm

71-172102	71-172103	71-172104
premolar with ext 3.8 mm	tall molar 6.4 mm	tall molar with ext 6.4 mm

Use Sectional matrix rings that confine the restorative material under pressure while the material is being cured

Composition
A. Tines (to hold the matrix tightly in place)
B. Ring placement forceps (hinged forceps that are designed to fit and securely grasp the G-rings)
C. Oval matrix bands

D. Sectional matrix system in place for mesio-occluso-distal (MOD) restoration
E. Different sizes of bands are available

Notes Bands are available in different sizes and shapes to accommodate restorations, including adult and pediatric bands and extended bands for deep cervical restorations.

Wedges and Wedge Wands

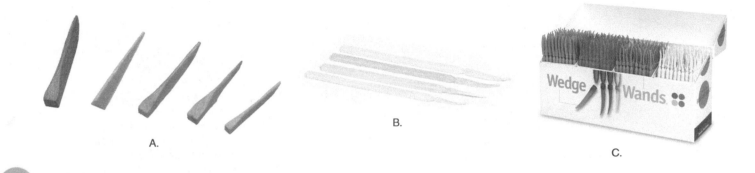

A.

B.

C.

Use
- To tightly hold matrix band in place along the gingival margins of Classes II, III, and IV preparations
- To prevent excess filling material from escaping between the tooth and the matrix band
- To ensure good contact with the adjacent tooth after the band has been removed

Composition
- Small, triangular piece of wood or plastic
  A. Sample of wooden wedges.
  B. Sample of light cure-through wedges.
  C. Wedge wands: The wand is one-piece flexible plastic wedge that separates after application.

Wedges and Wedge Wands *Continued*

Notes
- A variety of shapes and sizes are available.
- Wedges are either natural, clear, or colored.
- They usually come in an assortment kit with various sizes.
- Colors mark the different sizes within the kit.
- Wedges can be flexible or curved or can have an attached handle.
- The difference between the wedges and the wedge wands is the detachable handle. Removal of the wedge from the wand is done by applying gentle force on the waffle-like neck of the wand.
- Wedges are available as cure-through.

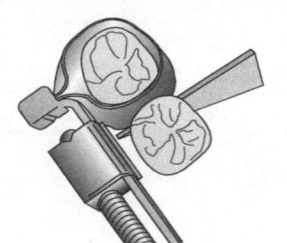

Cement Mixing Spatula

Use	To mix dental cements and materials
Composition	Single-ended flat spatula and handle
Notes	• The spatula is flexible or rigid and allows proper manipulation of materials.
	• It is made of stainless steel.
	• The spatula is sterilizable.
	• The edge of the spatula can be used to gather the materials for use.
	• They are available in a range of sizes.

Cavity Liners and Low-Strength Bases

Cavity liners and low-strength bases are used for cavity preparations where there is little or no dentin to cover the pulp. They have a variety of uses, including protecting and soothing the pulp. Some stimulate the formation of secondary dentin and some contain fluoride to strengthen the tooth.

Cavity liners and low-strength bases come in the forms of powder/liquid, two paste systems, single tube, and syringes with disposable tips.

Fuji Lining LC

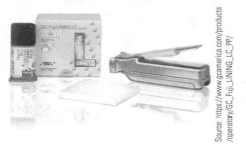

Source: https://www.gcamerica.com/products/operatory/GC_Fuji_LINING_LC_PP/

Use	Permanent durable lining or low-strength base under all types of restorations
Composition	• Silicate glass powder containing calcium, aluminum, and fluoride (calcium fluoroaluminosilicate glass) • Liquid: aqueous solution of polyacrylic acid
Properties	• Light-cured material • Releases fluoride

• Radiopaque material
• Biocompatible to reduce sensitivity
• Bonds mechanically and chemically to the tooth structure
• Also comes in paste form

Precautions Eye and skin irritation is possible; if contact occurs, rinse immediately.

Fuji Lining LC *Continued*

Mixing and Setting Times
- Mixing time is 5 to 10 seconds for the first portion and 10 to 15 seconds for the second portion, for a total not to exceed 20 seconds.
- Material is light-cured for approximately 30 seconds to set. (Time depends on strength of curing light.)
- Avoid long exposure to overhead light once the material is mixed.

Directions

1. Gather materials: powder and liquid, powder-dispensing scoop specific to this product (or paste cartridge and dispenser), paper pad, 2 × 2 gauze, and placement instrument.
2. Tooth should be isolated with rubber dam or cotton rolls.
3. Rinse and dry the cavity preparation.
4. Dispense one level scoop of powder (scoop comes with kit). Replace the cap on the powder.
5. Divide the powder into two sections on the paper pad. Dispense one drop of liquid by holding the bottle vertically upside down. Replace the cap on the liquid.
6. Incorporate the first portion into the liquid by mixing for 5 to 10 seconds.
7. Add the second portion, and mix the whole for 10 to 15 seconds. Total mixing time should not exceed 20 seconds.
8. Secure paste cartridge in the dispenser and dispense pastes onto the paper pad. Blend until the mixture is smooth and uniform.
9. Apply the mixture into the cavity preparation with a small applicator or suitable lining instrument.
10. Pass the instrument/applicator to the dentist and hold the paper pad and a gauze sponge close to the patient's chin for easy access during placement of the lining cement.
11. Once the material has been placed, light-cure for 30 seconds.

Vitrebond Plus

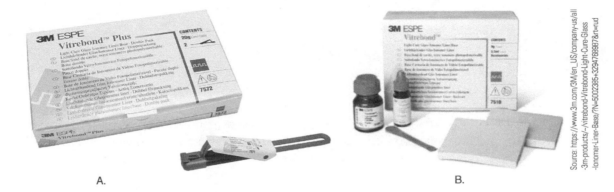

A.

B.

Use	• Permanent liner/base • Prevention of microleakage • Aids in reducing the effects of polymerization shrinkage of the restorative materials • Seals dentin to reduce postoperative sensitivity
Composition	Resin-modified glass ionomer paste and liquid form
Properties	• This product bonds strongly to dentin. • It has a "clicker" dispensing system for easy use. • It comes in a combination of powder and liquid.

• Vitrebond releases fluoride.
• It has good consistency and sets quickly.
   A. Auto cartridge dispenser
   B. Powder/Liquid

Precautions Eye and skin irritation is possible; if contact occurs, rinse immediately.

Mixing and Setting Times Mix for 10 to 15 seconds. Light-cure for 20 seconds.

Vitrebond Plus *Continued*

Directions

1. Gather materials: dual-barrel "clicker" dispensing gun or powder/liquid, cement spatula, paper pad, 2 × 2 gauze, and placement instrument.
2. Tooth should be isolated with rubber dam or cotton rolls.
3. Rinse and dry the cavity preparation.
4. Dispense a small amount of material onto a paper pad.
5. Gather the material with the cement spatula and mix for 10 to 15 seconds until the mix is uniform in color.
6. Pass the placement instrument to the dentist and hold the paper pad close to the patient's chin.
7. Once the material is in place, light-cure for 20 seconds.

Small-Balled Instrument (Dycal Instrument)

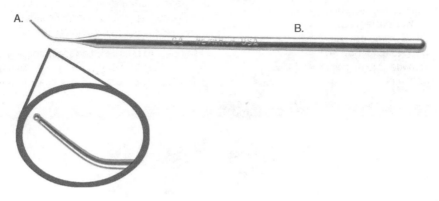

Use	Mix and place two-paste calcium hydroxide material or glass ionomer liner into the cavity preparation
Composition	• Small-balled tip • Straight handle
Notes	• It is available with a short or long handle. **A.** Mixing tip **B.** Dycal instrument

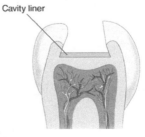

Cavity liner

Dycal-Two-Paste System

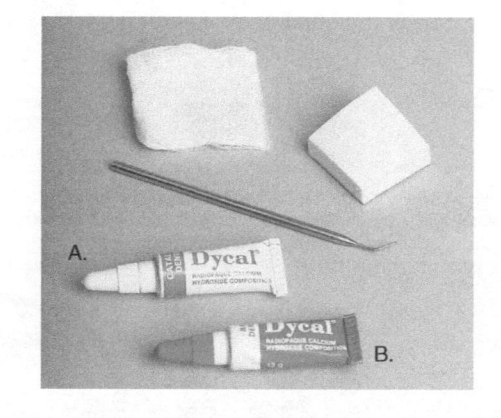

| Use | • Low-strength liner under any restorations, cements, and other base materials |
| | • Applied with indirect or direct pulp-capping procedures |

Use

- Low-strength liner under any restorations, cements, and other base materials
- Applied with indirect or direct pulp-capping procedures

Composition

- Base: zinc oxide, 1,3-butylene glycol disalicylate, calcium phosphate, calcium tungstate, and iron oxide pigments
- Catalyst: calcium hydroxide, *N*-ethyl-*o/p*-toluenesulfonamide, zinc oxide, titanium dioxide, zinc stearate, and iron oxide pigments (dentin shade only)
  - **A.** Dycal catalyst
  - **B.** Dycal base

Properties

- Rigid, self-setting material

- Therapeutic effect on the pulp.
- Alkaline pH between 9 and 11 stimulates the formation of secondary dentin when the material is in direct contact with the pulp.
- Some thermal insulating properties.
- Minimal strength to support the forces of condensation.

Precautions

- Some patients may be sensitive to calcium hydroxide cements.
- Avoid eye contact; if contact occurs, flush eyes immediately with flowing water.

Dycal-Two-Paste System *Continued*

Mixing and Setting Times
- Mix within 10 seconds.
- Mixed material will set in 2½ to 3½ minutes.
- Moisture and higher temperatures will decrease the working time and cause the material to set faster.

Directions

1. Gather materials: base and catalyst tubes, small paper pad, 2 × 2 gauze, and placement instrument (Dycal instrument or explorer).
2. Dispense equal amounts of the base and the catalyst onto the mixing pad provided.
3. Stir the two pastes together using the Dycal instrument or an explorer.
4. Mix until a uniform color has been achieved (about 10 seconds).
5. Wipe off the Dycal instrument with a gauze sponge and pass to the dentist.
6. Hold the small paper pad with the mixed material close to the patient's chin within easy reach for the dentist.
7. Have a gauze sponge ready to remove any excess material during the application.

Prisma VLC Dycal

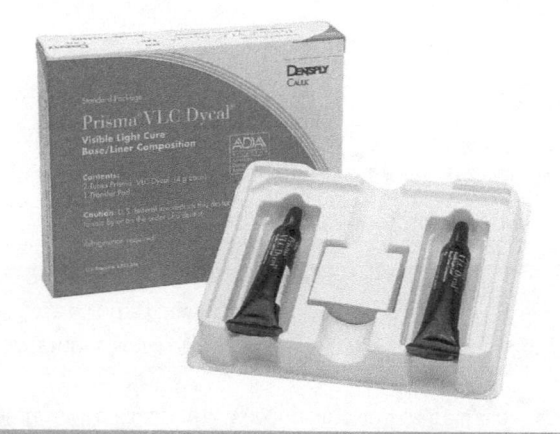

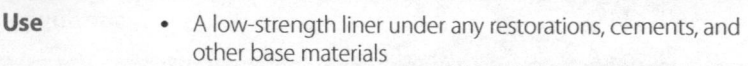

Use	• A low-strength liner under any restorations, cements, and other base materials
	• Applied with indirect or direct pulp capping procedures
Composition	Similar to two-paste calcium hydroxide with polymerizable monomers
Properties	• Light-cured material.
	• Requires no mixing.
	• Must be refrigerated to prolong shelf life.
	• Radiopaque.

• Therapeutic effect on the pulp.
• Alkaline pH between 9 and 11 stimulates the formation of secondary dentin when the material is in direct contact with the pulp.
• Some thermal insulating properties.
• Minimal strength to support the forces of condensation.
• Very low water solubility compared to two-paste calcium hydroxide.

Prisma VLC Dycal *Continued*

Precautions
- Some patients may be sensitive to calcium hydroxide cements.
- Avoid eye contact; if contact occurs, flush eyes immediately with flowing water.

Mixing and Setting Times No mixing required. Setting time depends on strength of curing light, but a minimum of 20 seconds is required.

Directions

1. Dispense Prisma VLC Dycal on a small paper pad and cover to avoid exposure to light. Allow the material to warm to room temperature.
2. Rinse and dry the cavity preparation.
3. Uncover the material, pass the Dycal instrument to the dentist, and hold the paper pad under the patient's chin within easy reach for the dentist.
4. Have a gauze sponge ready to remove any excess material during the application.
5. Prepare the curing unit and then cure the material for a minimum of 20 seconds, holding the light source within 2 mm of the material. If the curing unit is between 2 mm and 5 mm from the surface, cure the material for 30 seconds.

Plastic Filling Instrument (PFI)

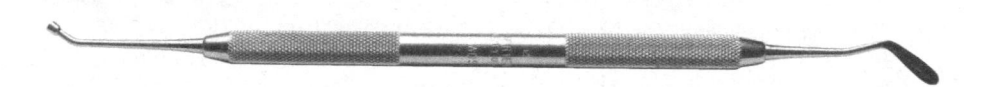

Use	• To place and condense pliable restorative materials
	• To place cement bases in the cavity preparation
Composition	• Usually double-ended
	• Paddle end to place materials
	• Small condenser end or different-shaped paddle end
Notes	• PFIs are available in various sizes, angles, and shapes.
	• They are used for placement of intermediate and temporary materials.

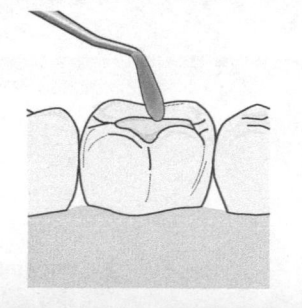

Cavity Varnish

Cavity varnish is a material that is used as a protective barrier between the restoration and the prepared tooth. It seals the dentin tubules from irritating chemicals found in restorative materials and cements. Varnish sometimes comes with a solvent to thin the varnish when it becomes too thick for placement.

Cavity varnish is used in some cavity preparations, but many dentists prefer to use a bonding agent that has multiple functions.

Copalite

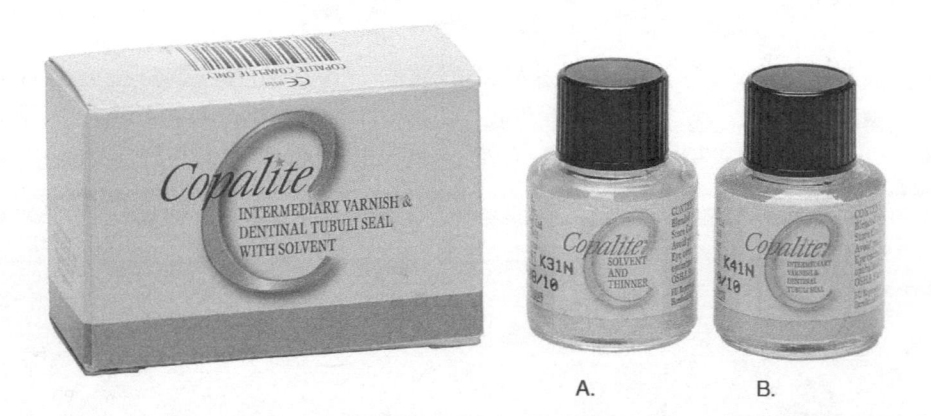

A.   B.

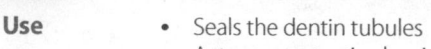

Use	• Seals the dentin tubules • Acts as a protective barrier
Composition	• Natural resins • Organic solvents (ether alcohol, acetone, or chloroform) **A.** Solvent **B.** Varnish
Properties	• Has a strong odor • Does not exhibit any strength • Does not provide any thermal insulation • Insoluble in the oral fluids

• Reduces microleakage
• Prevents penetration of acids from cements and restorative materials
• Nonacidic and nonirritating
• Solvent in the varnish will evaporate, so it is important to keep the bottle tightly capped when not in use.

Precautions
• Copalite may irritate the eyes, skin, and oral mucosa.
• This material has a strong odor and may cause respiratory difficulties upon inhalation.
• It should not be ingested.
• Product is flammable. Keep away from open flame

Copalite *Continued*

Mixing and Setting Times No mixing required. Setting time: 5 to 10 seconds, or just long enough for the layers to dry.

Directions

1. Clean and dry the cavity preparation.
2. Prepare two applicator brushes, cotton-tipped applicators, or small cotton pellets.
3. Remove the cap from the varnish and dip the applicators into the varnish until they are moistened.
4. Replace the cap on the varnish because it has a strong odor and to prevent evaporation of solvent.
5. Dab off the excess varnish on a gauze 2 × 2.
6. One layer of varnish is placed on dentin in the cavity preparation and then allowed to dry.
7. Apply the second coat using the second applicator in the same manner and allow it to dry.

Copal Cavity Varnish

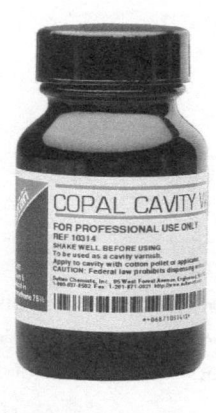

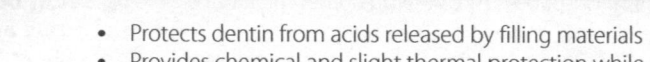

Use	• Protects dentin from acids released by filling materials
	• Provides chemical and slight thermal protection while eliminating air pockets
Composition	• Copal resins
	• 75% dichloromethane
Properties	• Needs no thinner
	• Does not exhibit any strength
	• Insoluble in the oral fluids

• Reduces microleakage
• Prevents penetration of acids from cements and restorative materials
• Nonacidic and nonirritating

Precautions
• This product may irritate the eyes, skin, and oral mucosa.
• Inhalation—this material has a strong odor.
• It should not be ingested.
• Product is flammable. Keep away from open flame.

Copal Cavity Varnish *Continued*

Mixing and Setting Times
- Comes in single bottle—no mixing required
- Setting time: 5 to 10 seconds just long enough for the layers to dry

Directions

1. Clean and dry the cavity preparation.
2. Prepare two applicator brushes, cotton-tipped applicators, or small cotton pellets.
3. Remove the cap from the varnish and dip the applicators into the varnish until they are moistened.
4. Replace the cap on the varnish because of the strong odor.
5. Dab off the excess varnish on a gauze pad.
6. One layer of varnish is placed on dentin in the cavity preparation and allowed to dry.
7. Apply the second coat using the second applicator in the same manner and allow it to dry.

Core Buildup Materials

A core buildup is a treatment performed on teeth that have very little crown structure left after the cavity preparation. The teeth are built up to support and provide retention for a permanent restoration such as a porcelain crown.

Miracle Mix

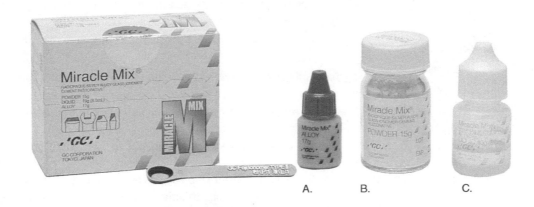

A.   B.   C.

Use
- Crown and core buildup
- Block-outs and repairs

Composition
- 100% fine silver alloy
- Glass ionomer cement
- Fluoride
- **A.** Alloy
- **B.** Glass Ionomer Powder
- **C.** Liquid

Properties
- Long-lasting
- Strong direct bond
- Color contrast with tooth structure

- Has high fluoride release to reduce secondary decay
- Easy to mix and place
- Won't stain or discolor surrounding teeth
- Shrinks and expands at the same rate as tooth structure
- Powder/liquid form and easy-to-use capsules

Precautions
- Eye and skin irritation is possible; if contact occurs, rinse immediately.
- Some patients are allergic to glass ionomer cements.

Mixing and Setting Times
- Powder/liquid: Mixing time is 35 to 40 seconds.
- Capsules: Preparation time is 10 to 15 seconds.
- Setting time is 4 to 5 minutes for both forms.

Miracle Mix *Continued*

Directions

Powder/Liquid

1. When using for the first time, pour the Miracle Mix alloy into the bottle of Miracle Mix powder and shake thoroughly.
2. Lightly tap the bottle for accurate dispensing of the powder.
3. Using the scoop that comes in the package, dispense two or three level scoops of powder onto a paper pad.
4. Divide the powder into two equal parts.
5. Hold the liquid bottle vertically and squeeze to dispense two drops of liquid.
6. Mix the first portion with all the liquid for 15 to 20 seconds.
7. Incorporate the second portion and mix thoroughly for 20 seconds.
8. Mix will be thick and putty-like.
9. Transfer the cement to the dentist using a syringe or plastic filling instrument (PFI).

Capsule

1. Tap the capsule on a flat surface to fluff the powder.
2. To activate, press the button on the bottom of the capsule.
3. Place the capsule in a high-speed amalgamator and triturate for 10 seconds.
4. Remove the capsule from the amalgamator and place it into the applier for delivery.

LuxaCore Dual Smartmix

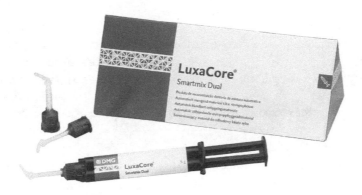

Use	One-step automix core buildup material
Composition	72% filled composite resin material
Properties	

- Compact, self-contained syringe for a consistent mix every time
- No mixing, no air bubbles, and no wasted material
- Light-cured, self-cured, and dual-cured
- Strong resin material
- Releases fluoride to protect against secondary caries

- Syringe delivery for easy use and less chance of cross-contamination
- Comes in three colors: Natural A3 for optimal esthetics, blue for contrast with the tooth, and white for perfect balance of contrast and esthetics
- Increased work time
- Radiopaque
- Composite viscosity to prevent material from slumping before it cures

LuxaCore Dual Smartmix *Continued*

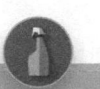

Precautions	• May cause skin and eye irritation; if contact occurs, rinse immediately.
	• Prolonged exposure may cause respiratory irritation.
	• If ingested, rinse mouth out with water and contact a physician.
Mixing and Setting Times	• No mixing required
	• Setting time: Light-cure according to size of buildup—20 to 40 seconds

Directions

1. Prepare, rinse, and dry the tooth.

2. Prepare the Smartmix handheld double-barreled syringe by removing the storage cap.

3. Place a small core tip or an intraoral tip.

4. Dispense a small amount of material on a paper pad or gauze to ensure that material is mixed.

5. Pass the syringe to the dentist and have a PFI ready.

6. Once the material is placed, pass the curing light or light-cure the material when the dentist indicates he/she is ready. Depending on the depth of the core material, the curing time will vary.

Encore Core Paste

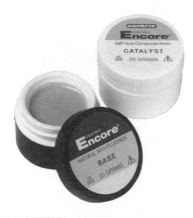

Use	Core buildup material
Composition	• Self-cured composite material • Two-paste system used with a syringe for placement
Properties	• High compressive strength • Cuts like dentin to reduce ditching • Comes with and without fluoride • Radiopaque • Comes in two shades: natural and white • No slumping, therefore no matrix needed

Precautions	• Product may be irritating to the skin and eyes. • It should not be ingested. • It may cause irritation on inhalation; keep area well ventilated.
Mixing and Setting Times	• Mixing time is 10 to 15 seconds. Working time is 2½ minutes. • Setting time is 4 to 5 minutes.

Encore Core Paste *Continued*

Directions

1. Prepare the tooth and apply the bonding agents.
2. Using one end of the spatula, take a small portion of the base.
3. Using the other end of the spatula, take a small and equal portion of the catalyst. Be sure not to cross-contaminate the two jars of material.
4. Blend the two materials together into a uniform mixture. Working time at this point is 2½ minutes.
5. Place the material into the Centrix C-R syringe tube. Fill halfway.
6. Place the plug in the end of the tube.
7. Place the syringe tube into the syringe barrel and dispense a small amount of material to test the flow.
8. Pass the syringe to the dentist for placement.

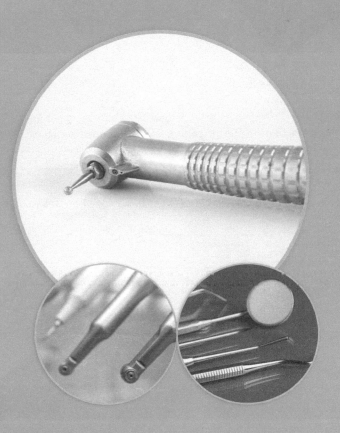

CHAPTER 10

Amalgam Bonding, Amalgam, Amalgam Instruments and Equipment

Bonding Agents

Bonding agents are used to attach restorative materials to the enamel or dentin of the tooth. There are many varieties of materials; they are self-curing, light-cured, or dual-cured. Most often they require conditioning or etching prior to placement. Some are unidose, meaning the etchant and the bonding agent are placed at the same time, whereas others require the etchant to be placed as a separate step.

Amalgambond Plus Adhesive System

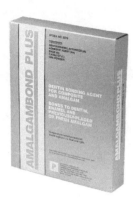

Use
- Chemical bonding of amalgams and composites to dentin, enamel
- Pulp capping

Composition Low-viscosity composite resin

Properties
- Provides a high-power bond
- Reduces the needs for pins
- Reduces sensitivity
- No need to place varnish or liners
- Reduces microleakage
- Self-curing

Precautions
- It may be irritating to the skin and eyes.
- It should not be ingested.
- It may be irritating on inhalation.

Mixing and Setting Time
- Mix the base and catalyst for 3 to 5 seconds.
- Allow the dentin activator to dry for 30 seconds.
- Allow the adhesive agent to dry for 30 seconds.
- Allow the base and catalyst to dry for 60 to 90 seconds before placing composite material.

Amalgambond Plus Adhesive System *Continued*

Directions

1. Rinse and dry the preparation completely.
2. Dispense one or two drops of dentin activator into the mixing well.
3. Brush the activator on the dentin for 10 seconds; to etch the enamel, leave on for 30 seconds.
4. Wash and dry the area.
5. Dispense one or two drops of adhesive agent into a clean mixing well.
6. Brush a thin layer of the adhesive onto the activated dentin surface.
7. Air-dry the surface to achieve an even, thin layer of coverage.
8. Leave for 30 seconds.
9. If placing an alloy restoration, place capsule into the amalgamator.
10. Dispense two drops of base and one drop of catalyst into a clean mixing well.
11. Mix thoroughly for 3 to 5 seconds.
12. Brush a thin, even layer onto the cavity preparation.
13. Mix and place the amalgam immediately before the adhesive dries. If placing a composite, allow the adhesive to dry for about 60 to 90 seconds before placing the composite.

Dental Amalgam—Permite

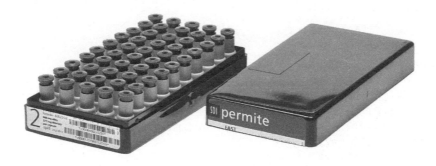

Use	Posterior restorations
Composition	• Nongamma 2 admix alloy—high silver content, copper, and tin • Mercury
Properties	• High strength • Highly polishable • Excellent handling qualities • Very low microleakage • Capsule design releases consistent mixes

- Not as affected by moisture as other preparations
- Less exposure to mercury vapor due to reduction in procedure time
- Comes in four settings: slow, regular, fast, and extra-carving time (ECT)
- Comes in one, two, three, and five spills

Precautions
- Material can cause irritation to the skin and eyes.
- Material may be irritating to respiratory system if powder is inhaled.
- If ingested, it may cause irritation, vomiting, and diarrhea.

Dental Amalgam—Permite *Continued*

Mixing and Setting Time
- Mixing time depends on type of amalgamator.
- Setting time is 2½ to 6 minutes, depending on type of mix.
- Carving time is 5½ to 9 minutes, depending on type of mix.

Directions

1. The tooth is prepared and the necessary liners, bonding agents, and matrix are placed.
2. The amalgam capsule is self-activating, so it is simply placed in the amalgamator.

3. The mixing and trituration speed is set according to the manufacturer's instructions.
4. Follow the guidelines to achieve the proper amalgam mix consistency.
5. The amalgam mix is removed from the capsule and placed into an amalgam well, dappen dish, or squeeze cloth for loading into an amalgam carrier.
6. Load both ends of the carrier and pass to the dentist for placement and condensation.
7. Repeat loading the carrier as the dentist requires.
8. Place the amalgam scraps in a well-sealed container. Regulations for disposal must be followed.

Dental Amalgam—Tytin Spherical Alloy

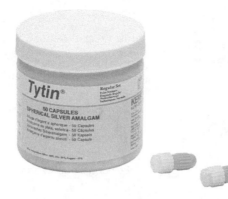

Use	Posterior restorative material
Composition	• Ternary alloy with high copper content • Spherical particles of silver, tin, and copper • Low mercury content
Properties	• Excellent clinical performance. • Higher in strength and lower in creep than other amalgams. • Very smooth surface. • Easy to place and carve and accepts immediate polishing; 8 minutes in Class I restorations.

- Comes in slow and regular set and single, double, and triple spill.
- Each capsule is guaranteed to have the perfect ratio with pouched mercury.
- Reliable and consistent mixes.
- Works with any amalgamator.
- Self-activating.
- Color-coded.

Precautions
- Material can cause irritation to the skin and eyes.
- Material may be irritating to respiratory system if powder is inhaled.
- If ingested, it may cause irritation, vomiting, and diarrhea.

Dental Amalgam—Tytin Spherical Alloy *Continued*

Mixing and Setting Time

- Mixing time—follow the manufacturer's instructions (7 to 8½ seconds).
- Setting time is 4 to 5 minutes for the initial set.

Directions

1. The tooth is prepared and the necessary liners, bonding agents, and matrix are placed.
2. The amalgam capsule is self-activating, so it is simply placed in the amalgamator.
3. The mixing and trituration speed is set according to manufacturer's instructions.

4. Follow the guidelines to achieve the proper amalgam mix consistency.
5. The amalgam mix is removed from the capsule and placed into an amalgam well, dappen dish, or squeeze cloth for loading into an amalgam carrier.
6. Load both ends of the carrier and pass to the dentist for placement and condensation.
7. Repeat loading the carrier as the dentist requires.
8. Place the amalgam scraps in a well-sealed container. Regulations for disposal must be followed.

Dental Amalgam—Valiant Amalgam, Valiant Ph.D, Valiant Snap-Set

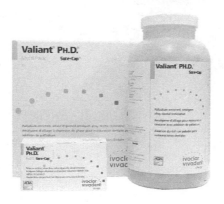

Use   Posterior restorative material Classes I and II

Composition
- Valiant and Valiant Snap-Set—Spherical amalgam alloy with high copper content and palladium added plus mercury
- Valiant Ph.D Amalgam—Phase-dispersed amalgam with palladium enriched and with lower mercury content

Properties
- High early strengths.
- Corrosion resistant.
- Smooth carving and burnishing.
- Specially designed capsules that are ultrasonically welded for increased safety and efficiency.
- Valiant Snap-Set has a faster setting time.
- Valiant Ph.D has a finer particle size for smoother carving, faster wetting, faster setting, and denser amalgam mass.
- All come in single, double, and triple spills.

Precautions
- Material can cause irritation to the skin and eyes.
- Material may be irritating to the respiratory system if powder is inhaled.
- If ingested, call a physician immediately.

Dental Amalgam—Valiant Amalgam, Valiant Ph.D, Valiant Snap-Set *Continued*

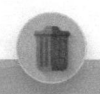

**Mixing and
Setting Time**
- Mixing time—follow the manufacturer's instructions (7 to 8½ seconds).
- Setting time is 4 to 5 minutes for initial set.

Directions

1. The tooth is prepared, and the necessary liners, bonding agents, and matrix are placed.
2. The amalgam capsule is self-activating, so it is simply placed in the amalgamator.
3. The mixing and trituration speed is set according to manufacturer's instructions.
4. Follow the guidelines to achieve the proper amalgam mix consistency.
5. The amalgam mix is removed from the capsule and placed into an amalgam well, dappen dish, or squeeze cloth for loading into an amalgam carrier.
6. Load both ends of the carrier and pass to the dentist for placement and condensation.
7. Repeat loading the carrier as the dentist requires.
8. Place the amalgam scraps in a well-sealed container. Regulations for disposal must be followed.

Best Management Practices for Amalgam Waste, Handling and Disposal

1. Use chairside traps, vacuum pump filters, and amalgam separators to retain amalgam and recycle their contents. Do not rinse devices containing amalgam over drains and sinks.

2. Use precapsulated alloys and stock a variety of capsule sizes.

3. The preferred method of loading amalgam into an amalgam carrier includes an amalgam well, dappen dish, or squeeze cloth.

4. Recycle used disposable amalgam capsule. Do not put capsules in biohazard containers.

5. Salvage, store, and recycle noncontact material (scrap amalgam). Do not place in biohazard, infectious waste, or regular garbage containers.

6. Salvage contact amalgam pieces from restorations after removal and recycle their contents. Do not place in biohazard, infectious waste, or regular waster.

Best Management Practices for Amalgam Waste, Handling and Disposal *Continued*

7. Recycle teeth that contain amalgam restorations. Do not dispose in biohazard, infectious waste, or regular garbage containers.

8. Manage amalgam waste by recycling as much as possible. Do not flush amalgam waste down the drain or toilet.

9. Use line cleaners that minimize dissolution of amalgam. Do not use bleach or chlorine-containing cleaners to flush water lines.

Source: https://www.ada.org/en/member-center/oral-health-topics/amalgam-separators

Amalgamators

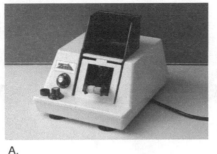

A.

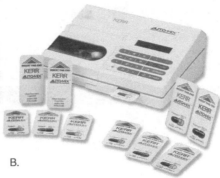

B.

Use	• Mechanical means to combine dental alloy and mercury into dental amalgam: restorative material • To mix various precapsulated dental cements, both permanent and temporary
Composition	Equipment that comes with cradles to hold amalgam capsules, cradle cover, a timer, and speed control **A.** Dental amalgamator with manual controls **B.** Dental amalgamator with programmable computerized mixing system
Notes	• Amalgam capsules contain dental alloy, mercury, a membrane separating the two components, and a pestle to mix the amalgam. • Capsules are placed in a cradle (some have to be twisted or pushed to activate), and the cover is closed before beginning. • The process of mixing is also called trituration or amalgamation. • Follow the manufacturer's directions for time and speed settings.

Amalgam Wells and Squeeze Cloths

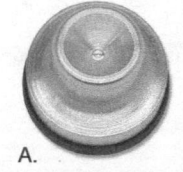

A.

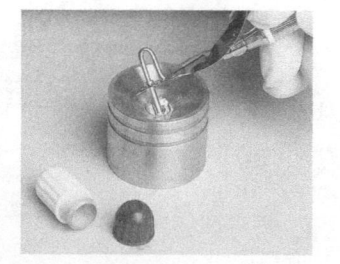

B.

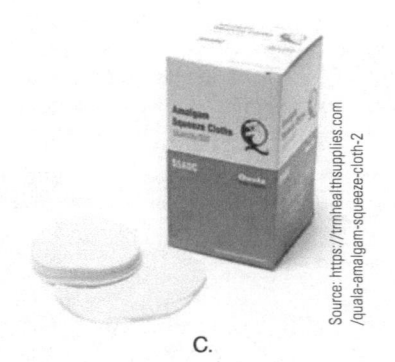

C.

Source: https://rmhealthsupplies.com /quala-amalgam-squeeze-cloth-2

Use	• To hold the pliable amalgam just after trituration • To load the amalgam into the carrier
Composition	Metal or glass dished-out containers designed for easy use with the amalgam carrier **A.** Metal amalgam well **B.** Placing the amalgam into the carrier from the amalgam well **C.** Squeeze cloth
Notes	• Different shapes and designs. • Metal are sterilized, squeeze cloth and dappen dish are disposed of.

Amalgam Carriers

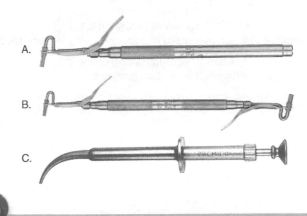

A.

B.

C.

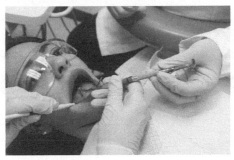

D.

Use To carry and dispense amalgam into the cavity preparation; the back-action condenser

Composition An instrument with a hollow tube on one or both ends that amalgam is placed into and then dispensed into the cavity prep with a spring action:
  A. May be single-ended.
  B. May be double-ended.

C. An amalgam gun is a single-ended carrier made of high-grade plastic or metal.
D. Passing of the amalgam carrier

Notes
• Double-ended carriers have a small and large end.
• Most carriers are made of stainless steel; some have Teflon or coated barrels to prevent clogging.

Amalgam Condensers and Back-Action Condensers

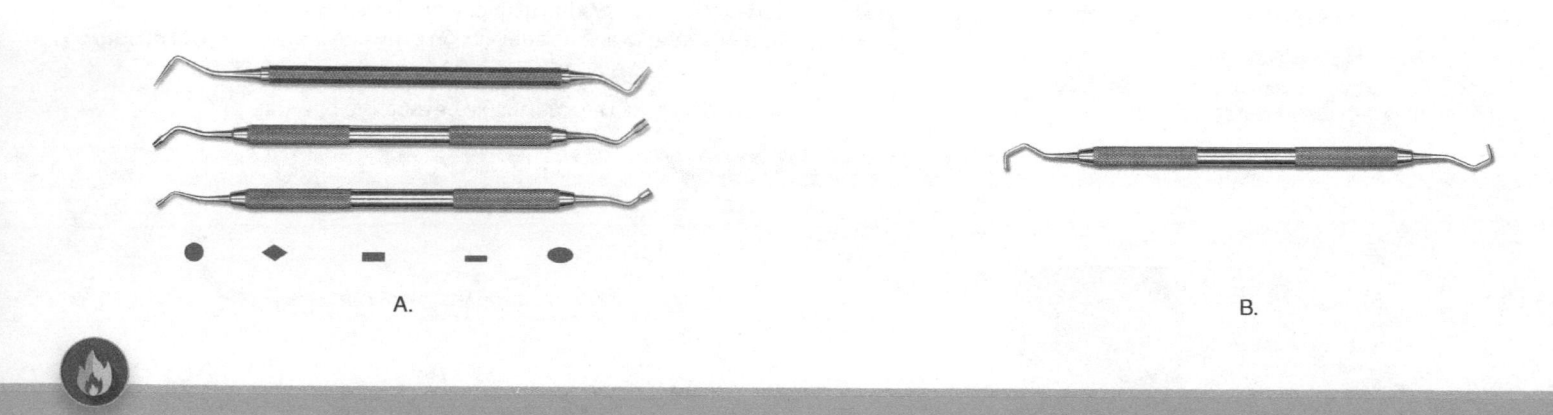

A.

B.

Use
To pack and condense amalgam into the cavity preparation; back-action gets in difficult-to-reach areas

Composition
- An instrument that has an end similar to a hammer that packs the amalgam into the preparation
- Single- or double-ended
- **A.** Various shapes of amalgam condensers
- **B.** Back-action condenser

Notes
- Condensers are diverse in design to be functional in the locations and designs of cavity preparations.

- Working ends may be plain (smooth) or serrated.
- Sometimes called "pluggers."
- Double-ended condensers have one small end and one large end.
- Variety of shapes of the working ends: round, diamond, rectangular, and ovoid condenser (shown in red).
- The shank has two or three angles.

Ball Burnisher and Football Burnisher

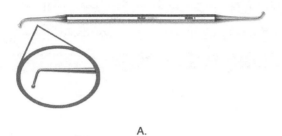

A.

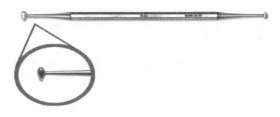

B.

Use	• To smooth rough margins of a restoration • To shape metal matrix bands
Composition	An instrument that has a rounded ball tip or a football-shaped tip used to smooth materials that are in the preparation. **A.** Ball Burnisher **B.** Football Burnisher

Notes	• Double- or single-ended. • On the double-ended ball or football burnisher, the ends may be different sizes.

Beavertail Burnisher and T-Ball Burnisher

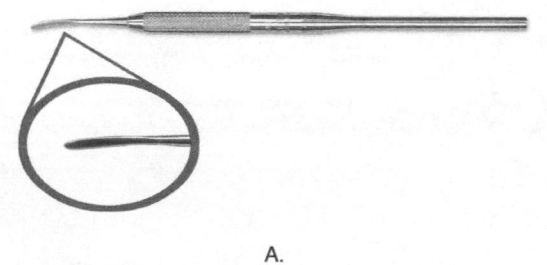

A.

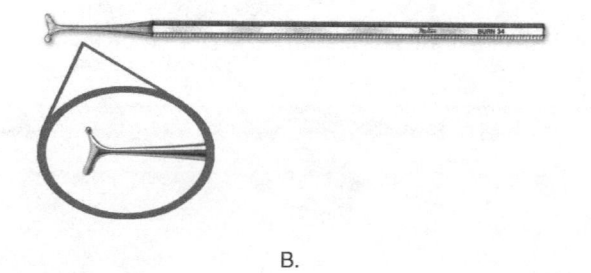

B.

Use
- To smooth rough margins of amalgam restorations.
- To shape metal matrix bands.
- The beavertail is used to tuck or invert the dental dam material around the teeth.
- The T-ball is used to slightly separate the teeth when contacts are very tight.

Composition
- An instrument that has a flat beavertail-shaped tip used to smooth materials that are in the preparation.

- An instrument that has a T-shaped end with a ball on one extension and a blade on the other used to smooth materials that are in the preparation.

A. Beavertail Burnisher
B. T-ball Burnisher

Notes
- Double- or single-ended.
- The T-ball burnisher comes in different sizes and is single-ended.

Acorn Burnisher

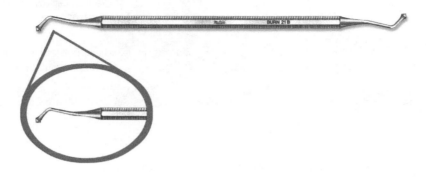

Use
- To smooth amalgam or composite restorations after placement
- To begin carving of amalgam or composite restorations by placing the initial grooves

Composition An instrument that has an acorn-shaped end used to smooth materials that are in the preparation.

Notes
- Single- or double-ended.
- On double-ended acorn ball burnishers, the ends may be different sizes.

Hollenback Carver and Half-Hollenback Carver

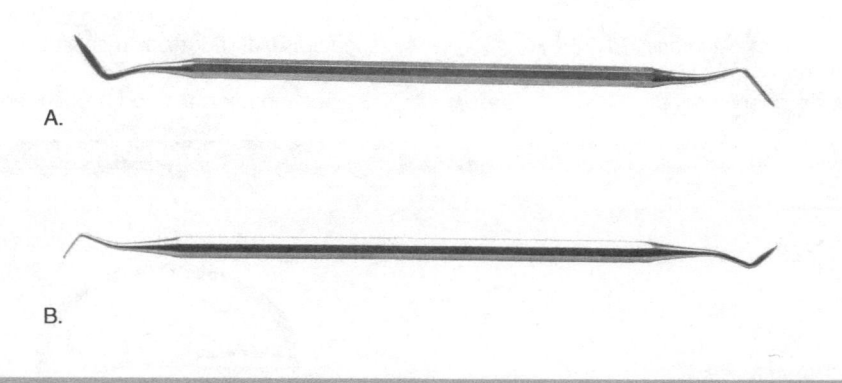

A.

B.

Use
- To remove excess restorative material
- To carve and shape occlusal and interproximal anatomy

Composition
A. Hollenback carver
B. Half-Hollenback carver (same shape blades as the Hollenback carver, just smaller in size)

Notes
- Double-ended: working ends positioned at different angles
- Available in different sizes

Cleoid-Discoid Carver

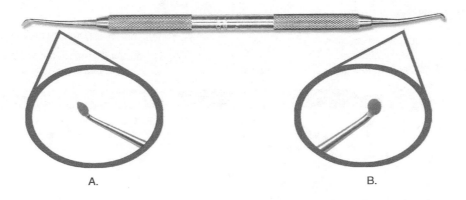

A.

B.

Use	• To remove excess restorative material • To carve and shape the occlusal anatomy
Composition	• Double-ended instrument with two different shaped ends • Cleoid end: looks like a claw or a spade and is pointed • Discoid end: round end; looks like a disc

A. Cleoid side of carver
B. Discoid side of carver

Notes

• Places the pits, fissures, and the anatomy in the restoration.
• If the bite is high, it is used to reduce the restoration material.

T-3 Carver

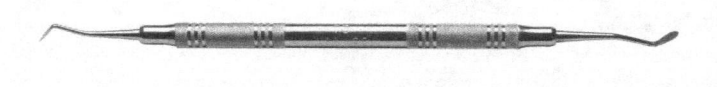

A.

Use
- To remove excess restorative material
- To carve and shape the occlusal anatomy

Composition Double-ended: one end is shaped like a disc and the other end is a blade.
A. T-3 Carver

Notes
- Places the pits, fissures, and the anatomy in the restoration.
- If the bite is high, it is used to reduce the restoration material.
- Has the function of two different instruments in one instrument.

Gold Carving Knife

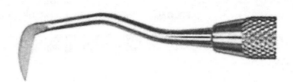

Use　To trim excess, carve and smooth amalgam, and composite filling materials in the interproximal surfaces

Composition • An instrument that has two or three angles in the shank that ends in a sharp knife blade; the ends appear at different angles.

Notes • Instruments are single- and double-ended.
• The instruments come in a variety of shapes and designs.
• The instrument is sometimes referred to as a gold finishing knife.

Interproximal Carver (IPC) Instrument

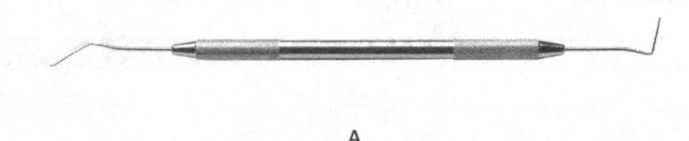

A.

Use To trim excess and carve and smooth amalgam and composite filling materials in the interproximal anatomy

Composition An instrument with long thin blades on each end placed at different angles.
A. Interproximal Carver

Notes
- The instruments come in a variety of shapes and designs.
- They are single- and double-ended.
- Thin blade aids in getting into the interproximal area to carve.

Tanner Carver

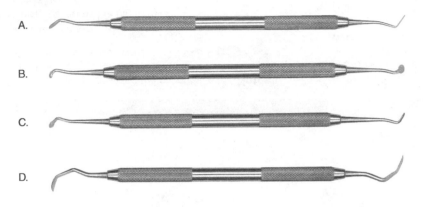

A.

B.

C.

D.

Use
To carve and shape the occlusal anatomy of an amalgam restoration

Composition
- An instrument with many different types of shapes on the working ends used to carve the occlusal anatomy.
- Instruments have a specific number reflecting the different shapes on each working end.
- **A.** #3 Tanner Carver
- **B.** #4 Tanner Carver
- **C.** #5 Tanner Carver
- **D.** #6 Tanner Carver

Notes
- Instrument is double-ended.
- The two ends are different in shapes, such as a spade on one end and a disc on the other.
- The ends may also be configured as a blade with each end at a different angle.

Articulating Forceps and Articulating Paper

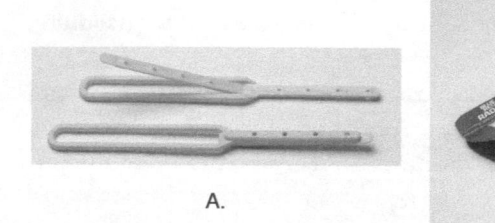

A.

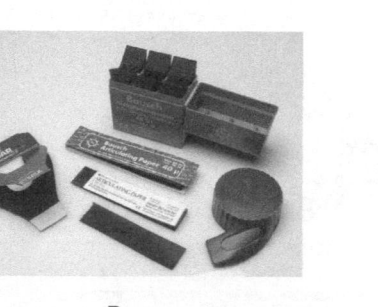

B.

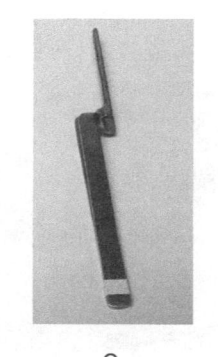

C.

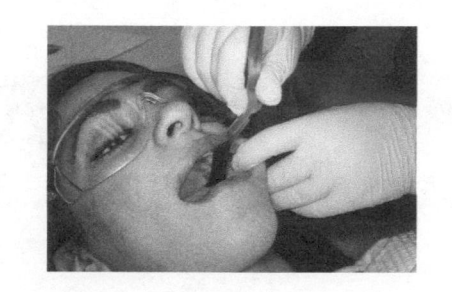

D.

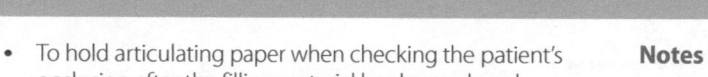

Use
- To hold articulating paper when checking the patient's occlusion after the filling material has been placed
- To mark patient's occlusion and check bite

Composition
- Handle with long beaks that secure the articulating paper
- Paper of various thickness, from ultrathin to thick
- Comes in rolls or individual strips
- **A.** Disposable Articulating Forcep
- **B.** Articulating Paper
- **C.** Metal Articulating Forceps
- **D.** Placement for Articulating Forceps

Notes
- Instrument may be made of stainless steel; this type is opened and closed by placing pressure on the handle to allow for articulating paper to be inserted and removed. May also be made of disposable plastic; in this type the articulating paper is held in position by closing and securing the beaks.
- Articulating paper comes in blue, red, black, and green. It is available on rolls, as individual strips, and in horseshoe shapes.
- Articulating paper can be stored in easy-access dispensers.
- Articulating paper is coated with liquid colors on both sides to facilitate accurate marking of occlusal contact and interferences.

Amalgam Tray Setup

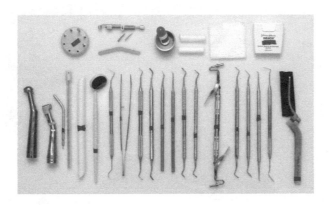

Composition
- Top of the tray: burs in bur block; matrix band, Tofflemire retainer, and wedges; amalgam well; amalgam capsules; cotton rolls; gauze sponges; floss.
- Bottom of the tray: high- and low-speed handpieces, air-water syringe, saliva ejector, high-volume evacuator (HVE) tip, mouth mirror, explorer, cotton pliers, spoon excavator, hatchet, binangle chisel, hoe, mesial and distal gingival margin trimmers, amalgam carrier, amalgam condenser, Hollenback carver, cleoid-discoid carver, ICP carver, articulating paper forceps, and articulating paper.
- Off-tray items include anesthetic, rubber dam, amalgamator, liners, and bases.

CHAPTER 11

Composite Instruments and Equipment

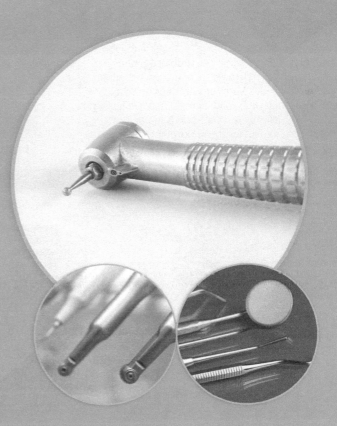

Composite Shade Guide

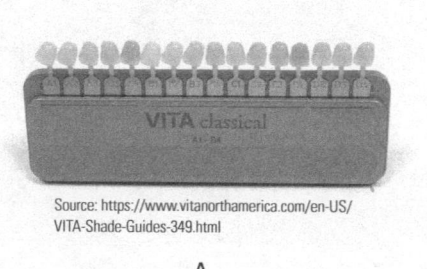

Source: https://www.vitanorthamerica.com/en-US/
VITA-Shade-Guides-349.html

A.

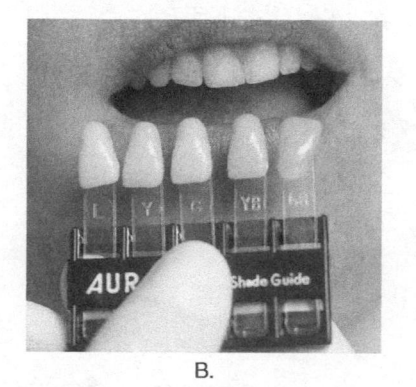

B.

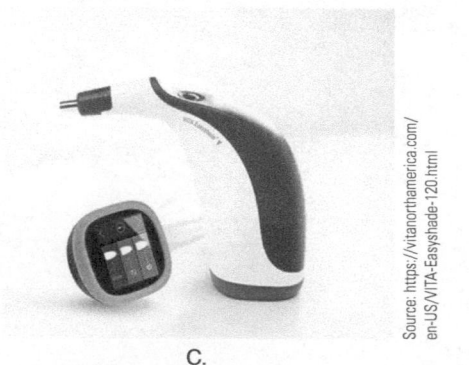

C.

Source: https://vitanorthamerica.com/
en-US/VITA-Easyshade-120.html

Use To obtain correct shade for composite restoration to match patient's current tooth shade

Composition A guide with multiple tooth shades on removable tabs that are labeled to indicate shade with letters and numbers
A. Vita shade guide shown
B. Obtaining a shade under natural light at the beginning of the procedure
C. VITA Easyshade V digital spectrophotometer

Notes
- A different shade may be used for the gingival third, the middle third, and/or the incisal third of the restoration.
- Many different shade guides are available.
- Digital or electric shade guides can select an overall single tooth shade or can select separate shades for the gingival, middle, and incisal thirds. The digital device can send the information about the shade to dental laboratories.
- Shade guides often come with composite kits.

Well for Composite Material

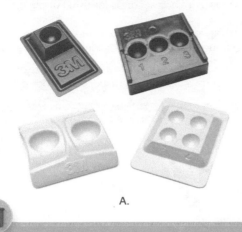

A.

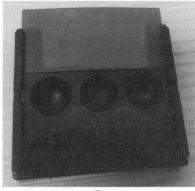

B.

Use To hold etchant, bonding, or composite material

Composition
- Disposable or autoclavable holder with different wells.
- Many have orange covers to block the materials from light, which initiates setting.
- **A.** Variety of composite wells
- **B.** Composite Well with light protection shield

Notes
- Wells are labeled with numbers or letters to designate different materials.
- Wells can be single, double, triple, or more.
- Wells often come with composite kits or materials.

Applicator

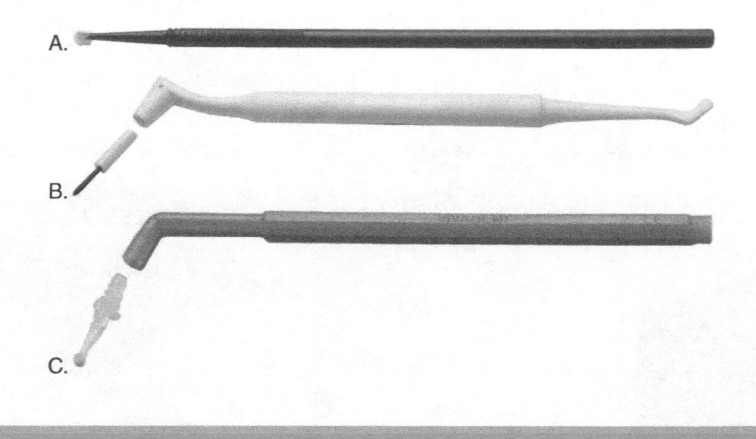

A.

B.

C.

Use   To apply conditioner, etchant, primer, and bonding material to cavity preparation

Composition
A. One-piece applicator, available in many colors and sizes to differentiate material being used. The working end bends.
B. Micro brush applicator, available in many sizes and styles.
C. Two-piece applicator, available in autoclavable handle and removable tip.

Notes
- Applicators or tips may be disposable.
- The comes in large quantities.
- There are several colors in each package.

Acid Etchant

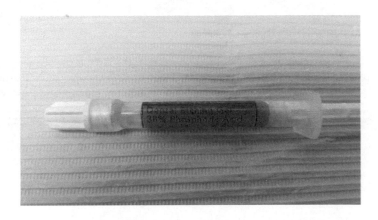

Use To enhance retention and bonding between tooth and dental materials

Composition Ranges from 30% to 40% phosphoric acid

Properties
- Used prior to bonding and applying restorative materials, dental cements, and pit and fissure sealants.
- Comes in liquid or gel.
- Comes in bottles or syringes.
- Applied with syringes with disposable tips.
- Applied with bottles by dispensing in a dappen dish and micro brush.
- Used on enamel and dentin.
- Follow manufacturers instructions for application time and rinsing.

Bonding Agents

Bonding agents are used to attach restorative materials to the enamel or dentin of the tooth. There are many varieties of materials; they are self-curing, light-cured, or dual-cured. Most often they require a conditioning or etching prior to placement. Some are unidose, meaning the etchant and the bonding agent are placed at the same time, whereas others require the etchant to be placed as a separate step.

Adper Prompt L-Pop Self-Etch Adhesive

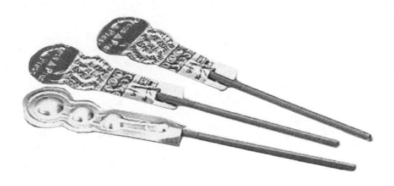

Use	Adhesive for direct restorative procedures

Composition
- Low-viscosity composite resin
- Di-HEMA phosphate
- Bisphenol a diglycidyl ether dimethacrylate
- Ethyl 4(dimethylamino)benzoate
- DL-camphorquinone

Properties
- Easy application
- Etches, primes, and bonds in one step
- Comes in a unit-dose delivery

Precautions
- May be irritating to the skin and eyes
- Should not be ingested
- No inhalation irritation

Mixing and Setting Time
- Mixing time is less than 5 seconds. (Refer to the directions.)
- Setting time is 10 seconds to light-cure.

Adper Prompt L-Pop Self-Etch Adhesive *Continued*

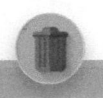

Directions

1. Tooth is rinsed and lightly dried.
2. Press on the red chamber to move the contents into the yellow chamber.
3. Fold the red chamber over the yellow chamber.
4. The yellow chamber will pop up to indicate the material has flowed into this area.
5. Push the applicator brush from the blue chamber into the yellow chamber.
6. Rotate the applicator brush and mix and churn the material to complete the mix.

7. Apply the material to the tooth by rubbing for 15 seconds.
8. Reapply until the surface is smooth and glossy.
9. The adhesive will appear a dull yellow.
10. Light-cure for 10 seconds.

Scotchbond Multi-Purpose Plus Dental Adhesive—Adper

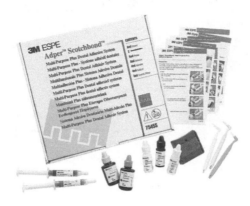

Use	• Dual-curing adhesive for bonding amalgams, composites, and porcelains • Bonding system for indirect restoration, including crowns, inlays, onlays, and orthodontic bands
Composition	• Primer contains HEMA • Adhesive contains HEMA and bis-GMA (low-viscosity composite resin)
Properties	• Excellent bond strength to a variety of surfaces • Fast and easy application

• Reduces microleakage and postoperative sensitivity
• Three-step system: etch, primer, and adhesive

Precautions	• May be irritating to the skin and eyes • Should not be ingested • No inhalation irritation
Mixing and Setting Time	• No mixing is required. • Material is light-cured for 10 seconds.

Scotchbond Multi-Purpose Plus Dental Adhesive—Adper *Continued*

Directions

1. Material works best if the tooth is isolated with a rubber dam.
2. Tooth is prepared, rinsed, and dried.
3. The etchant is applied to the enamel and dentin—wait 15 seconds.
4. Rinse thoroughly and then gently air-dry, leaving the tooth moist.
5. Apply Scotchbond Multi-Purpose Adhesive Primer to the enamel and dentin with an applicator brush.
6. Gently dry for 5 seconds; the surface should appear shiny.
7. Apply Scotchbond Multi-Purpose Adhesive to the enamel and dentin with an applicator brush.
8. Light-cure for 10 seconds.

OptiBond Solo Plus System

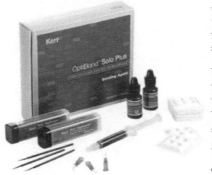

Source: https://www.kerrdental.com/en-eu/dental-restoration-products/optibond-solo-plus-dental-bonding-agents

Use	• Adhesive for direct and indirect bonding
	• Post and core applications
	• Different bonding applications—either unidose or self-curing bottle delivery
Composition	Micron-filled barium glass
Properties	• Two-step system: etch is one step and primer/adhesive is the second step
	• High bond strength to a variety of surfaces

	• Protects against sensitivity
	• Prevents microleakage
Precautions	• May be irritating to the skin and eyes.
	• Should not be ingested.
	• Inhalation irritation may occur.
Mixing and Setting Time	• If mixing is required, mix for 3 seconds.
	• Material is light-cured for 20 seconds.

OptiBond Solo Plus System *Continued*

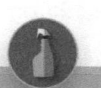

Directions   OptiBond Solo in Unidose (capsule or rocket) delivery

1. Etch the enamel and dentin for 15 seconds.
2. Rinse thoroughly and lightly air-dry.
3. Grip the unidose capsule at the wings and twist the sides in opposite directions.
4. Discard the larger end.
5. Dip an applicator tip into the opening and mix for 3 seconds.
6. Apply OptiBond Solo Plus for 15 seconds.
7. Air-dry for 3 seconds.
8. Light-cure for 20 seconds.

OptiBond Solo Plus in Bottles

1. Etch the enamel and dentin for 15 seconds.
2. Rinse thoroughly and lightly air-dry.
3. Place one drop of OptiBond Solo Plus into the mixing well and mix for 3 seconds.
4. Apply for 15 seconds.
5. Air-dry gently for 3 seconds.
6. Light-cure for 20 seconds.

Prime & Bond NT Adhesive

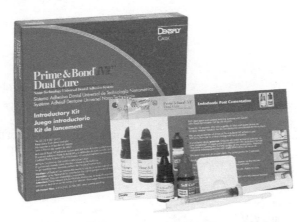

Use
- Direct composites and compomers
- Veneers
- Repairs on composites, ceramics, and metal
- Adhesive bonding of direct amalgam bonding

Composition
- Dimethacrylate and trimethacrylate resin and acetone
- Highly nanofilled composite

Properties
- Two-step system: etch is one step and primer/adhesive is the second step.
- Superior bond.
- Protection against microleakage.
- Better surface coverage and penetration into dentin.
- High bond strength.

Prime & Bond NT Adhesive *Continued*

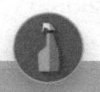

Precautions
- May be irritating to the skin and eyes
- Should not be ingested
- Inhalation irritation may occur

Mixing and Setting Time
- No mixing is required.
- Light-cure to set material.

Directions

1. Clean the cavity prep with a rubber cup and pumice or fluoride-free prophy paste and then rinse with water and air-dry.
2. Apply calcium hydroxide liner if necessary.
3. Condition/etch the tooth if required for 10 to 15 seconds and then rinse.
4. Gently air-dry; tooth can still be moist.
5. Open unidose or dispense Prime & Bond NT adhesive directly onto an applicator brush or dispense two or three drops into a dispensing well. Replace the cap immediately.
6. Apply the adhesive to the tooth generously so the surface is wet. Additional application may be needed to keep the surface wet for 20 seconds.
7. Gently air-dry for 5 seconds; the surface should be glossy. If not, repeat application of the adhesive.
8. Light-cure for 10 seconds and then place the restoration.

Composites—Filtek Supreme Plus—Nanocomposite Universal Restorative

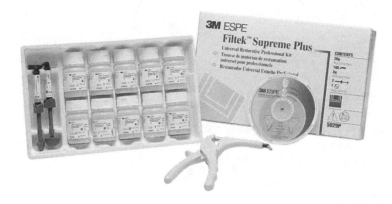

Use
- Designed for anterior and posterior restorations
- Core buildups
- Splinting
- Indirect restorations, including inlays, onlays, and veneers

Composition
- Nanocomposite
- Bis-GMA, UDMA, TEGDMA, and Bis-EMA resins
- Between 72.5% and 78.5% filler

Properties
- Highly regarded physical properties.
- Excellent clinical properties.
- Visible-light–activated material.
- Comes in a variety of shades that blend easily.
- Nonslumping and nonsticky.
- Strong and dependable.
- Wear comparable to enamel.
- Also available as Filtek Supreme Plus Flowable.
- Most shades are radiopaque.

Composites—Filtek Supreme Plus—Nanocomposite Universal Restorative *Continued*

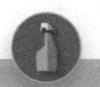

Precautions
- May cause eye irritation
- May cause skin irritation
- May cause problems if ingested

Mixing and Setting Time
- No mixing is required.
- Material is light-cured to set.

Directions

1. Before the tooth is prepared, select the shade under natural light.
2. The tooth is then prepared by the dentist.
3. A liner may be placed and then the matrix positioned.
4. Follow manufacturer's instructions regarding etching, priming and adhesive application, and curing.

5. Dispense the composite as follows:
   i. Syringe: Dispense necessary amount of material from the syringe onto a pad. If the material is not used immediately, protect it from light until used. Material is placed with a plastic filling instrument (PFI) in incremental layers.

   ii. Single-dose capsules: Place capsule into 3M-ESPE Restorative Dispenser, remove the cap, and pass to the dentist for placement.

6. Composite is placed in layers and light-cured after each layer.

Point 4 Optimized Particle Hybrid Composite System

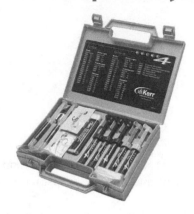

Use	Suitable for all classes of cavity preparations
Composition	Composite resin with 76% inorganic filler

Properties
- All shades are radiopaque.
- Polishes to a smooth, lustrous finish.
- Hybrid strength.
- Bridges the gap between the microfill and hybrid composites.
- Quick and easy to use.
- True chameleon effect; blends with adjacent teeth.

Precautions
- May be irritating to the skin with repeated and prolonged exposure
- Irritating to the eyes
- May be irritating if inhaled repeatedly
- Should not be ingested

Mixing and Setting Times
- No mixing is required.
- Material is light-cured to set.

Point 4 Optimized Particle Hybrid Composite System *Continued*

Directions

1. Prepare the etchant syringe and place the etchant in the cavity preparation for 15 seconds.
2. Rinse and dry lightly.
3. Apply OptiBond Solo Plus on enamel and dentin for 15 seconds using a gentle brushing motion. Lightly air-dry for 3 seconds and light-cure for 20 seconds.
4. Place the unidose base tip in the dispensing gun and pass to the dentist. Light-cure each layer for 20 seconds.
5. Place the unidose translucency tip in the dispensing gun and pass to the dentist. After placement, light-cure for 20 seconds.

Tetric EvoFlow—Flowable

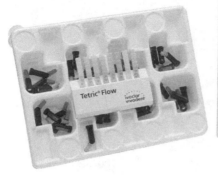

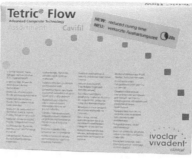

Use	• Initial layer/first increment in Classes I and II composite restorations in permanent teeth • Restorations in deciduous teeth
Composition	Monomer matrix of Bis-GMA, urethane, dimethacrylate, and triethylene glycol dimethacrylate, and 68% inorganic filler particles

Properties	• Low viscosity permits optimal wetting of the tooth. • A variety of shades are available for outstanding esthetics.
Precautions	• May be irritating to the skin • Irritating to the eyes
Mixing and Setting Times	• Material comes in syringe form. • Material is light-cured to set.

Tetric EvoFlow—Flowable *Continued*

Directions

1. Prepare the tooth and place the pulp protection and bonding agent according to manufacturer's instructions.
2. Tetric EvoFlow applicator tips are placed on the T syringe.
3. The material is applied directly into the cavity preparation.
4. Light-cure each increment for 20 seconds.

Esthet X HD—Micro Matrix Nanohybrid Composite

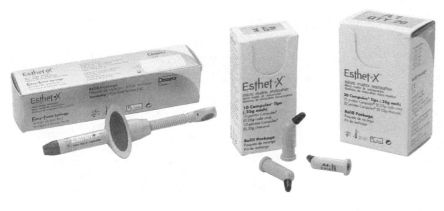
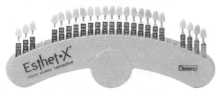

Use
- Esthetic restorative material for all cavity classes
- For primary and permanent dentition

Composition
- Dimethacrylate resin (urethane-modified bis-GMA)
- Inorganic fillers (including silica, barium boron fluoroaluminosilicate glass)
- Colorants

Properties
- Outstanding physical properties
- Long working time
- High fracture toughness for strength and durability

- Radiopaque
- High wear resistance
- Adapts well to margins
- No patient sensitivity
- Low shrinkage
- Brilliant polish
- Optimal handling
- Comes with detailed shade guide
- Optimized 31 shades and 3 opacities

Esthet X HD—Micro Matrix Nanohybrid Composite *Continued*

Precautions
- Can be irritating to eyes and skin
- No inhalation irritation
- Probably not harmful if ingested

Mixing and Setting Times
- No mixing is required. Materials come in single-dose compules or easy-twist syringe.
- Materials are light-cured to set.

Directions

1. Select appropriate shade.
2. Apply suitable dentinal bonding agent following manufacturers instructions.
3. Apply the opacious layer in no more than 2-mm increments and cure for 20 seconds.
4. Apply the regular body layer in no more than 2-mm increments and cure for 20 seconds.
5. Apply the translucent enamel layer in no more than 2-mm increments and cure for 20 seconds.
6. Finish and polish the restoration using discs, cups, and burs.

Premise Nano filled and Premise Flowable Composite

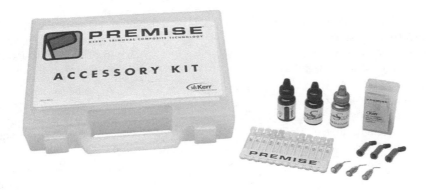

Use
- Universal for all restoration on the anterior and posterior teeth.
- Flowable form is also used as a pit and fissure sealant and for repair of enamel defects, repair of porcelain restorations, minor occlusal buildups in nonstress areas, and incisal abrasions.

Composition
- Resin: ethoxylated bis-GMA, triethylene glycol dimethacrylate, light-cured initiators, and stabilizers
- Three fillers: prepolymerizable filler, barium glass, and silica nanoparticles (84% filler)
- Polymerizable organophosphate dispersant

Properties
- Universal material—ultralow shrinkage
- Universal application with strength for the posterior teeth and esthetics for anterior teeth
- Three different fillers to improve this nanorestorative material
- Unmatched handling
- Comes in a variety of shades, including body shades, translucent shades, and packable shades
- High polish and gloss characteristics
- Flowable material flows easily but holds its shape; excellent mechanical strength, low shrinkage, and high polishability and wearability

Premise Nano filled and Premise Flowable Composite *Continued*

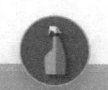

Precautions
- Prolonged or repeated exposure may cause irritation to the skin
- May cause irritation to the eyes
- Prolonged or excessive inhalation may cause irritation to the respiratory tract
- May be harmful if swallowed

Mixing and Setting Time
- No mixing is required. The universal comes in unidose tips and the flowable comes in a syringe.
- Both materials are light-cured to set.

Directions
Universal Premise
1. Apply self-etching bonding system following manufacturer's instructions.
2. Place the unidose tip of the selected shade into the dispensing gun.

3. Pass to the dentist and prepare the curing light.
4. Light-cure for 5 to 20 seconds, depending on the curing light, after each increment is placed.
5. When finished, remove the unidose tip from the gun and dispose of it.

Flowable Premise
1. Apply self-etching bonding system following manufacturer's instructions.
2. Place disposable tip on selected shade of Premise Flowable and secure.
3. Pass to the dentist and prepare the curing light.
4. The dentist will flow the material into the cavity preparation and place in layers. Light-cure for 5 to 20 seconds, depending on the curing light.
5. Restoration is finished and polished.

Heliomolar HB—Packable Microfilled Restorative Material

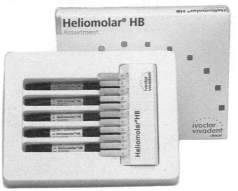
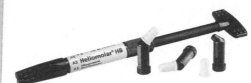

Use	• Microfill composite for the posterior region
	• Restorations in primary teeth

Composition
- Monomer matrix of bis-GMA, urethane dimethacrylate, and decanediol dimethacrylate.
- Fillers include copolymer, silicone dioxide, and ytterbium trifluoride.
- Total amount of inorganic fillers is approximately 66%.
- Catalysts, stabilizers, and pigments.

Properties
- Highly viscous packable material
- Nine shades to choose from
- Highly radiopaque
- Low wear value
- Polishes to a long-lasting high gloss

Precautions
- May be irritating to the eyes and the skin.
- No problems anticipated if small amount of material is ingested.
- Move to fresh air if it causes respiratory irritation.

Heliomolar HB—Packable Microfilled Restorative Material *Continued*

Mixing and Setting Time
- No mixing is required. Material comes in a syringe or a Cavifill.
- Material is light-cured for 20 seconds for each increment.

Directions

1. The tooth is conditioned/etched, and bonding agent is applied following manufacturer's instructions.
2. Prepare and coat the cavity with a layer of Heliomolar flow.
3. Heliomolar comes in a Cavifill.
4. Cavifills—place the selected shade of Cavifill and place it into the dispensing gun.

5. Secure the Cavifill and remove the tip. Pass to the dentist for placement.
6. Heliomolar is placed in increments, and after placement each increment is light-cured for 20 seconds.
7. Several shades may be used to achieve the desired results.

Tetric EvaCeram—Nanohybrid Composite

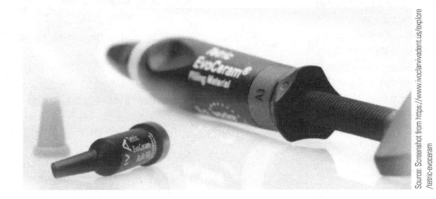

Source: Screenshot from https://www.ivoclarvivadent.us/explore
/tetric-evoceram

Use
- All classes of anterior and posterior restorations (Classes I, II, III, IV, and V)
- Veneering of discolored anterior teeth
- Preventive restoration in premolars and molars
- Splinting of mobile teeth
- Extended fissure sealing in premolars and molars

Composition
- Monomer matrix of bis-GMA, urethane dimethacrylate, and triethylene glycol dimethacrylate
- Fillers of barium glass, ytterbium trifluoride, highly dispersed silicon dioxide, and spherical mixed dioxide (81% fill)
- Catalysts, stabilizers, and pigments

Tetric EvaCeram—Nanohybrid Composite *Continued*

Properties
- Good polishability
- Good radiopacity
- Continuous fluoride release
- High shade stability
- Easy handling
- Thirteen shades, including one translucent and three opaque dentin shades

Precautions
- May be irritating to the eyes and the skin.
- No problems anticipated if small amount of material is ingested.
- Move to fresh air if it causes respiratory irritation.

Mixing and Setting Time
- No mixing is required. Material comes in a syringe or a Cavifill.
- Material is light-cured for 40 seconds for each increment.

Directions

1. Apply conditioner and bonding agent according to manufacturer's directions. Recommended to use product from the same manufacturer.
2. Tetric comes in either a syringe or a Cavifill. Prepare the syringe by removing the cap and dispensing the selected shade onto a pad.
3. Hold the paper pad and pass the plugger/condensing composite instrument.
4. Cavifill—Place the selected shade of Tetric and place it into the dispensing gun.
5. Secure the Cavifill in the dispensing gun and then remove the tip. Pass to the dentist for placement.
6. Tetric is placed in increments, and after placement each increment is light-cured for 40 seconds.
7. Several shades may be used to achieve the desired results of matching the tooth coloring.

Glacier—Microfilled Hybrid Composite

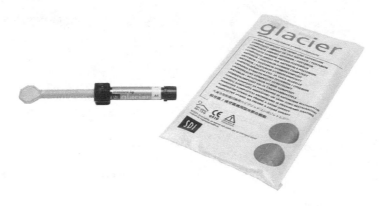

Use	• Anterior and posterior esthetic restorations (Classes I, II, III, IV, and V) • Veneers • Inlays/onlays • Core buildups
Composition	• Microfilled hybrid composite with strontium glass and amorphous silica • Initiators, stabilizers, and pigments
Properties	• High compressive strength • Radiopaque • Low shrinkage that reduces sensitivity and microleakage • Wear resistant • Nonstick and nonslumping • Polishes to a high luster
Precautions	• May be irritating to the eyes and the skin. • No problems anticipated if small amount of material is ingested. • Move to fresh air if it causes respiratory irritation.

Glacier—Microfilled Hybrid Composite *Continued*

Mixing and Setting Times
- Material comes in a syringe or Complets (compules). No mixing is required.
- Glacier is light-cured to set.

Directions

1. Etch the tooth for 20 seconds with 37% phosphoric etchant.

2. Rinse the tooth thoroughly and then remove excess moisture, leaving the tooth moist.

3. Apply a bonding agent according to manufacturer's instruction and light-cure for 20 seconds.

4. Gently blow-dry for 2 seconds until glossy, then light-cure for 20 seconds.

5. Prepare the syringe of the selected shade by removing the cap and placing a dispensing tip on the end. If using the Complets (compules), place the Complets in the applicator and snap to secure. Remove the end from the Complets.

6. Pass to the dentist for placement. Light-cure for 20 seconds after each increment is placed.

7. Restoration is ready to finish and polish.

Dyract Flow Flowable Compomer

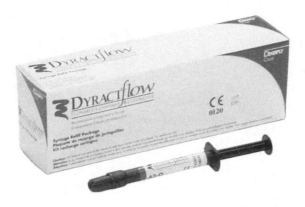

Use Direct esthetic restoration indicated for all cavity classifications (Classes I through V) as a base/liner

Composition
- Polymerizable dimethacrylate resin—urethane dimethacrylate resin, trimethacrylate resin, carboxylic-acid-modified dimethacrylate, triethylene glycol dimethacrylate, camphorquinone, ethyl 4-(dimethylamino)benzoate, and butylated hydroxy toluene.
- UV stabilizer.
- Strontium aluminum fluoro silicate glass.
- Colorants are inorganic iron oxides.

Properties
- Improved physical properties—less sticky handling and increased working time
- Excellent wear resistance
- Fluoride release
- Shortened curing time
- Easier finishing and polishing to a high luster restoration
- Comes in a variety of shades
- Also comes in a flowable composition

Dyract Flow Flowable Compomer *Continued*

Precautions
- May be irritating to the eyes.
- May cause irritation to the skin.
- Material is probably not harmful if swallowed.

Mixing and Setting Time
- No mixing is required. Dyract comes in individual compule tips.
- Material is light-cured for 10 to 20 seconds.

Directions

1. Place two to three drops of self-etching adhesive into clean mixing well.
2. Apply generous amount with small applicator and scrub for 15 seconds, then repeat.
3. Spread the adhesive and then gently spread with air until there is no more flow of the material—about 5 seconds.
4. Light-cure at least 10 seconds and then immediately place the restoration.

Compoglass F—Compomer-Based Restorative Material

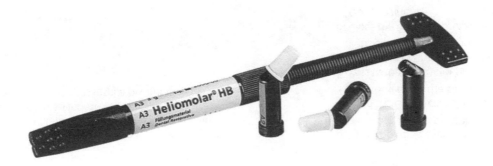

Use
- Restoration for deciduous teeth
- Class V (cervical caries, root erosion, and wedge-shaped defects)
- Class III restorations
- Intermediate Classes I and II restorations

Composition
- Monomer matrix of urethane dimethacrylate, tetraethylene glycol dimethacrylate, and cycloaliphatic dicarboxylic acid dimethacrylate. Inorganic fillers—Ba-fluorosilicate glass, mixed oxides, and ytterbium trifluoride (77% inorganic fillers).
- Catalysts, stabilizers, and pigments.

Compoglass F—Compomer-Based Restorative Material *Continued*

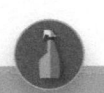

Properties
- Advantages of glass ionomer cements and light-cured composites
- Radiopaque
- Polishable
- High fluoride release
- High abrasion resistance
- Excellent bonding to enamel and dentin

Precautions
- Flush with water if material gets into the eyes.
- May cause skin irritation—wash with water and soap.
- No known problems if ingested.
- Move to fresh air if it causes respiratory irritation.

Mixing and Setting Times
- No mixing is required.
- Light-cure to set.

Directions

1. It is recommended to use a bonding agent from Ivoclar Vivadent.
2. Apply primer to the cavity preparation using a small applicator tip. Brush on for 30 seconds and then disperse excess liquid with strong stream of air until mobile liquid has disappeared.
3. Apply bonding agent with applicator tip. Using a gentle airstream, disperse evenly and light-cure for 10 seconds.
4. Load the Cavifill capsule into the dispensing gun and secure. Remove the cap.
5. Pass to the dentist for placement with an instrument such as an PFI. Material will be placed in increments and light-cured for 40 seconds after each is placed.
6. Close the Cavifill capsule after placement. Restoration is ready to finish.

GC Fuji IX GP-Glass Ionomer Restorative Material

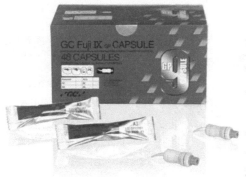

Source: https://www.gcamerica.com/products/operatory/GC_Fuji_IX_GP/

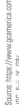

Use	• Geriatric and pediatric restorations (Classes I and II)
	• Final restoration in nonstress areas
	• Core-buildups
	• Class V and root surface restorations
	• Long-term temporaries

Composition
- Glass ionomer
- Liquid: polyacrylic acid
- Powder: polyacrylic acid and aluminosilicate glass

Properties
- Easy to handle and packable
- Chemically bonds to tooth structure
- Cures extremely hard and is very wear resistant
- Fluoride release
- Nonsticky
- High compressive and flexural strength
- Placed and finished similar to amalgam

GC Fuji IX GP-Glass Ionomer Restorative Material *Continued*

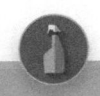

Precautions
- If ingested do not induce vomiting, give water and seek medical attention.
- May be irritating to the eyes—flush with water for 15 minutes.
- May be irritating to the skin—wash with soap and water.

Mixing and Setting Time
- Two-minute working time.
- Self-cures in 2.5 minutes (4.5 minutes from start).

Directions

1. Rinse the cavity preparation and air-dry gently.
2. Shade the capsule or tap on a hard surface to loosen the powder.
3. Push the plunger in until it is even with the capsule or immediately place capsule in the GC metal capsule activator and compress handle until it clicks. This activates the capsule.

4. Immediately place the activated capsule into an amalgamator and triturate for 10 seconds +/− the designated amount of time depending on the amalgamator/mixer.
5. Immediately remove the capsule from the amalgamator and place in the GC applier. Compress the handle for two clicks to be sure the material is ready. Remove the tip and pass to the dentist for placement.

Ketac Fil Plus Aplicap—Glass Ionomer Restorative Material

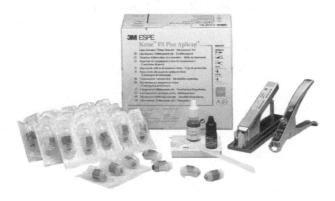

Use
- Ideal for pediatric and geriatric patients
- Classes III and V restorations
- Cervical defects
- Small Class I
- Core buildups

Composition
- Glass ionomer
- Powder: glass powder
- Liquid: water, polyethylene, polycarbonic acid, and tartaric acid

Properties
- High compressive strength
- Minimal abrasion
- Excellent surface hardness
- Fluoride release
- Bulk placement
- Chemical bonds to enamel and dentin
- Eight shades
- Tooth-like coefficient of thermal expansion, thus less shrinkage and microleakage
- Radiopaque

Ketac Fil Plus Aplicap—Glass Ionomer Restorative Material *Continued*

Precautions
- May be irritating to the skin and eyes
- Should not be ingested
- May cause upper respiratory irritation

Mixing and Setting Time
- Activating the Aplicap–2 seconds.
- Mix the Aplicap for 8 to 10 seconds in a rotary mixer or an amalgamator.
- Processing from start of mix is 1.5 minutes.
- Setting from start of mix is 7 minutes.

Directions

1. Prepare tooth according to manufacturer's instructions.
2. Rinse and gently dry the cavity preparation. Do not overdry.
3. Activate the Aplicap by placing it in the Aplicap Activator and squeezing the handle.
4. Remove Aplicap and immediately place in rotary mixer or amalgamator for 8 to 10 seconds.
5. Remove Aplicap and place in Applier. Raise the dispensing tip and pass to the dentist for placement. Pass a placement instrument.

Composite Syringes and Cartridges

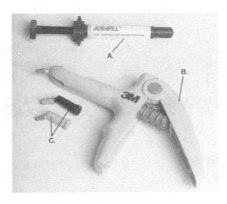

Use   Packaged one-paste composite systems that come in a syringe or a single-dose cartridge that is used with a syringe to place the material in the cavity preparation or on the composite well/paper pad for delivery with the composite placement instrument

Composition   **A.** Composite one-paste syringe for several applications
B. Composite syringe
C. Single-dosage cartridges to be used with the composite syringe

Notes   • These come in many shades.
• Shade guides accompany each composite system.

Composite Placement Instrument

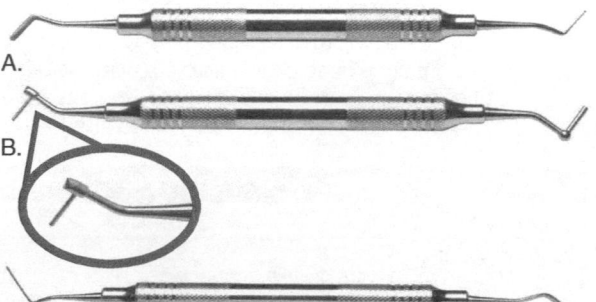

A.

B.

C.

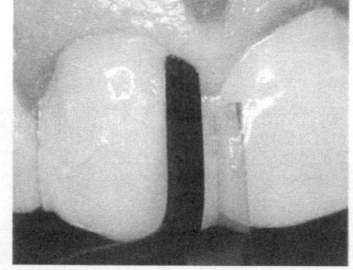

D.

Use
- To carry composite material to and from cavity preparation
- To place and condense composite material in the cavity preparation
- To rough carve composite material after it has been placed in the cavity preparation

Composition Double-ended instrument with different angles and working ends
  A. Placement and contouring instrument
  B. Condensing instrument

C. Placement and contouring instrument
D. The working end of a placement instrument on the tooth

Notes
- These are available in a variety of shapes, angles, and sizes.
- They are available in metal or plastic.
- Each end of the instrument is used differently: One end is used to place the material; the other end is used to contour and rough carve the material.

Composite Burnisher

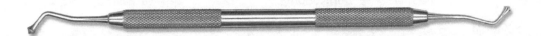

Use	• To smooth, contour, and form occlusal anatomy in composite restorations • To attain the anatomical grooves, pits, and fissures	**Notes**	The composite burnisher is available in titanium–nitride coating or gold–titanium–nitride coating, which resists scratching and discoloration of composite material. The nonstick surface of the tip of the instrument allows for a smooth surface.
Composition	• Double-ended instrument. • Different angle on each end of the instrument. • The tip is often shaped like an acorn.		

Curing Light with Protective Shield

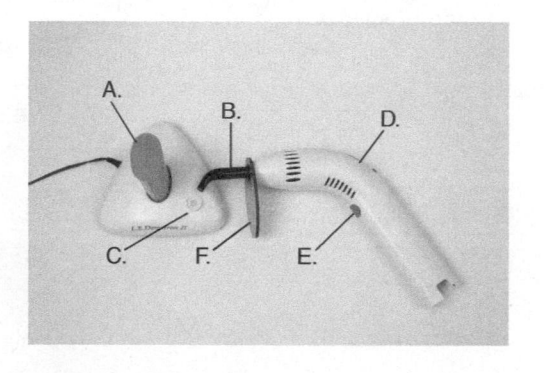

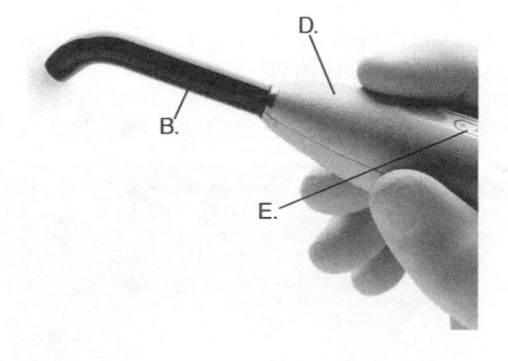

Use
- Used to "cure" or "set" light-cured materials
- Shield is to protect the operator and auxiliary's eyes during the curing of dental materials

Composition
- **A.** Battery pack
- **B.** Wands or tips
- **C.** Radiometer
- **D.** Motor
- **E.** Triggers to activate the light
- **F.** Protective shield

Curing Light with Protective Shield *Continued*

Notes

- The curing light can be battery powered, as shown, or electric, where the light is attached to the motor with a cord.
- Some curing lights have digital display countdown timers and preset curing times.
- The dental materials that are to be cured must be cured in increments of 2 mm or less to ensure complete setting.
- A testing device (radiometer) or meter is used to evaluate the accuracy of the curing light (see C in figure).
- Most curing lights come with a shield attached. The shields can be disinfected.
- Glasses and handheld or paddle devices can be used with orange- or green-colored lenses to protect the operator's eyes.

Curing Light Meter

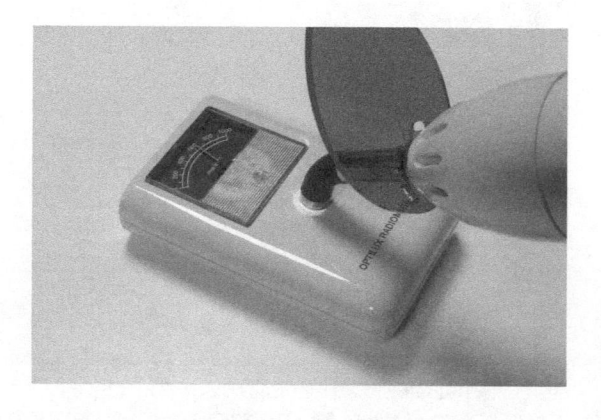

Use To test the curing lights to ensure that the correct level of power is emitted

Composition Radiometer with area for curing light tip placement to check accuracy of the output; a gauge on the radiometer is present to show the reading.

Notes
- Lights should be tested following manufacturers directions.
- There are radiometers for both halogen and light-emitting diode (LED) curing lights.
- If the material does not appear to be setting, the light should be tested immediately.
- The curing lights are continually improving, and newer devices are available for testing.

Composite Polishers

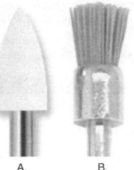
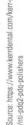

Source: https://www.kerrdental.com/kerr-rotary/nti-pdq2-pdq-polishers

A.   B.

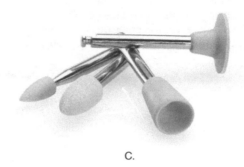

Source: https://www.ivoclarvivadent.com/en/p/all/products/clinical-accessories-instruments/polishing-systems/astropol

C.

Use   To contour, refine, and polish the composite restorative material

Composition
- Metal-centered discs that adapt to the mandrel
- Snap-on discs impregnated with synthetic material of various grits, shown by different colors
- **A.** Polishing Point
- **B.** Polishing Brush
- **C.** Astropol assortment of polishers and high-gloss polishing system

Notes
- Composite polishers are available in a range of grits, from extrafine to coarse.
- They are often color-coded according to grit.
- They are available in a variety of shapes and sizes.
- The discs are disposable; some come with disposable mandrels.
- The darker the color of the disc, the more abrasive it is.
- Points and cups come in different grits and sizes and can be sterilizable or disposable.

Finishing Strip

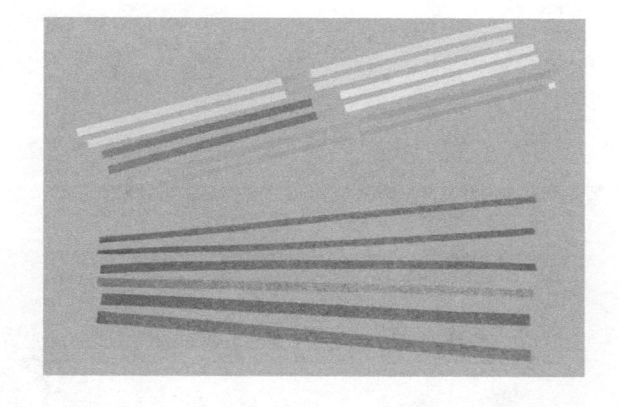

Use　To smooth and finish the interproximal surfaces of composite restorations

Composition　Strips of synthetic fabric that are abrasive to remove excess restorative material from the interproximal area

Notes
- Finish strips are available in different grit consistencies.
- Many have no abrasive material in the center of the strip. This allows the operator to slide the strip between the teeth without removing tooth structure and/or the proximal of the restoration.

Composite Procedure Tray

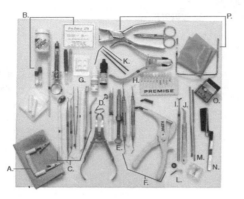

Composite Restoration with Tetric Microhybrid Material

Use
- To assist in cavity preparation and placement and the finishing of a composite restoration
- This procedure is performed by the dentist and the dental assistant at chairside.

Composition Basic set up is shown:
A. Bib and clip
B. Anesthetic: topical applicators, carpules, needle shield, syringe, and needle

C. Basic setup: mirror, explorer, spoon excavator, cotton pliers, evacuation (HEV) tip, saliva ejector, and three way syringe tip
D. Matrices with placement forceps
E. Etchant
F. Composite, composite placement instruments, and composite dispensing gun
G. Composite well
H. Shade guide
I. T-ball burnisher

Composite Procedure Tray *Continued*

J. #12 blade and scalpel

K. Etchant applicator tips, bonding applicator tips, primer, and adhesive

L. Composite finishing discs

M. Composite finishing strip

N. Articulating paper and forceps

O. Burs and bur block (handpieces not shown)

P. Dental dam, dental dam frame, dental dam forceps, dental dam punch, crown and collar scissors

Directions

1. Select the shade under natural light before the procedure begins. The tooth should be clean.

2. The anesthetic is given and the dental dam is placed for isolation.

3. The dentist prepares the cavity to receive the restoration material.

4. The dental assistant places a liner if required. Check composite instructions for type of material to select. Assistant mixes the material, usually calcium hydroxide or glass ionomer liner, and holds the pad, applicator, and a 2×2 gauze near the patient's chin. After each application wipe the instrument. Light-cure if required.

5. Place the matrix and the wedge.

6. Place a dispensing tip on the etchant syringe and place the etchant for 10 to 20 seconds. Wash and rinse the tooth thoroughly for 20 to 30 seconds.

7. Gently remove any excess moisture using air.

8. Using a small application brush or cotton-tipped applicator, place the bonding agent, gently dry to remove any moisture, and then light-cure for approximately 10 seconds.

Note

An all in one etchant/bonding agent may also be used. This material is placed in one step. Prepare the selected shades of Tetric (Tetric comes in either Cavifills or the syringe.

Composite Procedure Tray *Continued*

9. Secure the Cavifills in the dispensing gun and then remove the tip or remove the cap from the Tetric syringe and dispense some material onto a paper pad. Pass to the dentist for placement.

10. Tetric is placed in increments and each increment is light-cured after placement for 40 seconds.

11. Several shades may be used to achieve the desired results of matching the tooth coloring.

12. Remove the wedge and matrix strip and pass an explorer to the dentist.

13. Rubber dam may be removed at this point, according to the dentist's preference.

14. Prepare and pass high-speed handpiece with fine diamond and/or finishing burs to remove the excess material.

15. Pass finishing strip to finish the proximal surfaces.

16. Pass articulating forceps/paper to the dentist to check the occlusion.

17. Pass the low-speed handpiece with silicone polishers, polishing discs, and polishing strips.

18. Rinse and evacuate.

CHAPTER 12

Endodontic Instruments and Materials

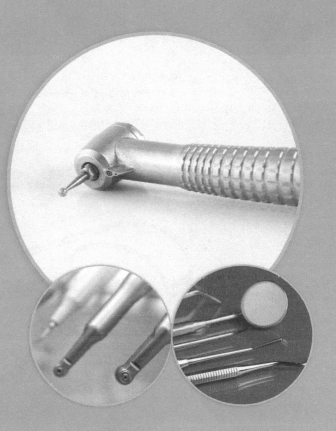

Pulp Tester and Vitality Scanner

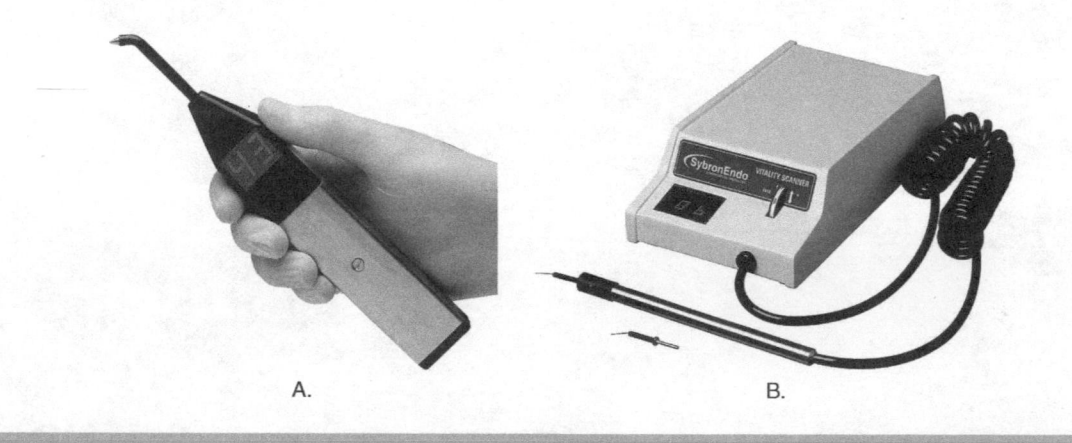

A.

B.

Use	To test each tooth for vitality
Properties	• The vitality scanner unit includes long, short, and mini probe tips.
	• Grounding lead with lip clip
	• There are two types:
	A. Battery operated
	B. Electronic with digital display
Notes	• They deliver high-frequency stimuli to the tooth, which cause a reaction if the tooth is vital.

- The impulse is slowly increased until the patient indicates sensitivity.
- With some units, toothpaste is applied to the coronal surface of the tooth where the probe tip is placed. The toothpaste acts as a conductor.
- Some units give readouts on the vitality of the tooth.

Endo Ice

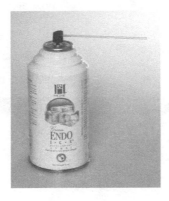

Use   To test pulp vitality

Composition Tetrafluoroethane

Properties
- Fast and easy method for testing pulp vitality
- Much colder than ice or ethyl chloride
- Spearmint-scented
- Directional spray extension

Precautions
- After inhalation: Get fresh air.
- After skin contact: Wash with water for 15 minutes.
- After eye contact: Flush with water for 15 minutes.
- After swallowing: Drink water to dilute. Do not induce vomiting.
- If irritation persists, contact a physician with all of the above information.

Mixing and Setting Time   No mixing or setting time required.

Directions

1. Place spray extension into the cap securely.
2. Have cotton-tipped applicator or cotton pellet ready.
3. Spray the applicator or pellet and hand to the dentist to apply to the tooth.

Endodontic X-Ray Film Holder

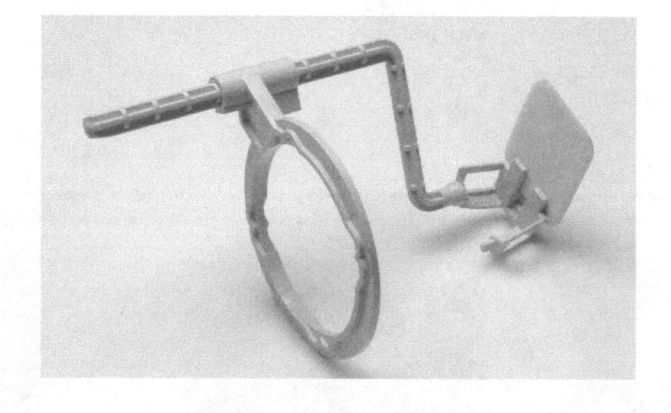

Use	Film holder designed specifically for endodontic radiographs
Composition	Rod with a ring specially designed to hold the radiograph sensor and obtain a quality x-ray of an endodontic tooth showing the apex
Notes	• The film holder can be used to expose radiographs on the maxillary and mandibular teeth in both the anterior and posterior areas.

- The endodontic film holder allows for an x-ray to be exposed with a reamer in place.
- It is designed to fit over rubber dam clamps and endodontic files.
- The x-ray holder is used to take endodontic measurements.
- This is available for digital or manual use and is radiolucent on the radiograph.

Tooth Slooth

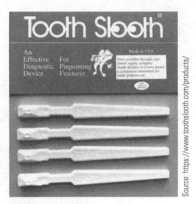

Source: https://www.toothslooth.com/products/

Use

- Helps locate cracked teeth that normally cannot be detected clinically or radiographically.
- Small indentation of instrument delivers force of bite to one cusp at a time.
- Easy to use on lingual cusps.
- Speeds diagnosis and minimizes patient discomfort.
- Eliminates the use of unpredictable and inaccurate testing objects such as orangewood sticks, cotton rolls, and rubber wheels.
- Eliminates patient discomfort and helps the patient understand the need for treatment.

Properties   Sterilizable

Endodontic Handpiece

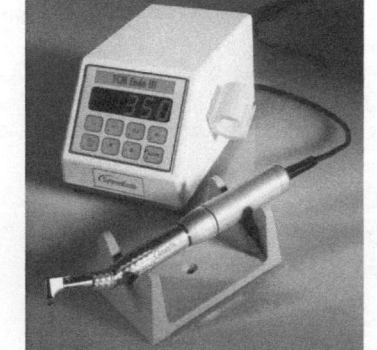

Use
- To open the occlusal surface of the tooth to locate the tooth canal
- To mechanically clean and enlarge the root canal
- To place the endodontic sealer in the canal

Properties
- A slow-speed electric torque motor with foot control with display controls to set speed and torque level
- Area for endodontic attachments

Notes
- The endodontic handpiece attaches to a slow-speed handpiece.
- It consistently and evenly supplies quarter-turn motion.
- It is used with reamers, files, and Peeso and Lentulo spirals during endodontic procedures.

Apex Locator

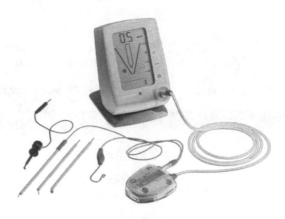

Use　　　To locate the apex of the tooth and display the information on a digital readout

Properties　An electronic unit with display screen that shows the length of the apex through multiple-frequency technology

Notes
- Many units have visual readouts and audible alerts.
- The unit attaches to a reamer or file and is placed in the canal.
- It can work in either wet or dry environments.

Endodontic Explorer and Endodontic Spoon Excavator

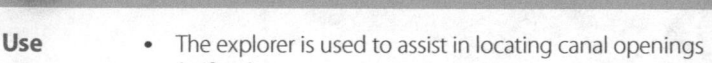

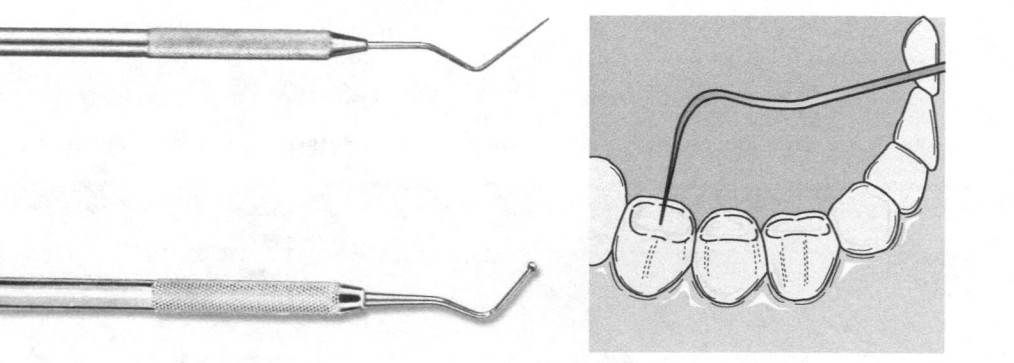

Use	• The explorer is used to assist in locating canal openings (orifices). • The spoon excavator is used to reach into the coronal portion of the tooth; to reach the bottom of the pulp chamber; and to remove deep caries, pulp tissue, and temporary cement.
Properties	• The explorer has long tapered ends that have sharp points allowing for exploration and finding the canals.
Notes	• The spoon excavator has a very long shank to reach into the pulp chamber. • The instruments are double ended. • The stiff-ended explorer is designed specifically for endodontic procedures. • It is available in a variety of sizes.

Broaches

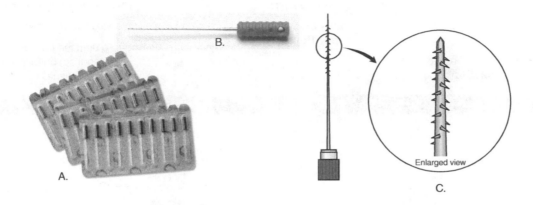

A.

B.

C.

Enlarged view

Use	To remove soft tissue from the pulp canal (extirpate)
Properties	Fine metal wire with tiny, sharp projections or barbs along the instrument shaft
	A. Packages of barbed broaches in various diameters
	B. Single-barbed broach
	C. Close-up drawing of a barbed broach
Notes	• Broaches come in individual sterile cell packs.
	• Broaches are discarded after one use.

- Barbed broaches are supplied in various diameters, ranging from xxxx-fine to coarse.
- Color-coded plastic handles make proper size selection easier.
- It also comes with a notched (latch) end to be used with an endodontic handpiece.

C.L. Canal Lubricant

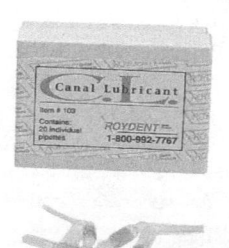

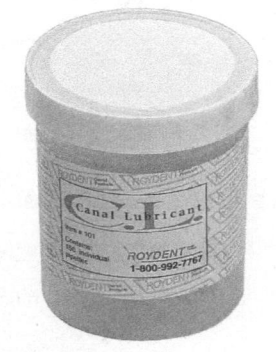

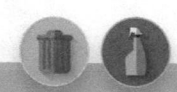

Use
- Chelates root canal walls
- Aids in enlarging the root canals
- Assists in instrumentation by lubricating the canals

Composition 17% ethylenediaminetetraacetic acid in aqueous gel

Properties
- This product lubricates the canal.
- It also softens calcifications in the root canals.

Precaution
- Inhalation: none
- Eyes: may cause transient irritation
- Skin: nonirritating
- Ingestion: none expected with this product with normal conditions of use

Mixing and Setting Time No mixing or setting time is required.

Directions

1. C.L. Canal Lubricant comes in pipettes for easy dispensing.
2. With the material in pipettes it can be placed directly in the canal or a reamer, or file can be used to place the lubricant into the canal.
3. Holding the pipette, cut the tip off. The pipette is then

RC-Prep Root Canal Preparation Cream

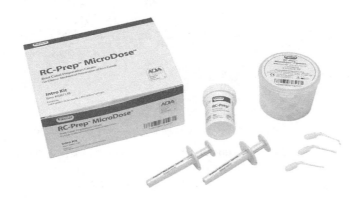

Use   Chemomechanical preparation for root canals

Composition   Glycol, urea peroxide, and ethylenediamine tetraacetic acid (EDTA) in special water-soluble preparation

Properties
- Removes calcifications from the root canal
- Lubricates the canal for efficient instrumentation
- Used with apex locators for reliable readings
- Allows for efficient use of reamers and files
- Prevents instruments from binding
- Easy to use
- Also comes in a microdose form

Precautions
- Skin: There may be irritation and redness. Remove contaminated clothing and wash with soap and water.
- Eyes: There may be pain and redness, and eyes may water. Vision may blur. Rinse with water for 15 minutes and seek medical assistance.
- Ingestion: There may be soreness and redness in the mouth and throat. Nausea and stomach pain may occur. Wash out mouth with water, give water to drink, and seek medical assistance.
- Inhalation: There may be irritation in the throat and a feeling of tightness in the chest. Remove from exposure area.

RC-Prep Root Canal Preparation Cream *Continued*

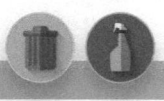

Mixing and Setting Time No mixing is required.

Directions

1. RC-Prep comes in jars, pumps, or syringes.

2. With the material in the jars and pumps, a reamer, file, or root canal filler is used to place the RC-Prep into the canal. Dispense a small amount of the RC-Prep on a pad and then coat the reamer, file, or root canal filler with the material.

3. With the syringe, the material is placed directly into the canal with the tip of the syringe.

4. When the material reacts with the sodium hypochlorite, it lifts debris from the canal.

SlickGel ES Root Canal Preparation Cream

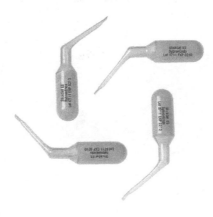

Use	Aids in the negotiation of root canals
Composition	EDTA, urea peroxide, proplyene glycol, and polyethylene glycol

Properties
- The product's highly effervescent action produces vigorous bubbling.
- It chemically removes the smear layer.
- It helps prevent blockage during shaping and cleaning.
- It lubricates the canal, which aids in negotiation.
- It aids in softening calcifications in the root canal.
- It is easy to use.
- It comes in microdose polytubes that do not require disinfection after each use, reducing cross-contamination; these are disposable.
- Its solution is smooth, not grainy.

Precautions
- Eyes: Flush with water for 15 minutes.
- Skin: Wash thoroughly with soap and water.
- Ingestion: Drink two glasses of water and seek medical attention.

SlickGel ES Root Canal Preparation Cream *Continued*

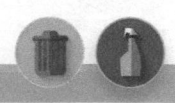

Mixing and Setting Time No mixing or setting time is required.

Directions

1. SlickGel comes in microdose polytubes.
2. When the dentist is ready, the assistant cuts the end of a unidose polytube and passes it to the dentist.
3. The dentist places the tip of the polytube into the root canal and squeezes.
4. At the end of the procedure, the polytube is thrown away.

K-Type Files

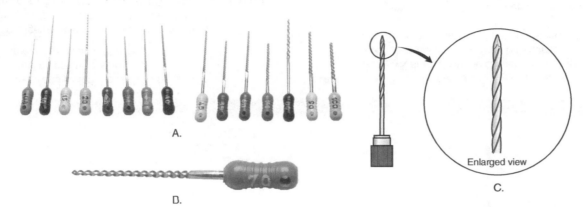

A.

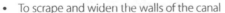

D.

Enlarged view

C.

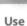

Use	• To scrape and widen the walls of the canal • To remove necrotic tissue

Properties	• Stainless steel with a tightly twisted design
	• Handles are color-coded according to size
	  A. Variety of K-type files
	  B. Single K-type file
	  C. Close-up of tip of the K-type file

Notes	• K-type files are twisted into the canal. • They are also available in nickel–titanium for more flexibility. • They also come with a notched (latch) end to be used with an endodontic handpiece. • They are available in various diameters to match the width of the canals. • Different lengths are available, for example, 21 mm, 25 mm, 28 mm, and 31 mm.

Hedstrom Files

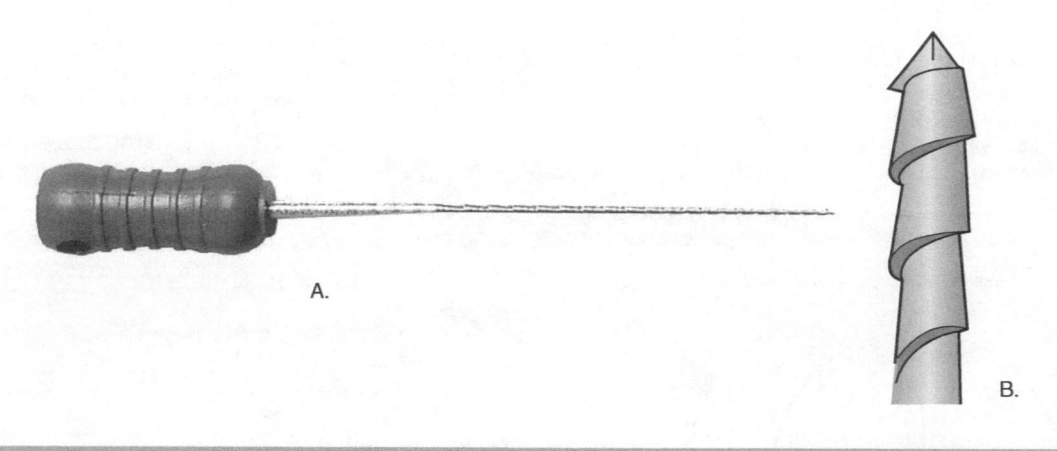

A.

B.

Use
- To scrape and widen the walls of the canal
- To remove necrotic tissue
- To smooth the walls of the canal

Properties
- The edges are very sharp and cut aggressively.
- The handles are color-coded according to size.
- Also comes with a notched (latch) end to be used with an endodontic handpiece
  A. Hedstrom file
  B. Close-up of the tip of a Hedstrom file

Notes
- These files are used only in a push-and-pull motion so they will not bind in the canal.
- They are manufactured by a different process.
- They are shaped like pine trees and appear to look like a stack of cones.
- Available in various diameters to match the width of canals.
- Different lengths are available, for example, 21 mm, 25 mm, 28 mm, and 31 mm.

Flex Files

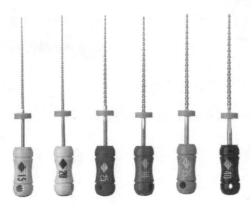

Use
- For curved and narrow canals
- To scrape and widen the walls of the canal
- To remove necrotic tissue

Properties
- Made of stainless steel or nickel–titanium.
- Handles are color-coded according to size.
- They also come with a notched (latch) end to be used with an endodontic handpiece.

Notes
- Flex files are crafted for optimal balance of flexibility, strength, and sharpness.
- They are available in various diameters to match the width of canals.
- Different lengths are available, for example, 21 mm and 25 mm.

Reamer

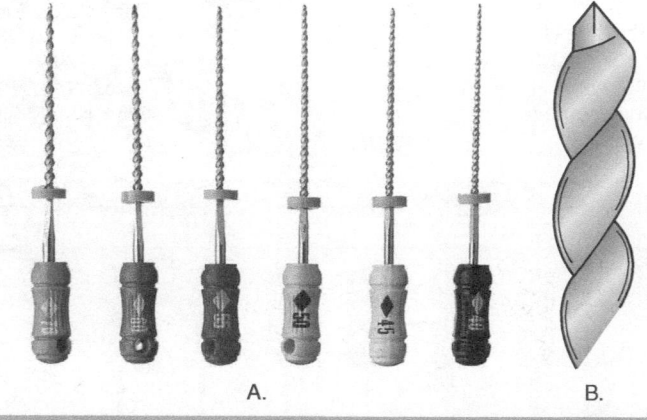

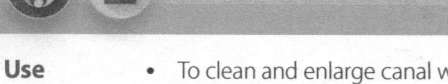

A. Selection of reamers in various diameters

B. Close-up view showing spiral cutting edges

Use
- To clean and enlarge canal walls
- To smooth canal walls

Properties
- Have twisted shanks like the files, but the blades are spaced much farther apart
- The handles are color-coded and numbered according to size, similar to the files.
- Also comes with a notched (latch) end to be used with an endodontic handpiece
    - **A.** Selection of reamers in various diameters
    - **B.** Close-up view showing spiral cutting edges

Notes
- Reamers are used with a twisting ("reaming") motion.
- They are similar to K-type files, but have fewer twists; therefore, the cutting edges are further apart.
- Different lengths are available, for example, 21 mm, 25 mm, 28 mm, and 31 mm.

Gates-Glidden Drills

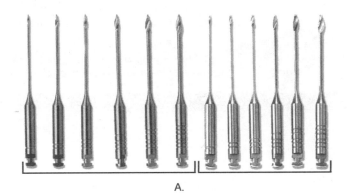

A.

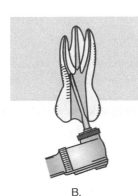

B.

Use	• To prepare the opening access in the coronal portion of the canal • To widen the upper portion of the canal for better access
Properties	Long-shanked bur with various-sized cutting ends **A.** Various-sized Gates-Glidden drills **B.** Line art showing Gates-Glidden drill in canal of tooth
Notes	• The latch-type bur is used with a contra-angle low-speed handpiece. • The cutting ends are elliptical (football-shaped).

• They are supplied in six sizes, marked by the number of grooves on the shank.
• Their sizes are compatible with all endodontic instruments.
• There are two lengths: longer for anterior teeth and shorter for posterior teeth.

Peeso Reamer

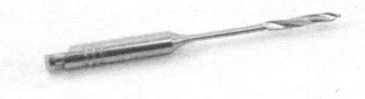

Use   The Peeso reamer is used to prepare the canal for a post and to reduce the curvature for the canal orifice for straight-line access.

Properties   The Peeso instrument is a latch-type reamer; it is used with a contra-angle attachment on a low-speed handpiece and has parallel cutting sides.

Notes   The Peeso reamer is supplied in various sizes; the shanks are marked with grooves to indicate the corresponding size.

Endo Organizers and Endodontic Measuring Device/Millimeter Ruler

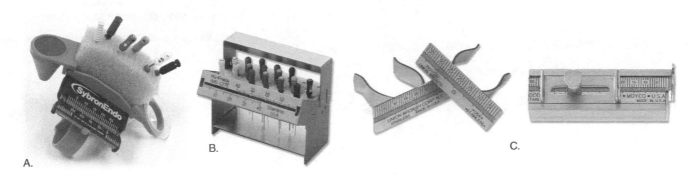

A.

B.

C.

Use	• To store and organize reamers and files • To measure length of endodontic reamer or file and mark with rubber stoppers
Properties	Measurement device with area to hold endodontic broaches, reamers, or files **A.** Ring plastic with disposable sponge endodontic organizer. **B.** Stainless steel endodontic organizer with ruler. **C.** Millimeter rulers with a finger clip or attached to an endodontic organizer. The ruler has an adjustable indicator that shows the length of the stop position.
Notes	• Some of the storage containers can be sterilized. • Some are designed to hold a range of intracanal instruments. • Large organizers often have measuring gauges for setting stops. • Finger rings are much smaller, holding only a few instruments at once. • They are available in stainless steel or plastic. • Some of the units can be sterilized. • The smaller handheld units often have disposable sponges.

Endodontic Measuring Stops

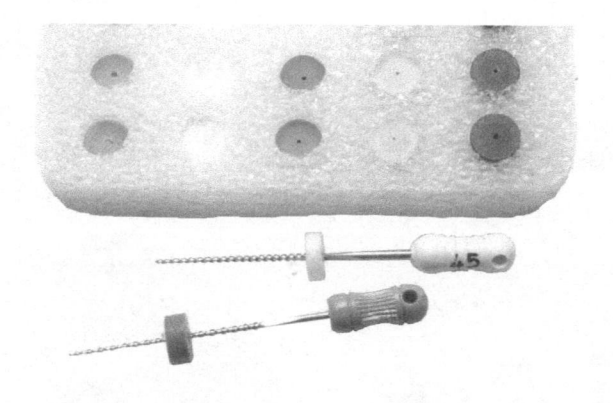

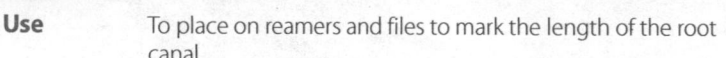

Use	To place on reamers and files to mark the length of the root canal
Properties	Small, circular, and silicone discs of various colors
Notes	• Endodontic measuring stops are also known as rubber stops or markers.
	• The length of the canal is determined by holding a file with a rubber stop against a radiograph and adjusting the stop to match the incisal or cusp edge.

• The marked file is then measured on a small-millimeter gauge.
• This number is recorded for reference and for marking other intracanal instruments.

Chairside Glass Bead Sterilizer

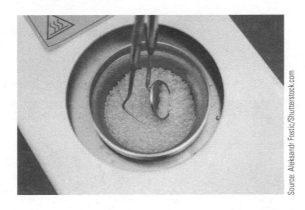

Source: Aleksandr Fostic/Shutterstock.com

Use	To sterilize reamers and files during the root canal procedure
Properties	Small, circular glass beads no larger than 1 mm

Notes
- Glass beads must be smaller than 1 mm to be effective in transferring heat.
- Temperature is between 424 and 474.8°F.

- This is the sterilization method used at a chairside root canal treatment.
- Instruments are left in for a minimum of 5 seconds.

Endodontic Irrigation Syringe/Luer Lock Syringe

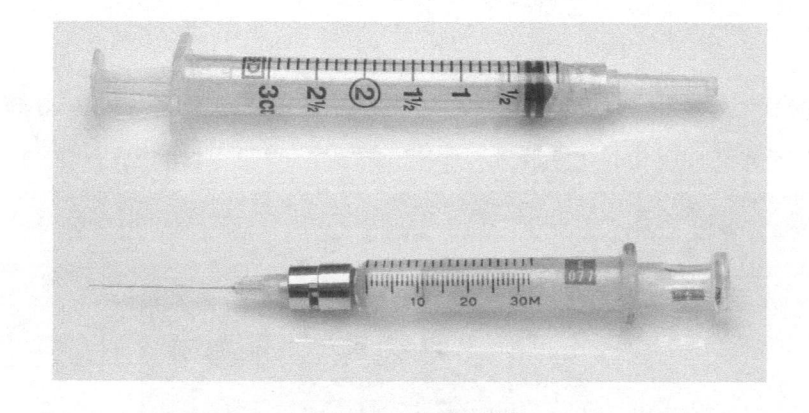

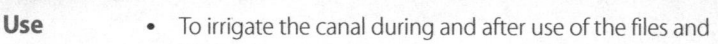

Use
- To irrigate the canal during and after use of the files and reamers
- To debride (cleanse) the canal

Properties
- Calibrated barrels come in different sizes, for example, 3 cc or 12 cc.
- Plunger.
- Needle: 23, 27, or 30 gauge.

Notes
- The plastic types are disposable.
- The glass types are sterilizable, with disposable tips.

Buckley Formo Cresol

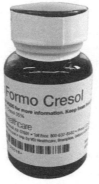
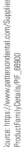

Source: https://www.pattersondental.com/Supplies/ProductFamilyDetails/PIF_66900

Use	Devitalize and sterilize infected pulp chambers and canals
Composition	• 35% Cresol • 19% Formaldehyde • 17.5% Glycerin
Properties	• Slightly less irritating to periapical tissues than other products • Lower content of formaldehyde than other products

Precautions
- Eye contact: Flush with plenty of running water.
- Skin irritation possible: Wash with soap and water and remove contaminated clothing.
- Ingestion—Quickly drink three or more glasses of milk or water.
- Inhalation—Move to fresh air and have qualified person restore and/or support breathing with oxygen.

Buckley Formo Cresol *Continued*

**Mixing and
Setting Time** No mixing or setting time is required.

Directions

1. Clean the tooth and root canal.
2. Use a cotton-tipped applicator or cotton pellets to apply the Formo Cresol.
3. Place the applicator in the Formo Cresol, remove excess liquid, and place in the canal.

Sodium Hypochlorite

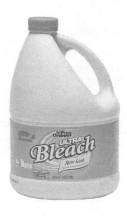

Use	To irrigate and debride root canals and to disinfect root canals during and after debridement
Properties	Aqueous 3% or 6% sodium hypochlorite
Notes	• Sodium hypochlorite is available in bottles and syringes and can use a Luer lock syringe.
	• The solution is 50/50 bleach and water.
	• Do not get on skin or clothing.
	• It is an antimicrobial agent.

Endodontic Locking Pliers

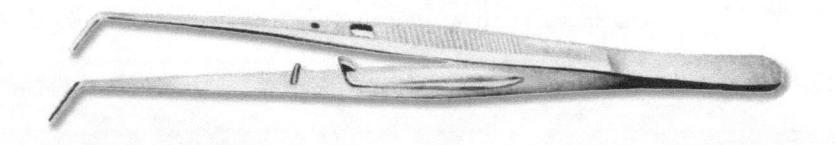

Use	To grasp and transport various materials to and from the oral cavity
Composition	• Locking handles to secure items for transfer, placement, and retrieval • Similar to tweezers; can be smooth or can have serrations on the ends of the beak
Notes	Some have grooved tips (as shown) to better grasp intracanal instruments and materials

Absorbent Paper Points

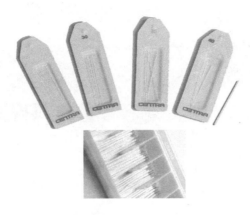

Use
- To dry canals (placed in the canal until canal is dry)
- To place medications in the canal
- To take cultures of the canal

Properties Paper points are absorbent and in the shape of a long narrow cone.

Notes
- Paper points are supplied in various sizes from x-fine to coarse.
- They are available in sterile and nonsterile.
- Some are color-coded to match the endodontic files.
- The sizes match the length and width of the canal.
- Several points are used to ensure that the canal is dry.

Lentulo Spiral

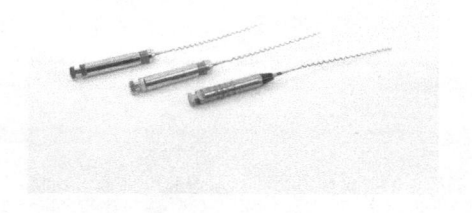

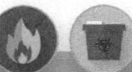

Use   The Lentulo spiral is used to place and evenly distribute root canal sealer or cement in the canal.

Properties   The Lentulo spiral is a long, twisted, and very flexible wire instrument.

Notes
- Spirals are used with low-speed handpieces and contra-angle attachments.
- If a Lentulo spiral becomes bent, it should not be reused.
- The Lentulo spiral attachment end is latched.

Gutta Percha

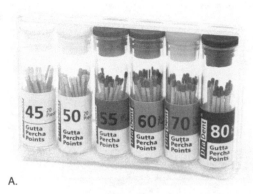

A.

B.

Use	To obturate (fill) the root canal after the canal has been opened and cleaned
Properties	• Thermoplastic material that is flexible at room temperature yet stiff enough to be placed in the root canal. • Comes in cones that are supplied in graduated sizes, from extrafine to large. • The gutta percha and cores can be heated with special heating units before being inserted into the canal. **A.** Various gutta percha kits **B.** Gutta percha shown in root canal prior to removing ends in crown of tooth

Notes
- Some are color-coded to match endodontic files called master cones.
- Some are radiopaque so they can be seen on radiographs.
- Thermal gutta percha endodontic obturation systems are also available; these systems include metal cores coated with gutta percha.

Apexit Endodontic Sealer/Cement

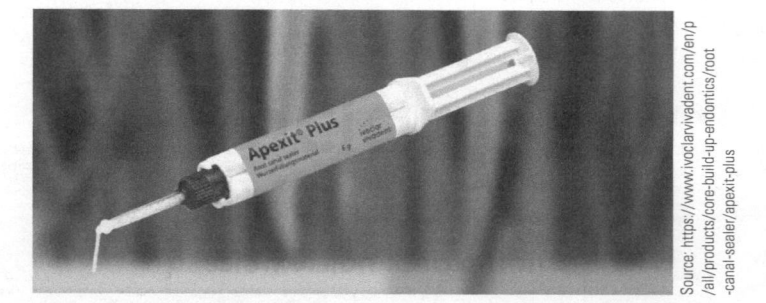

Source: https://www.ivoclarvivadent.com/en/p/all/products/core-build-up-endontics/root-canal-sealer/apexit-plus

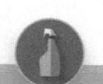

Use	Permanent obturation of root canals
Composition	Base and activator: calcium hydroxide, calcium oxide, inorganic fillers, colophony, and disalicylate
Properties	• High biocompatibility
	• Low water solubility
	• Mixes easily
	• Highly radiopaque
	• Nonshrinking

- Can be used with all obturating systems
- Flows easily into canals and adapts to the walls of the root canals
- Comes in automix syringes for easy handling

Precautions
- Eye irritation: Flush with water for 10 to 15 minutes.
- Skin irritation: Wash with soap and water.
- Ingestion: No hazards anticipated from swallowing small amount during incidental or normal handling.
- Inhalation: Move to fresh air.

Apexit Endodontic Sealer/Cement *Continued*

Mixing and Setting Time
- Automix syringes requiring no mixing.
- Working time is approximately 3 hours.

Directions

1. Remove the cap from the automix syringe by turning it a 1/4 turn counterclockwise.
2. Insert the mixing tip by pushing down until the notch of the tip is aligned with the double-push syringe.
3. Secure the mixing tip in place by gripping the colored base and turning a 1/4 turn clockwise.
4. The double-push syringe contains predosed amounts of Apexit Plus activator and base, which are automatically mixed and dispensed when the two materials are extruded.
5. The material is placed into the canal with a Lentulo spiral or an intraoral root canal tip.

Nogenol Root Canal Sealer

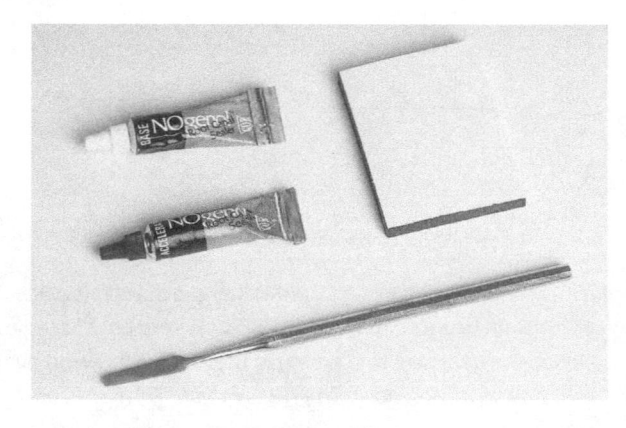

Use　　　　　Root canal sealer

Composition
- Base: salicylic acid
- Catalyst: zinc oxide, vegetable oil, barium sulfate, and bismuth oxychloride

Properties
- Biocompatible
- No eugenol
- Radiopaque
- Sets quickly in the mouth
- Two-paste system that is easy to mix and use
- Long working time
- Allows time for placement and manipulation of material
- Adheres to dry surface
- Seals and adapts to the tooth surface well
- Low solubility

Precautions
- Eye and skin irritation possible with prolonged exposure.
- Ingested:
  - Base: induce vomiting and seek medical attention.
  - Catalyst: Drink several glasses of water.
- Inhalation: Move to fresh air and seek medical attention.

Nogenol Root Canal Sealer *Continued*

Mixing and Setting Time
- Mixing time is 10 to 15 seconds.
- Setting time is 7 minutes in the mouth.

Directions

1. The dentist prepares the root canal according to routine procedure.
2. Prepare and pass paper points to dry the canal.
3. Extrude equal lengths of each paste on a paper pad. Approximately 3/4 of an inch of each paste.
4. Blend with a spatula for 10 to 15 seconds until mix is uniform in color and consistency.
5. Nogenol Root Canal Sealer has a long working time on the paper pad, but once placed in the mouth it will set in about 7 minutes.
6. Prepare a spreader or other endodontic instrument to place the sealer.
7. Prepare the gutta percha points or silver points to be coated with the sealer.

Sealapex Xpress Noneugenol Root Canal Sealer

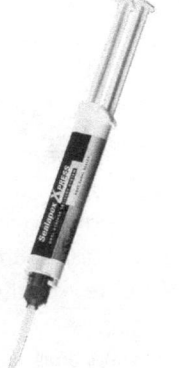

Use To seal the root canal after treatment

Composition • Isobutyl salicylate, silicone dioxide, bismuth trioxide, and titanium dioxide pigment
• Base: N-ethyl toluene, sulfonamide resin, silicone dioxide, zinc oxide, and calcium hydroxide

Properties • Noneugenol
• Nonirritating
• No manual mixing required

• Stimulates hard tissue formation
• One-to-one syringe ratio

Precautions • May be irritating to the eyes and skin.
• Inhalation may cause drowsiness. Move to fresh air.
• If ingested, consult a physician.

Mixing and Setting Time No mixing or setting time is required.

Sealapex Xpress Noneugenol Root Canal Sealer *Continued*

Directions

1. Remove the cap from the automix syringe by turning it 1/4 turn counterclockwise.
2. Insert the mixing tip by pushing down until the notch of the tip is aligned with the double-push syringe.
3. Secure the mixing tip in place by gripping the colored base and turning 1/4 turn clockwise.
4. The automix syringe contains predosed amounts of Sealapex Xpress catalyst and base, which are automatically mixed and dispensed with the two materials extruded.
5. The material is placed into the canal with a Lentulo spiral or an intraoral root canal tip.

Endodontic Spreaders

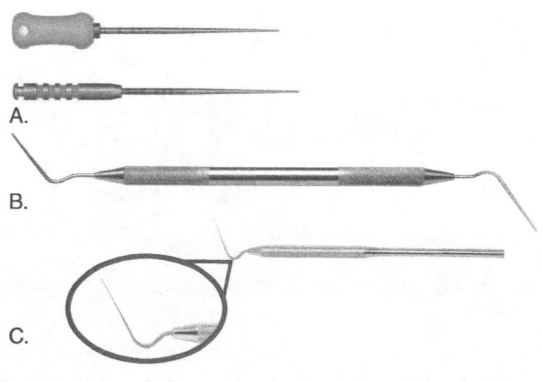

A.

B.

C.

Use
- To laterally condense materials when obturating (sealing/filling) the canal
- To adapt the gutta percha (root canal filling material) to the canal

Properties Spreaders are pointed on the ends.
- **A.** Finger spreaders, hand and slow-speed attached spreaders
- **B.** Double- and single-ended hand spreaders
- **C.** Close up of Endodontic Spreader

Notes
- Some spreaders have short handles that are rotated and held by the fingers; thus, they are called finger spreaders.
- Spreaders are single- or double-ended.
- They are sized to correspond to canal size.
- Rings in millimeter increments are found on the working end.

Endodontic Pluggers

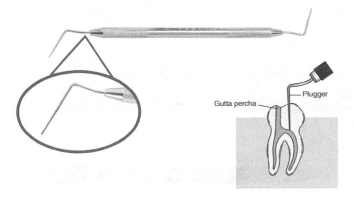

Use	To vertically condense material when obturating (sealing/filling) the canal
Properties	• Single-ended • Flat ends • Short and long handles
Notes	• Endodontic pluggers are available in various sizes to fit into canals.

Glick Endodontic Instruments

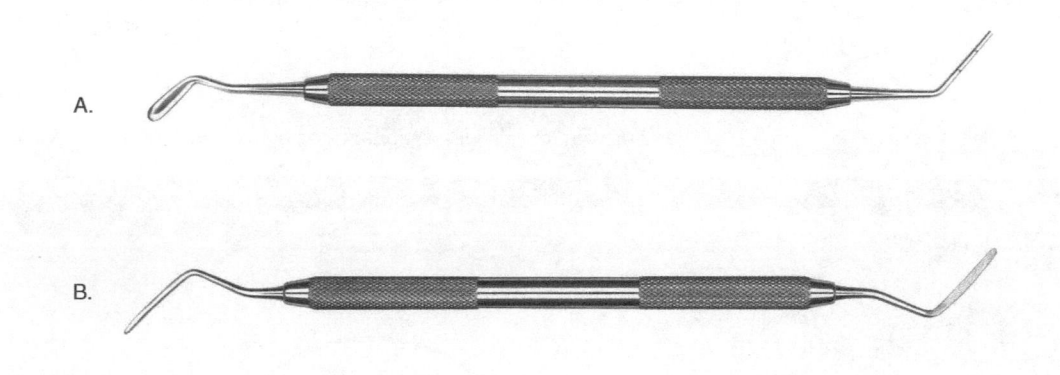

A.

B.

Use	• To remove excess gutta percha from the coronal portion of the canal by heating with a Bunsen burner
	• To condense the remaining gutta percha in the canal opening
Properties	• Doubled-ended
	A. #1 Glick
	B. #2 Glick
	• Long, tapered spoon on each end
Notes	• There may be millimeter rings on the plugger end.
	• They are available in a variety of working ends.

Bunsen Burner

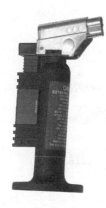

Use	To heat instruments such as a Glick to remove excess gutta percha and seal the root canal
Composition	Instrument that produces an open flame

Gutta Percha Obturation System

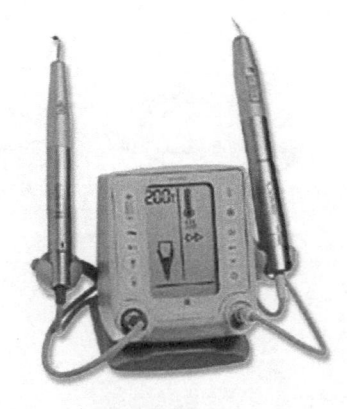

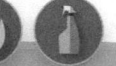

Use
- To soften the gutta percha before placing it in the canal
- To backfill, cauterize, and hot pulp test

Properties
- Unit with control console with a digital display, an extruder handpiece, and a second handpiece used for downfilling, backfilling, cauterizing, and hot pulp testing
- Has a temperature control

Notes
- Temperature can be controlled to adjust the viscosity of the gutta percha.
- Many types are available, with various function combinations.

Woodson Plastic Filling Instrument

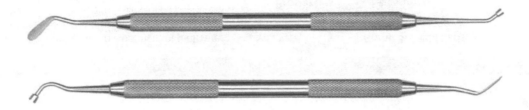

Use	• To pass and place (condense) various dental materials during cavity preparation • To place temporary restorative materials into cavity preparation
Composition	A double-ended instrument that has a condenser on one end and a blade on the other

Notes
• This comes in a variety of sizes and some variation of shapes.
• The angle of the blade may be rotated.

Temporary Restorative Materials: IRM (Intermediate Restorative Material) and IRM Caps

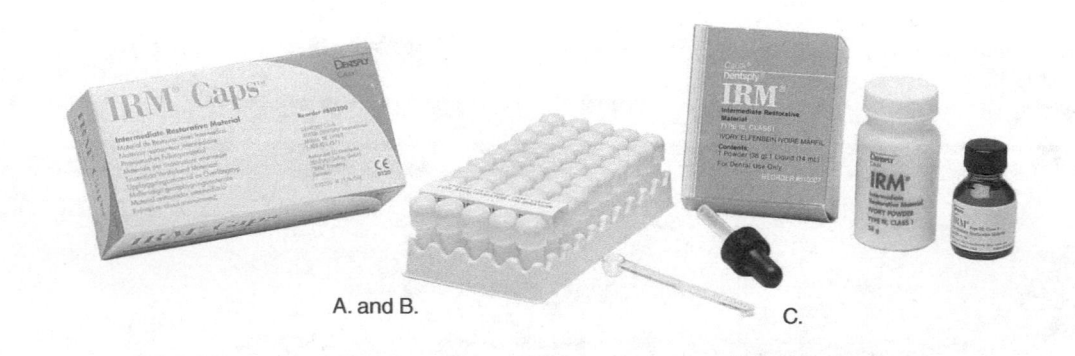

A. and B.　　　　　　　　C.

Use
- Restoration of primary teeth if permanent teeth are within 2 years after eruption
- Restorative emergencies and sealing of root canal opening
- Caries management for Classes I and II restorations lasting up to 1 year
- Public health care programs and dental school clinic application

Composition
- Powder: polymer-reinforced zinc oxide
- Liquid: eugenol material and acetic acid
- Comes in a powder/liquid and capsules

A. and B.　IRM Capsules
C.　IRM is Powder/ Liquid form

Properties
- Fairly strong.
- Low abrasion qualities.
- Low solubility.
- Prevents microleakage.
- Fairly easy to mix and clean up.
- Easy to place.
- Material can be carved with a small round bur when hardened, if necessary.

Temporary Restorative Materials: IRM (Intermediate Restorative Material) and IRM Caps *Continued*

Precautions
- May be irritating to the eyes and skin.
- Irritating to the respiratory system; move the affected person to fresh air.
- If ingested, contact a physician.

Mixing and Setting Time
- Mixing time for the powder/liquid is 1 minute.
- Mixing time for the capsule is 8 to 30 seconds, depending on the amalgamator. Mix at high speed.
- Setting time is 5 minutes from start to finish.

Directions

IRM Powder/Liquid
1. Prepare the tooth by rinsing and drying completely. Place a liner if needed.
2. Fluff the powder; using the scoop provided, measure one level scoop with the spatula and place on the paper pad.
3. Dispense one drop of liquid and replace the cap immediately to prevent evaporation. (When the liquid reaches the discard level marked on the bottle, it should be discarded.)

4. Bring half of the powder into the liquid and mix quickly and thoroughly.
5. Bring remaining powder into the mix in two or three increments and blend thoroughly with a spatula.
6. Once all the powder is in the mix, continue mixing for 5 to 10 seconds. Mix will become smooth and adaptable. Completely mix in 1 minute.
7. IRM is now ready to place.

IRM Caps

1. To activate the IRM capsule, hold it vertically by the bottom half and turn the top firmly until you feel a snap as the liquid is released.
2. Continue to tighten to be sure it is seated.
3. Place the capsule in an amalgamator and mix for the designated amount of time.
4. Once mixed, remove the bottom lid (called the press cap) and remove the mixed IRM.
5. It may be placed on a paper pad for dispensing or may be placed directly into the tooth.

Cavit and Cavit G

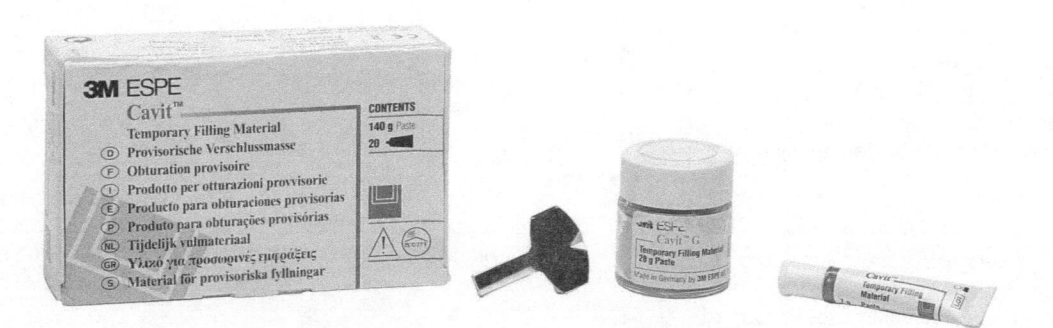

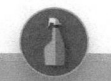

Use	Temporary filling material for Classes I and II and root canal openings
Composition	• Zinc oxide
	• Calcium sulfate
	• Barium sulfate and talc
	• Ethylene bis-diacetate and zinc sulfate
	• Polyvinyl acetate
Properties	• High surface hardness
	• Simple to apply
	• Slight expansion seals margins

• Light-cured
• Comes in a tube or jar

Precautions
• May be irritating to the eyes and skin.
• Irritating to the respiratory system; move exposed person to fresh air.
• If ingested, contact a physician.

Mixing and Setting Time
• No mixing is required.
• The hardening process begins within a few minutes, and the patient should be advised to avoid chewing pressure

Cavit and Cavit G *Continued*

Directions

1. Remove the cap and use the sharp end to puncture the metal end of the tube when used for the first time.

2. Squeeze from the bottom of the tube to extrude a small amount of material. Replace the cap immediately. Use a plastic filling instrument (PFI) to take the Cavit from the tube and place in the cavity. If additional material is required, use a clean instrument to remove what is needed.

3. Wipe the excess from the instrument with gauze and continue filling the cavity. The cavity should be moist. Once the material is placed, have the patient bite down and then remove the excess material.

4. The hardening process begins a few minutes after placement.

Cavit G is applied following the same steps.

Tempit Moisture-Activated Temporary Filling and Sealing Material

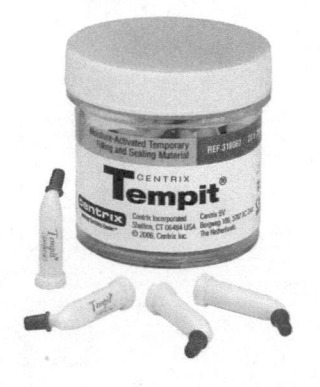

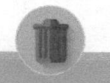

Use   For sealing access cavities during root canal procedures

Composition   Calcium sulfate and zinc oxide, glycol, ethyl methacrylate polymer, barium sulfate, and silica

Properties
- No mixing and no mess
- Sets in minutes
- Easy to remove
- Noneugenol formula

Precautions
- Eyes: Flush with copious amounts of water and seek medical attention.
- Skin irritation possible: Wash with soap and water.
- Ingestion: Not applicable.
- Inhalation: Not applicable.

Mixing and Setting Time
- No mixing is required.
- The setting time is 5 minutes or less.

Tempit Moisture-Activated Temporary Filling and Sealing Material *Continued*

Directions

1. Remove the cap from the syringe.
2. Place the tip securely on the end of the syringe.
3. Squeeze the syringe with slow steady pressure to ensure that it is functional.
4. Dispense a small amount on the pad, and then inject into the moist canal.
5. Tamp down with a moist instrument and dismiss the patient.
6. On the patient's return appointment, use an explorer to remove Tempit material.

Root Canal Therapy–Opening Appointment Tray Setup

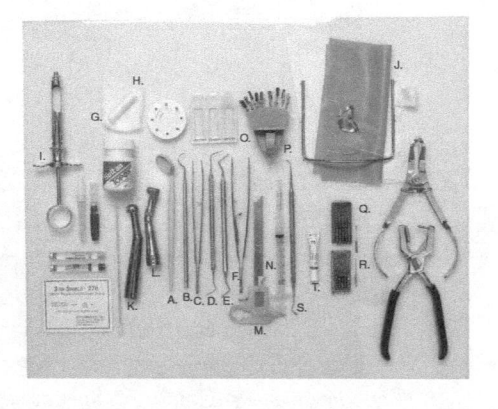

Properties

A. Mouth mirror
B. Explorer
C. Cotton pliers
D. Endodontic explorer
E. Endodontic spoon excavator
F. Locking cotton pliers
G. Cotton rolls
H. Gauze sponges
I. Anesthetic setup
J. Dental dam setup
K. High-speed handpiece

L. Low-speed handpiece
M. Millimeter ruler
N. Irrigating syringe and solution
O. Paper points
P. Barbed broach, assorted reamers and files with stops in endodontic organizer
Q. Peeso reamers
R. Gates-Glidden drills
S. Glick endodontic instrument
T. Temporary filling material

Root Canal Therapy–Closing Appointment Tray Setup

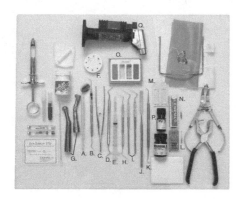

Properties

A. Mouth mirror
B. Endodontic explorer
C. Locking cotton pliers
D. Endodontic spoon excavator
E. Irrigating syringe
F. Burs
G. High- and low-speed handpieces
H. Spreaders
I. Pluggers

J. Spatula
K. Glick instrument
L. Gates-Glidden drills
M. Absorbent sterile paper points
N. Lentulo spiral
O. Gutta percha
P. Root canal sealer
Q. Heat source

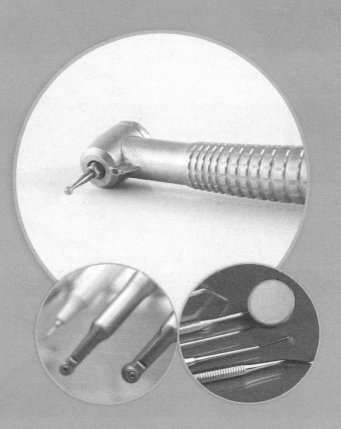

CHAPTER 13

Oral Maxillofacial Surgery Instruments and Materials

Surgical Scalpels (Surgical Knives)

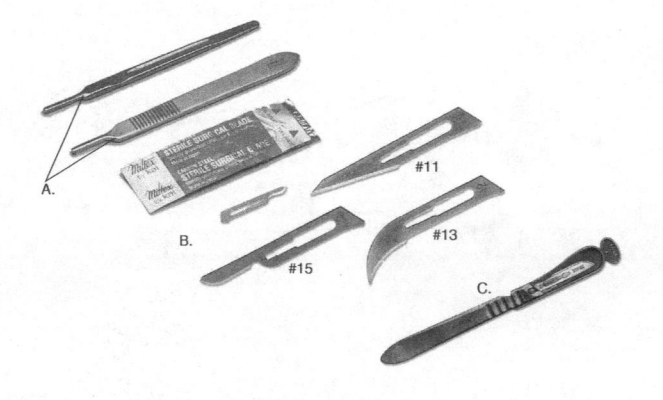

A.

B.

#11

#15

#13

C.

Use   To precisely incise or excise soft tissue with the least amount of trauma

Properties   **A.** Handles: These are slim and straight and are designed to accommodate detachable disposable blades. Handles are flat and often have a metric ruler on them. These are sterilized in an autoclave.

   B. Disposable blades (scalpel): These come in various shapes and sizes and are very sharp. They are supplied in sterile packages and disposed of in the sharps container after one use. Common blades are:

- #15 blade for surgical procedures.
- #11 blade to incise and drain.
- #13 blade incise and drain.

C. Disposable scalpels are also available. These have plastic handles with metal blades and are supplied in sterile packages and disposed of in the sharps container after one use.

Notes
- Scalpels are also known as Bard Parkers.
- They are made from stainless steel or are disposable.
- Scalpel and blades are used in surgery and periodontal surgical procedures as well as in finishing composite restorations.

Scalpel Blade Removal Device

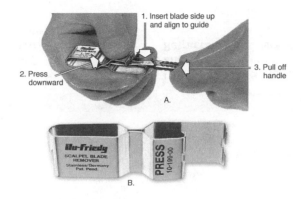

1. Insert blade side up and align to guide

2. Press downward

3. Pull off handle

A.

B.

Use	To remove the blades from the blade handle
Properties	Metal device with a slot into which the blade fits for safe removal
	A. Blade being placed in remover
	B. Scalpel blade remover

Notes
- Place the blade into the remover and to align with the notch.
- Press down on the blade remover.
- Slowly pull away the handle from the blade; the blade should remain within the remover.
- Discard the blade in a sharps container.

Tissue Forceps and Retractors (Lip, Tongue, and Cheek)

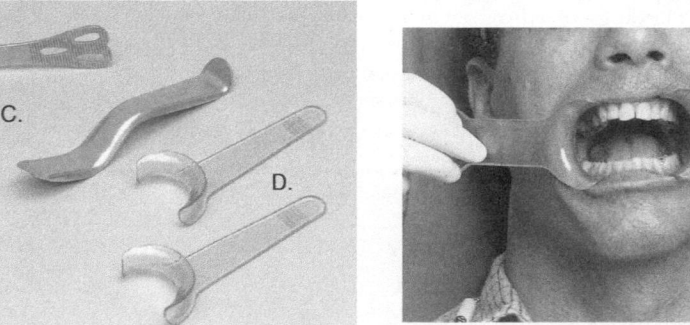

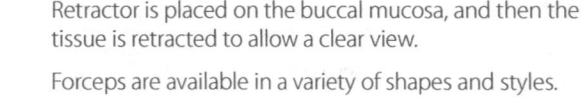

A.

B.

C.

D.

E.

Use	• To hold tissue back from the surgical site so that the operator's view is unobstructed • To hold the lip, tongue, and cheeks out of the way so the operator can view the site during the procedure	**Lip, Tongue, and Cheek Retractors**	**C.** Spoon- or blade-shaped at different angles for tongue and oral cavity **D.** Arch-shaped for cheeks and lips **E.** Patient shown with retractors placed
Properties			Retractor is placed on the buccal mucosa, and then the tissue is retracted to allow a clear view.
Tissue Forceps	**A.** Forceps (hinged types) **B.** Cotton-plier style and straight hand grasp instrument	**Notes**	Forceps are available in a variety of shapes and styles.
	The working end of both types has small teeth to assist in securely grasping the tissue.		

Mouth Gag

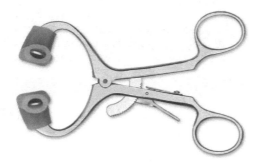

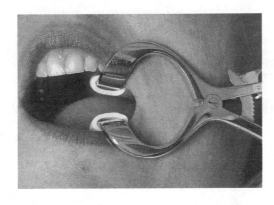

Use	• To prevent the patient's mouth from closing during a procedure
Properties	• Hinged device with ratchet release
	• Handles and beaks

Notes
- To apply, close the beaks and insert into the patient's mouth.
- Gently squeeze the handle; this opens the beaks and the patient's mouth.
- The forceps are locked in this position until the release is engaged.
- The mouth gag is supplied in pediatric, child, and adult sizes.

Hemostats and Needle Holders

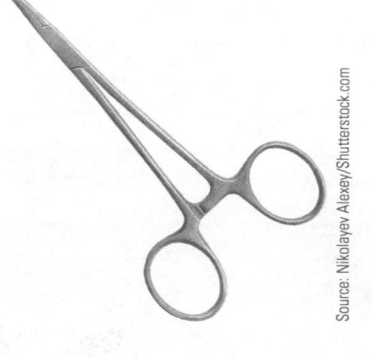

Source: Nikolayev Alexey/Shutterstock.com

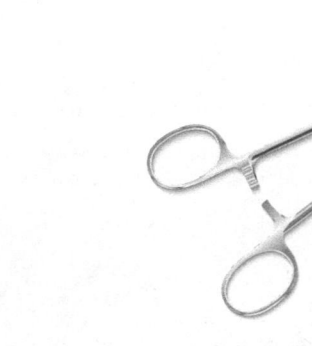

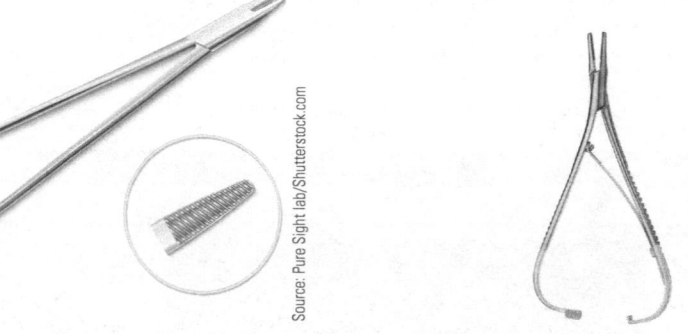

Source: Pure Sight lab/Shutterstock.com

Source: JethroT/Shutterstock.com

Use

- To retract tissue
- To remove small root tips
- To clamp off blood vessels
- To grasp loose objects
- To grasp and handle suture needle during suturing procedure

Properties

- Working ends are long, serrated, or grooved beaks.
- Locking handles can be manipulated with one hand.
- The beaks of the needle holder are shorter than those of the hemostat.

Notes

- The needle holder has fine serrations with a groove down the center of each beak to hold the suture needle.
- Hemostats and needle holders are available in various sizes.
- There are various types, including Kelly hemostats and Halstead Mosquito forceps.
- They are available with straight or curved beaks.

Suture Needle and Sutures

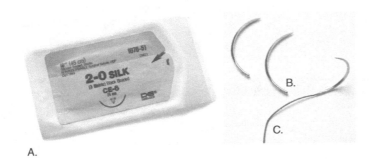

A.

B.

C.

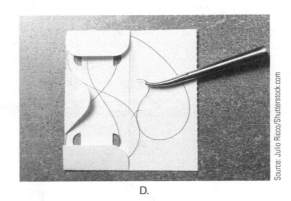

D.

Source: Julio Ricco/Shutterstock.com

Use	To suture (or close up with thread) the surgical site
Properties	**A.** Available in sterile package with suture attached to needle
	B. Suture needle
	C. Suture needle with suture attached
	D. Sterile suture package open with needle holder

Notes
- Available in a variety of suture needle sizes and different suture materials
- Resorbable sutures: chromic gut, gut plain, and polyglycolic
- Available in sterile packets
- Nonresorbable sutures: nylon, polyester, polypropylene, and silk (most popular)

Suture Scissors and Surgical Scissors

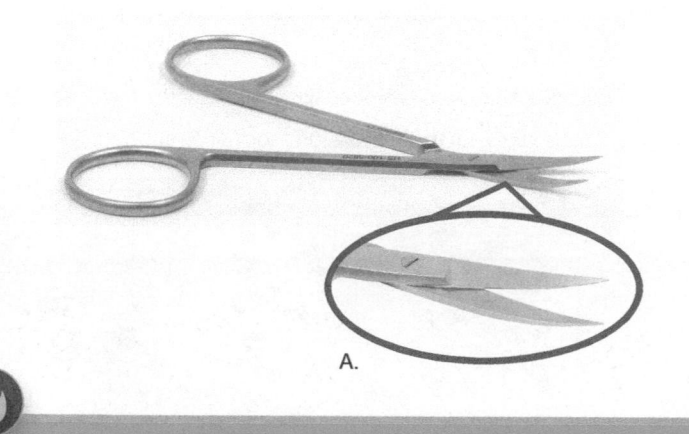

A.

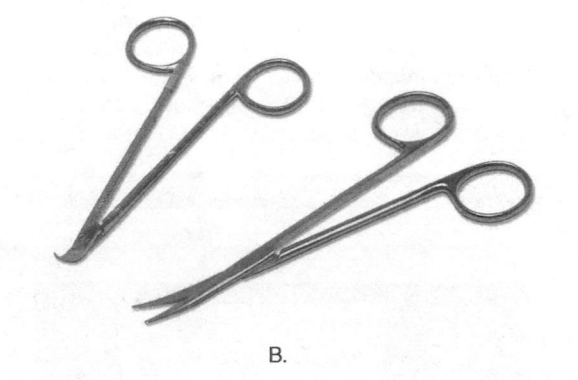

B.

Use	• To cut sutures
	• To trim soft tissue
Properties	• Stainless steel.
	• Suture scissors have a C-shaped notched area to slide under the suture and allow cutting to occur.
	• Surgical scissors have pointed beaks with straight or angled blades.

A. Suture Scissors
B. Surgical Scissors

Notes	• Supplied in various sizes and shapes.
	• Often one side of the cutting blades has a serrated area that holds the tissue while cutting.

Surgical Aspirating Tips

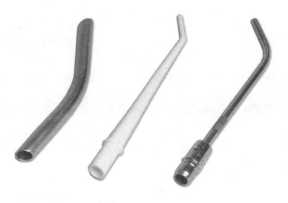

Use	To aspirate blood and debris from the surgical site and back of the oral cavity in sedated patients
Properties	Long tubes that are very slender or tapered to small openings that attach to high-volume suction
Notes	Made of plastic (disposable) or metal (sterilizable)

Surgical Curettes

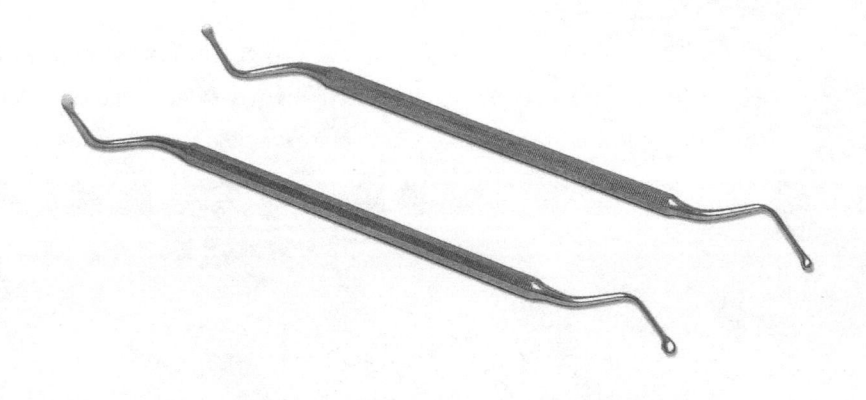

Use

For curettage and debridement of the tooth socket or diseased tissue

Properties

- Double-ended and have straight or curved shanks.
- The working end of the instrument is spoon-shaped.

Notes

They are available in various sizes.

Surgical Chisel and Mallet

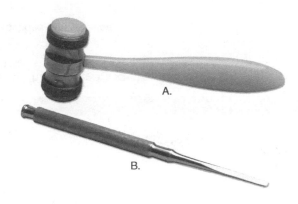

A.

B.

Use
- To gently tap the end of the chisel to split a tooth prior to removal.
- Surgical chisels are used to remove or shape bone.

Properties
A. Surgical mallet
B. Surgical chisel

Notes
- Surgical chisels are available beveled on one side or on both sides (bibeveled).
- Bibeveled chisels are used for splitting a tooth.
- Single-beveled chisels are used to remove and shape bone.

Surgical Bone File

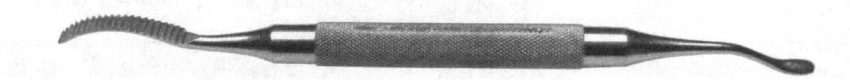

Use
- To trim and smooth bone after teeth have been extracted
- Used in a back-and-forth motion

Properties
- Usually double-ended.
- The working end is normally rounded with serrations.

Notes   They are available in various sizes and shapes.

Rongeur (RON-jeer)

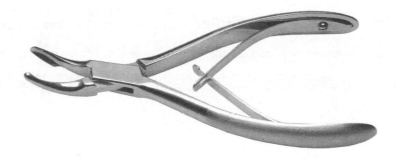

Use   To trim and shape the alveolar bone after extractions

Properties   • Hinged forceps with springs in the handle.
                 • Beaks have sharp cutting edges.

Notes   They are available in different sizes and shapes.

Periosteal Elevator

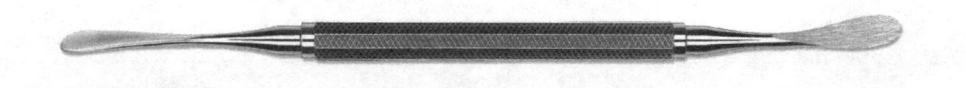

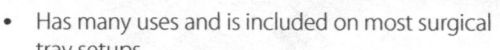

Use
- Has many uses and is included on most surgical tray setups
- Often used to detach the periosteum (bone covering) and gingival tissues from around the tooth prior to the use of extraction forceps
- Also used to reflect and lift the mucoperiosteum (mucosa and periosteum) from the bone

Properties
- Double-ended
- Various working-end combinations

Notes
- Often one end is pointed and the other end is rounded.
- They are available in various sizes and shapes.

Elevators

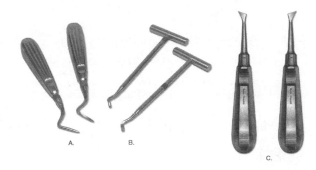

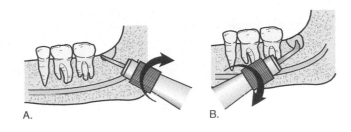

A.

B.

C.

Use	To loosen and remove teeth, retained roots, and root fragments
Properties	• Single-ended instruments with large bulbous or T-shaped handles to allow for a firm grip. • The working ends of elevators may be straight or angular and are often paired left and right. • Common designer elevators are:

A. Apical: root tip
B. Potts: T-bar
C. Cryers: root

Notes   Designed in different shapes and sizes

Root Tip Picks

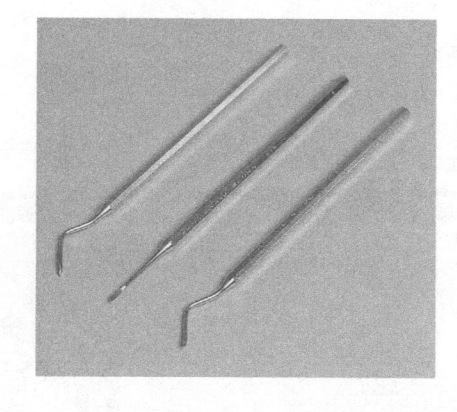

Use	To elevate and remove root tips and fragments
Properties	Slender instruments that have an elongated pointed working end

Notes

- They have either a slender or an enlarged handle.
- They are available as single- or double-ended instruments.
- Root tip picks are even thinner and longer than apical elevators.
- Root tip picks are paired left and right and are straight or angled.

Maxillary Extraction Anterior Forceps: #65 and #99C Maxillary Extraction Forceps

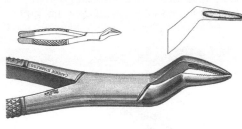

A.

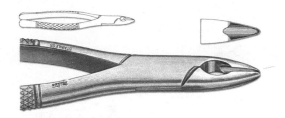

B.

Use	• To remove maxillary incisors and cuspids from the alveolar bone

Properties
• Handle
• Hinge
• Beak
A. #65 Maxillary anterior teeth and roots
B. #99C Maxillary anterior teeth

#150 Maxillary Anterior Extraction Forceps

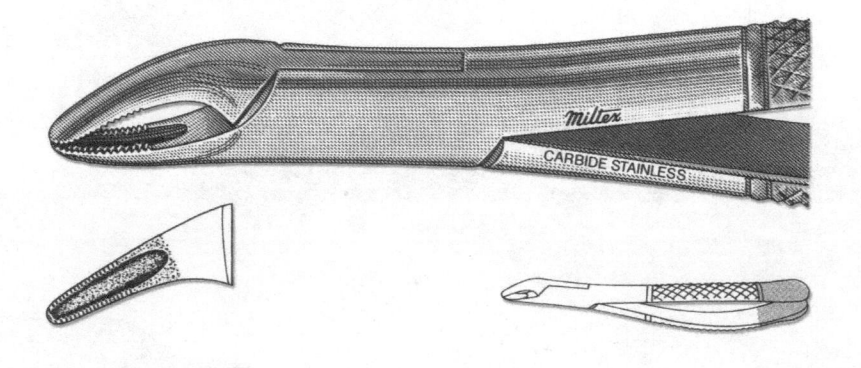

Use
- Termed "universal forceps," because they are used for both the right and left sides of the mouth
- To remove maxillary incisors, cuspids, bicuspids, and roots

Properties
- Handle
- Hinge
- Beak

#88R and #88L Maxillary Molar Extraction Forceps

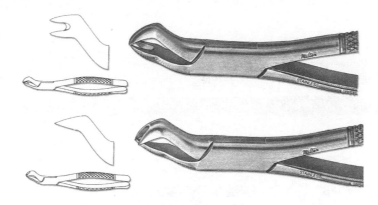

Use	To remove first and second maxillary molars
Properties	• Handle
	• Hinge
	• Beak

Notes
- Each instrument has a number imprinted on the handle and is labeled with an "L" for left or "R" for right.
- These forceps are designed according to the tooth morphology; the two-beaked sides of the forceps are used to surround the lingual root, and one single side is used to go between the buccal roots in the bifurcation.

#53R and #53L Maxillary Molar Extraction Forceps

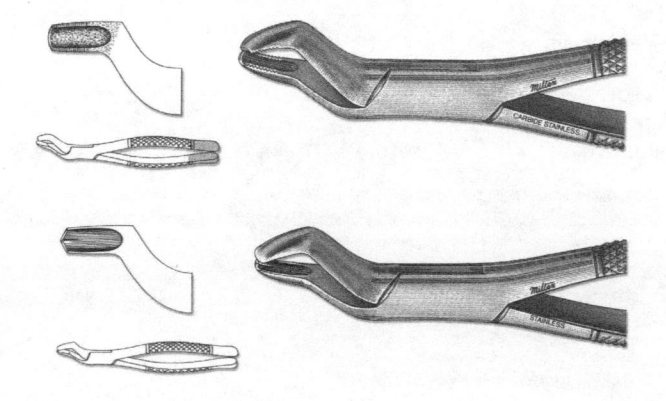

Use
To remove maxillary first and second molars

Properties
- Handle
- Hinge
- Beak

Notes
Each instrument has a number imprinted on the handle and is labeled with an "L" for left or "R" for right.

#210 Maxillary Extraction Third Molar Forceps

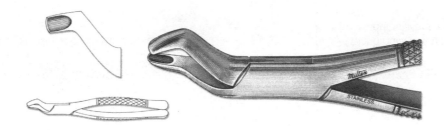

Use
- Termed "universal forceps," because they are used for both the right and left sides of the mouth
- Used to remove maxillary third molars

Properties
- Handle
- Hinge
- Beak

Mandibular Extraction Anterior Forceps: #24 and #203 Anterior Extraction Forceps

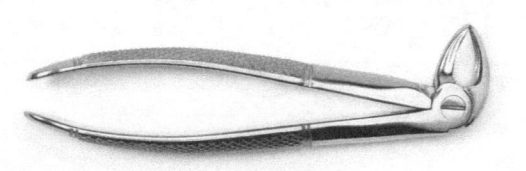

Source: JethroT/Shutterstock.com

A.

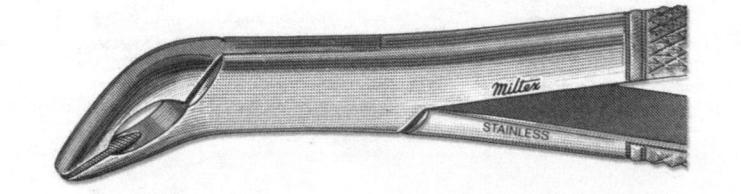

B.

Use	To remove mandibular incisors, bicuspids, cuspids, and roots
Properties	• Handle
	• Hinge
	• Beak

A. #24 Mandibular anterior teeth, also known as Bird Beaks

B. #203 Mandibular anterior teeth and root tips
- Handle
- Hinge
- Beak

#151 Mandibular Anterior Extraction Forceps

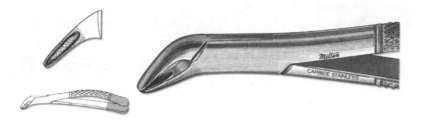

| **Use** | • Termed "universal forceps," because they are used for both the right and left sides of the mouth
• To remove mandibular incisors, cuspids, and roots | **Properties** | • Handle
• Hinge
• Beak |

Mandibular Molar Extraction Forceps: #23 and #17 Universal Mandibular Extraction Forceps

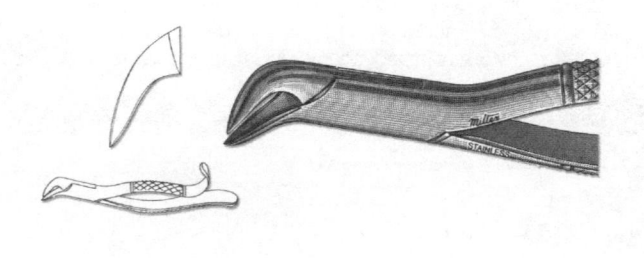

A.

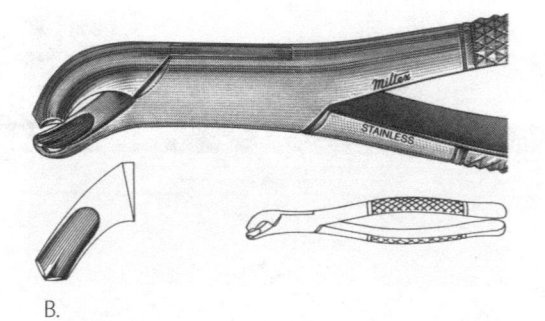

B.

Use	• To remove first and second molars • Termed "universal forceps," meaning used for the right and left sides of the mouth
Properties	• Handle • Hinge • Beak **A.** #23 Mandibular first and second molars, also known as Cow Horns **B.** #17 Mandibular first and second molars

Notes

• "Cow horn" forceps are so named because of the bend of the beaks, with a point at the end of each beak.
• Beaks have a formed point in the middle to go into the bifurcation (where the mesial and distal roots divide).
• They are available in right and left if the handle is curved (called the finger ring on the handle).

#222 Mandibular Third Molar Extraction Forceps

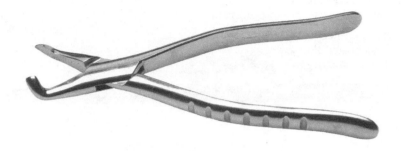

Use
- Termed "universal forceps," because they are used for both the right and left sides of the mouth
- Used to remove third molars

Properties
- Handle
- Hinge
- Beak

Alvogyl

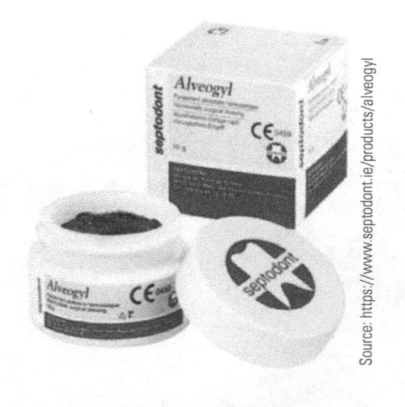

Source: https://www.septodont.ie/products/alveogyl

Use	• Dry socket treatment • Postextraction dressing
Composition	Eugenol, butamben, and iodoform
Properties	• One-step dressing • Rapidly alleviates pain • Soothing effect throughout healing process • Fibrous consistency for good adherence during healing

• Analgesic action
• Anesthetic action
• Antimicrobial action

Precautions
• May be irritating to the eyes and skin.
• Irritating to the respiratory system: Move to fresh air.
• If ingested, contact a physician.

Mixing and Setting Time No mixing is required.

Alvogyl *Continued*

Directions

1. Prepare socket or surgical site. Gently rinse socket with warm water then dry.
2. Remove the lid from the paste.
3. Remove the amount necessary to fill the socket.
4. Place material into the socket with a flat-bladed instrument and pack into place.
5. Tamp down to cover exposed bone.
6. Material remains in the socket as the socket heals.

Tray Setup for Simple Extraction

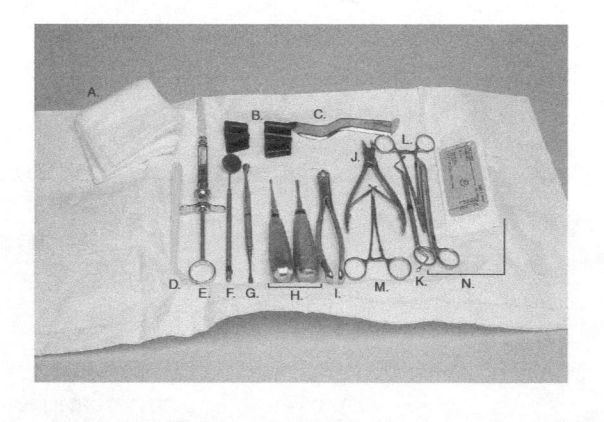

Properties

A. Gauze sponges
B. Mouth props
C. Retractor for the tongue and the cheek
D. Surgical high-volume evacuator (HVE) tip
E. Local anesthetic
F. Mouth mirror
G. Periosteal elevator
H. Straight elevators
I. Extraction forceps
J. Rongeurs

K. Surgical curette
L. Needle holder
M. Hemostat
N. Surgical scissors/suture setup

Tray Setup for Multiple Extractions and Alveoplasty

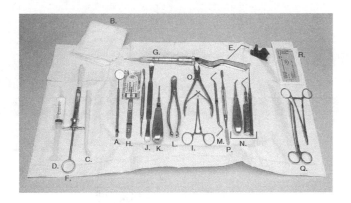

Properties

A. Mouth mirror
B. Gauze sponges
C. Surgical HVE tip
D. Luer Lock syringe and sterile saline solution
E. Retractor for the tongue and cheeks
F. Local anesthetic setup
G. Low-speed handpiece and surgical burs
H. Scalpel and blades
I. Hemostat and tissue retractors
J. Periosteal elevator

K. Straight elevator
L. Extraction forceps
M. Surgical curette
N. Elevators and root tip pick
O. Rongeurs
P. Bone file
Q. Surgical scissors and needle holder
R. Suture setup

Tray Setup for Suture Removal

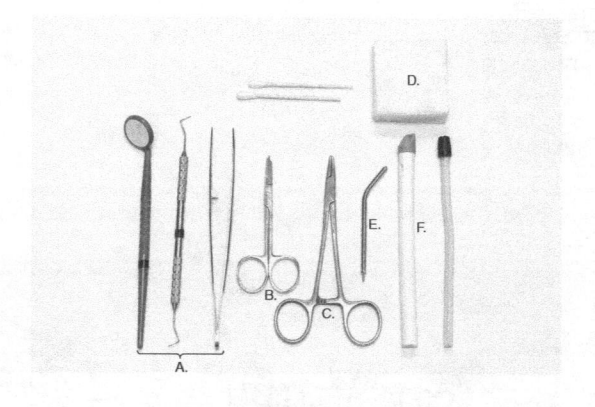

Properties   **A.** Basic setup, mouth mirror, explorer, and cotton pliers
    B. Suture scissors
    C. Hemostat
    D. Gauze sponges
    E. Air-water syringe tip
    F. HVE tip and/or saliva ejector

CHAPTER 14

Orthodontic Instruments and Materials

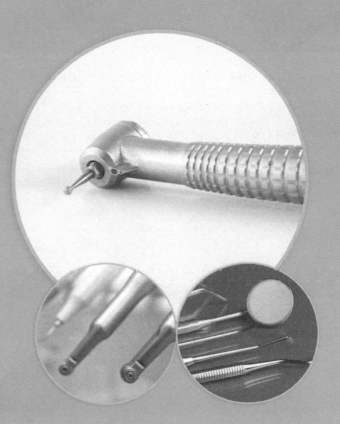

Orthodontic Lip and Cheek Retractors

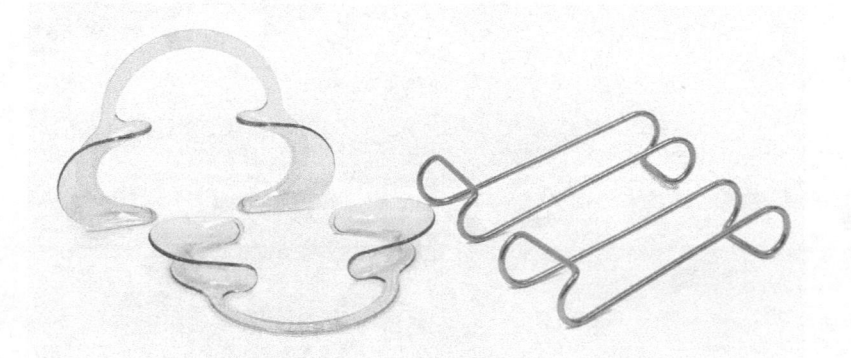

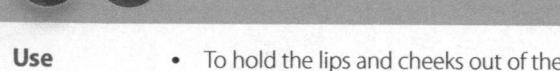

Use
- To hold the lips and cheeks out of the way during orthodontic treatment
- To retract the lips and cheeks out of the way during a photo shoot

Composition Two U-shaped guards, connected or separate, that are placed at the corners of the patient's mouth to retract the tissue out of the way of the operator

Notes
- They are available in a variety of styles and sizes.
- They are made from plastic or metal.

- Some are reusable (autoclavable) and others disposable.
- Camera systems used in oral photography sometimes come with lip and cheek retractors.
- They keep the entire field in view and dry.
- Many retractors come with tabs or handles that the dental assistant or patient uses to hold back the lips and cheeks.
- Some come with areas for placement of the saliva ejector.

Orthodontic Bands

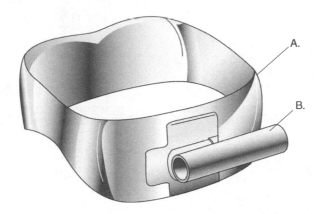

A.

B.

Use
- To cement around a tooth to hold and control tooth movement.
- Tubes, brackets, and attachments are fused and applied to the band to facilitate tooth movement.
- Used for holding arch wires.
- For placement of orthodontic headgear while patient is wearing it.

Composition
A. Stainless steel band to be placed on posterior teeth
B. Bracket and buccal tube placed on the band

Notes
- Orthodontic bands come in a variety of sizes and are cemented in place.
- They are used on the posterior teeth.
- They are disposable.
- They are anatomically designed to fit the tooth.
- Right and left anatomy and accurate gingival contouring bands are available.

Orthodontic Arch Wire

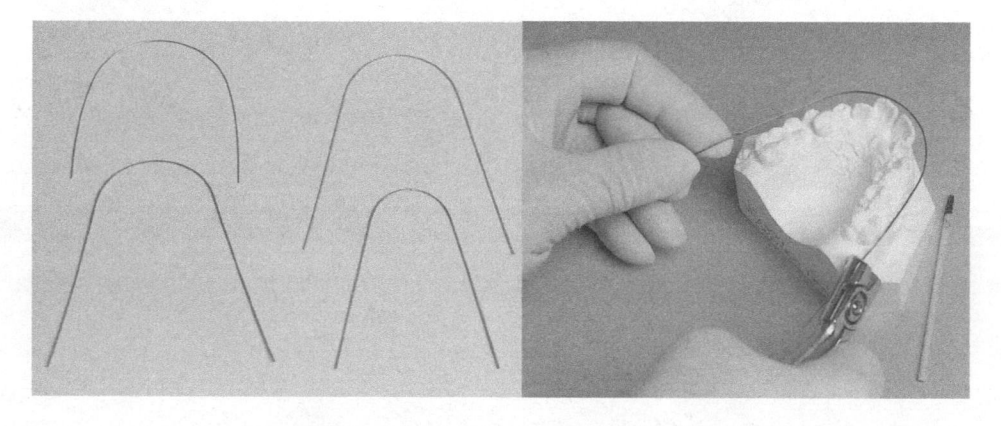

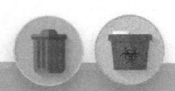

Use	To apply force to either move the teeth or to hold teeth in the desired positions
Composition	Nickel–titanium or stainless steel arch wires that fit the natural arch form
Notes	• Orthodontic arch wires are secured to the brackets by ligature ties or elastics.
	• They are supplied in different shapes: round, rectangular, etc.

- The different diameters and compositions alter the effect of the treatment.
- They should be disposed of in sharps containers.
- They are placed in the buccal tubes and brackets that have been secured to the tooth.
- Nickel–titanium memory wire is designed to hold its shape.

Orthodontic Brackets and Bracket Trays

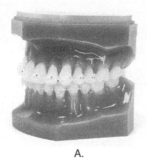

A.

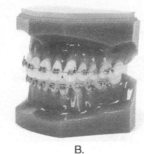

B.

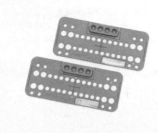

C.

Use
- To hold the arch wire in place.
- To transmit the force of the arch wire to move the teeth.
- Trays hold brackets and/or bands in order prior to their placement on the teeth.

Composition Anatomical brackets made to fit on the middle third of the teeth; each bracket has a slot to hold the arch wire.
- **A.** Clear brackets
- **B.** Metal brackets
- **C.** Compartmental trays to hold each bracket in anatomical order to prevent brackets from spilling

Notes
- Brackets are either welded to the bands or bonded directly to the teeth.
- Posterior brackets are made of stainless steel.
- Anterior brackets are made of stainless steel, ceramic, or acrylic materials.
- Some trays have adhesive backing to prevent spilling.

Self-Ligating Bracket System and Placement Instrument (Damon)

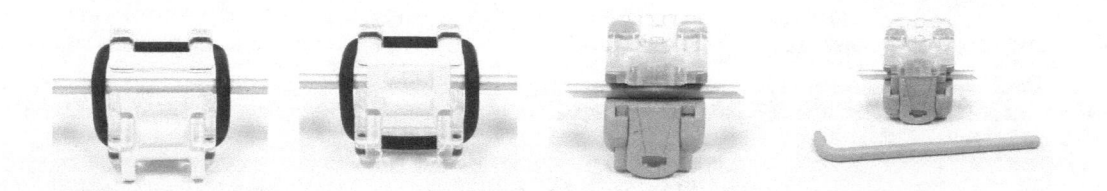

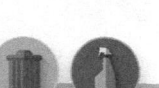

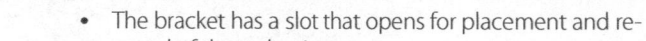

Use To hold and secure the arch wire to the brackets without the use of ligature wire or elastics

Composition **A.** Clear self-ligating Damon bracket
B. Metal self-ligating Damon bracket with placement instrument

Notes
- The bracket has a slot that opens for placement and removal of the arch wire.
- The self-ligating bracket holds the arch wire tighter to control movement, thereby reducing treatment time.
- Several styles of self-ligating brackets are available.

Separators

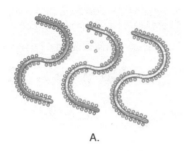

A.

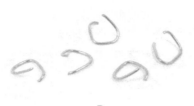

B.

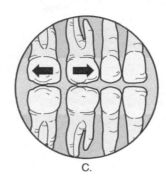

C.

Use	To separate the teeth to allow for placement of the orthodontic bands

Composition
A. Elastic separators that are placed in the contact area to force the teeth apart to accommodate the orthodontic band
B. Metal C-shaped springs that are placed in the interproximal area to gently force the teeth apart to make space for the orthodontic band
C. Drawing showing how the teeth are spread after placement of elastic separators

Notes
- Separators are placed a few days prior to band placement.
- Many different elastic separators are available.
- Many different-shaped metal separators are available.
- Brass wire is also used for separation of teeth.

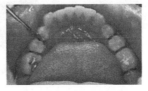

Force Module Separating Pliers (Elastic Separating Pliers)

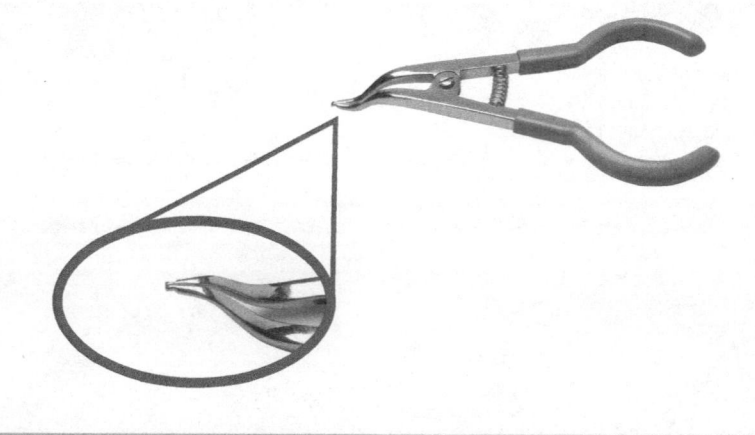

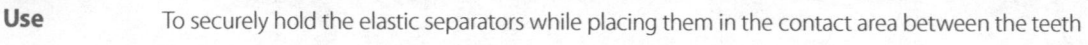

Use   To securely hold the elastic separators while placing them in the contact area between the teeth

Composition • Hinged instrument with spring action
                 • Small projections on each side to hold and grip the elastic separators
                 • Single-ended

Notes   • They are sterilizable.

Orthodontic Ligature Wire/Elastic Modules

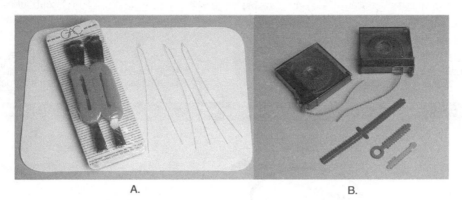

A.

B.

Use	To hold the arch wire to the brackets
Composition	**A.** Ligature wire is a very thin, flexible wire that comes in precut lengths or on spools.
	B. Elastic modules come in many colors to motivate patients to wear them, and come on sticks, canes, and chains.
Notes	• These are placed with the Coons ligature-tying pliers.
	• The elastic modules may be placed with an explorer or scaler.
	• They are sterilizable.

Coons Ligature-Tying Pliers and Mathieu Needle Holders

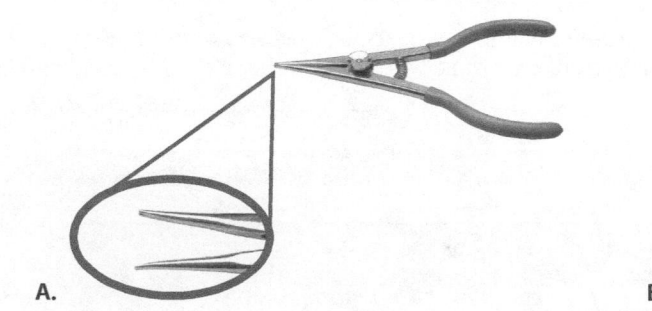

A.

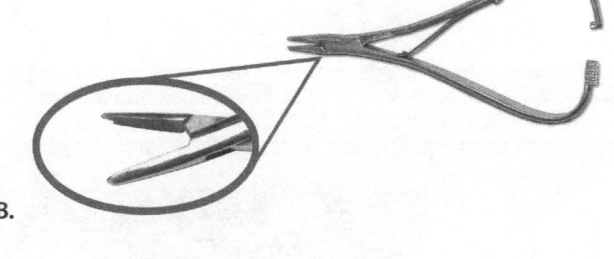

B.

Use
- Coons: To manipulate and tie the ligature wire
- Mathieu: To place elastic ligatures; to hold and place ligatures and separators

Composition **A.** Coons ligature tying pliers: A spring-loaded hinged instrument with two beaks at the working end; they are serrated for a tight grip.

B. Mathieu needle holders:
- Each beak end is notched to hold the ligature wire.
- This is also called an orthodontic hemostat.
- One action will lock and release these pliers.
- At the nonworking end or handle is a locking device.

Notes
- These are available in a variety of styles.
- They are sterilizable.

Ligature Director

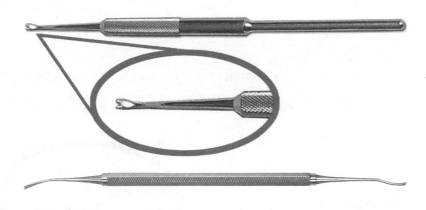

Use	To tuck twisted ligature wire ends into the interproximal spaces
Composition	A single- or double-ended instrument with the working end notched for placement of the ligature.
Notes	• Ligature directors are available with different types of working ends, with some resembling a plugger or scaler.
	• The working ends of the instrument are notched to secure and manipulate the ligature wire around the brackets.
	• They are sterilizable.

Pin and Ligature Cutter or Light Cutting Pliers

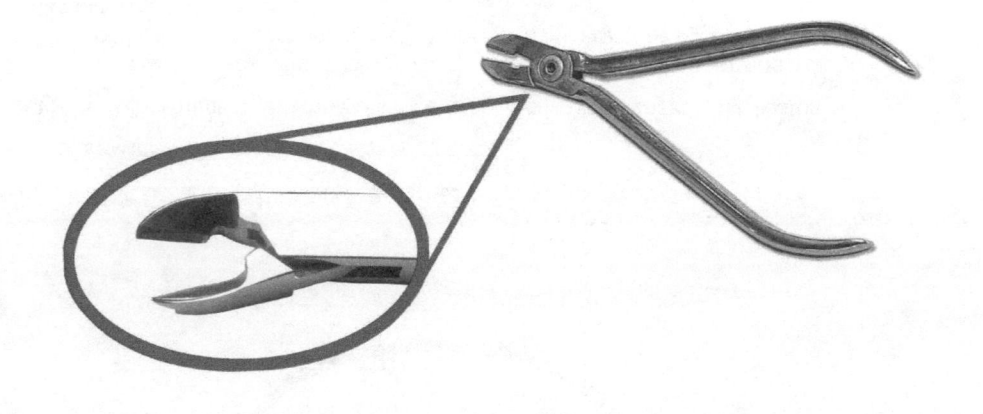

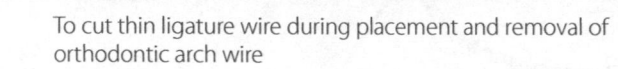

Use	To cut thin ligature wire during placement and removal of orthodontic arch wire
Composition	• A hinged instrument with cutting blade on working end. • Photo shows the back of the entire instrument with a close-up of the working-end top side.

Notes
- They are available in various sizes and shapes.
- They are available with straight, angled, or tapered working ends.
- They are sterilizable.

How (Howe) Pliers/Utility Pliers

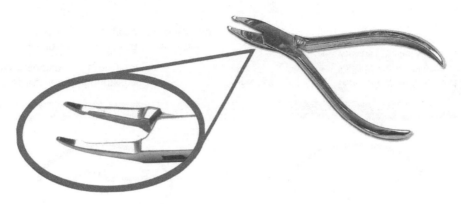

Use
- To manipulate, place, and remove the arch wire
- To check for loose appliances

Composition
- A hinged plier with serrated beaks
- Photo shows the back of the entire instrument with a close-up of the working-end top side

Notes
- They come with curved or straight beaks.
- The working ends are flat and serrated for tighter grip.
- They are sterilizable.

Band Seater/Plugger with Scaler

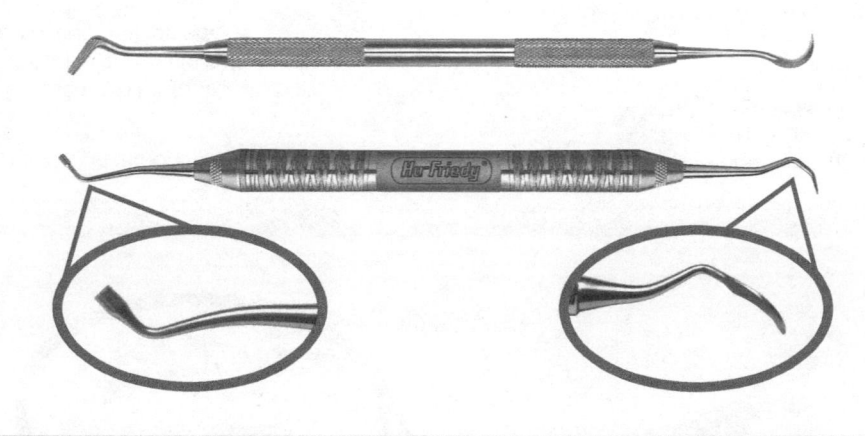

Use
- To place or seat posterior orthodontic bands
- To remove excess cement

Composition A straight double-ended instrument with an angled scaler on one end and a serrated angled plugger on the other end

Notes
- These are double-ended.
- Various shapes of condensers are available.
- Various types of scalers are available.
- They are sterilizable.

Bite Stick/Band Seater and Band Pusher

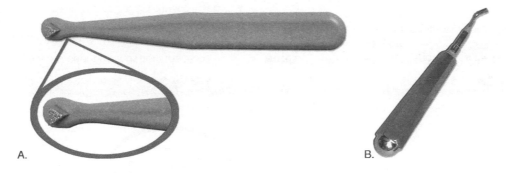

A.

B.

Use

To push and seat the orthodontic bands into place during the try-in and cementation appointments

Composition **A.** The bite stick is a straight plastic broad instrument with a triangular metal serrated insert on the working end. On the opposite side of the insert is a wide flat surface.

B. The band pusher is a large-handled metal instrument with a tapered-angled working end. The working end has a flat serrated tip.

Notes
- Force of occlusion is used to seat the band.
- This is also called a band biter.
- The instrument is single-ended.

- The instrument is a flat stick with small metal triangle on the working end that sits on the orthodontic band; the patient bites down on the flat opposite side.
- The band pusher has a large handle for a good grip to apply pressure on the orthodontic band.
- They are sterilizable.

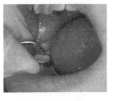

Posterior Band-Removing Pliers

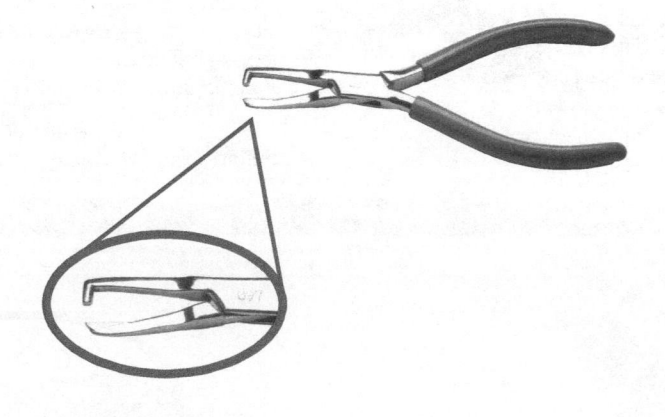

Use To remove posterior orthodontic bands from the teeth

Composition A hinged plier with different-shaped working ends: One beak has a round plastic cover to place on the occlusal surface of the teeth; the other beak has a small flat surface that is placed under the band near the gingival tissue or under the bracket on the band.

Notes
- Pressure is applied and the band is gently removed from the tooth.
- Some band-removing pliers have replaceable plastic tips.
- They are sterilizable.

Crimping Pliers

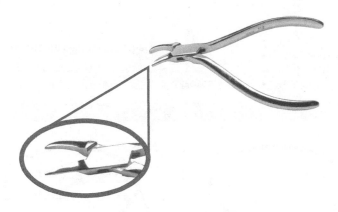

Use   To crimp and re-form crowns and orthodontic bands to adapt more tightly to the tooth

Composition   A hinged plier with beaks that curve and contour on the same plane

Notes

- One beak has a rounded end and the other is blunt.
- These are sometimes called crown- or band-crimping pliers.
- The band fits between the beaks to be shaped and contoured.
- They are sterilizable.

Contouring Ball Pliers

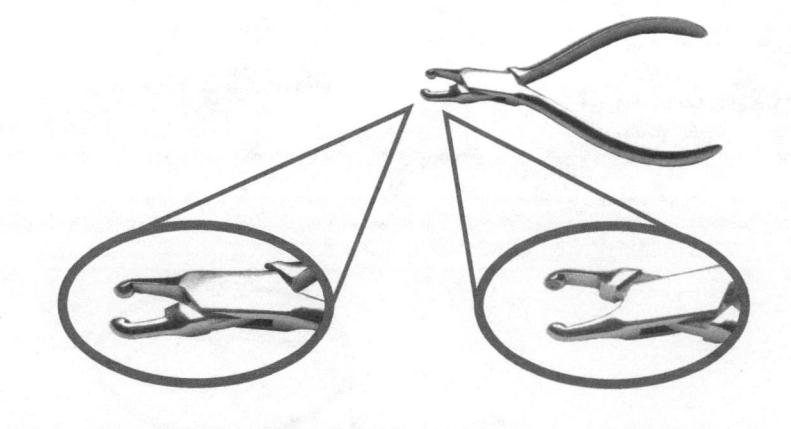

Use
- To contour orthodontic bands
- To contour stainless steel/aluminum crowns

Composition A hinged instrument with beaks: one is a ball and the other is a matching socket.

Notes
- These have matched ball and socket tips for contouring the bands.
- Large and small tips are available.
- They are sterilizable.

Bracket Forceps

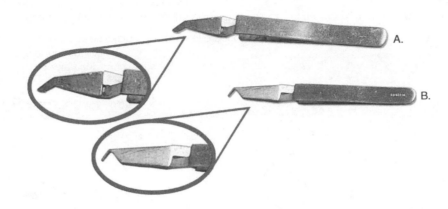

Use
- To hold and pass the brackets for placement and positioning
- To place the brackets on the tooth for bonding

Composition The instrument has handles that you pinch together to allow the tips to secure and release the brackets.
A. Posterior bracket forceps
B. Anterior bracket forceps

Notes They come in a range of sizes and shapes.

Bird-Beak Pliers and Three-Prong Pliers

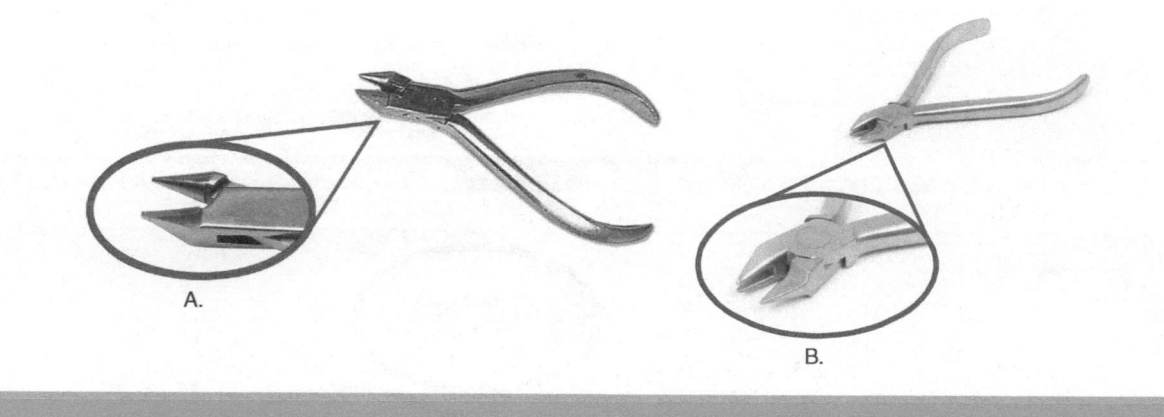

A.

B.

Use	**A.** Bird beak pliers:
	• To contour and bend wire, clasps, and loops
	• To form springs in orthodontic wire
	B. Three prong pliers: To adjust wire on retainers and other appliances with wire
Composition	**A.** Bird beak pliers: A hinged instrument that has two short working ends. One of the working ends is triangular in shape; the other working end is rounded in shape (bird beak).
	B. Three-prong pliers: One side has only one beak and the other side has two beaks (three-prong).
Notes	• They are sterilizable.

Weingart Utility Pliers

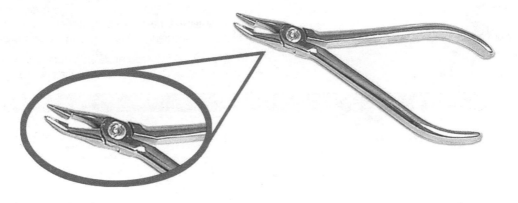

Use	• To place and remove arch wire • Also used for numerous other orthodontic functions
Composition	A hinged instrument with elongated serrated clasping tips
Notes	• These pliers are slim enough to fit between the bracket and the arch wire.

• They are very functional in manipulating orthodontic arch wire.
• The working ends are serrated and tapered.
• They are sterilizable.

Tweed-Loop Pliers

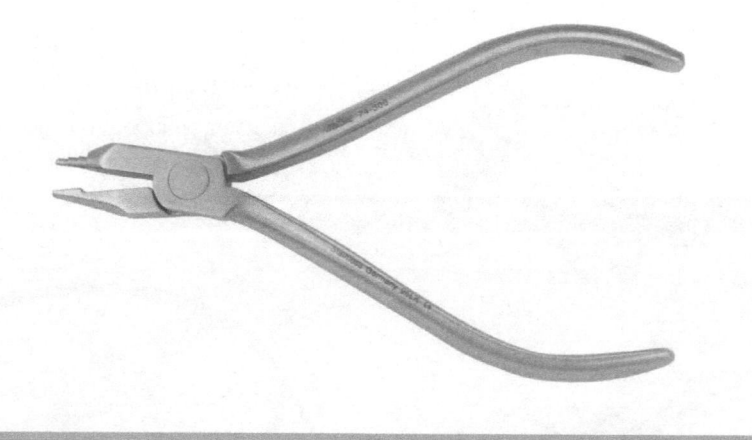

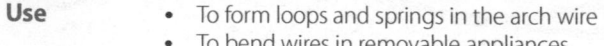

Use	• To form loops and springs in the arch wire
	• To bend wires in removable appliances
Composition	• A hinged instrument with two beaks. One beak has grooves in a graduated cone that assist in the bending of the wire and in forming the loops; the other beak has a flat serrated tip.
	• They are sterilizable.
Notes	• These come in a variety of styles.
	• They are sterilizable.

Arch-Bending Pliers

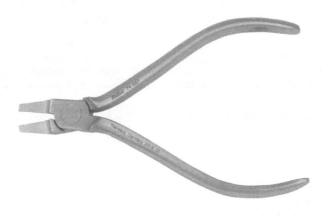

Use
- To bend arch wires
- Designed for placing first-, second-, and third-order bends

Composition A hinged instrument with two tapered ends that are flat

Notes
- One action will lock and release these pliers.
- These are available in a variety of styles.
- They are sterilizable.

Distal End-Cutting Pliers

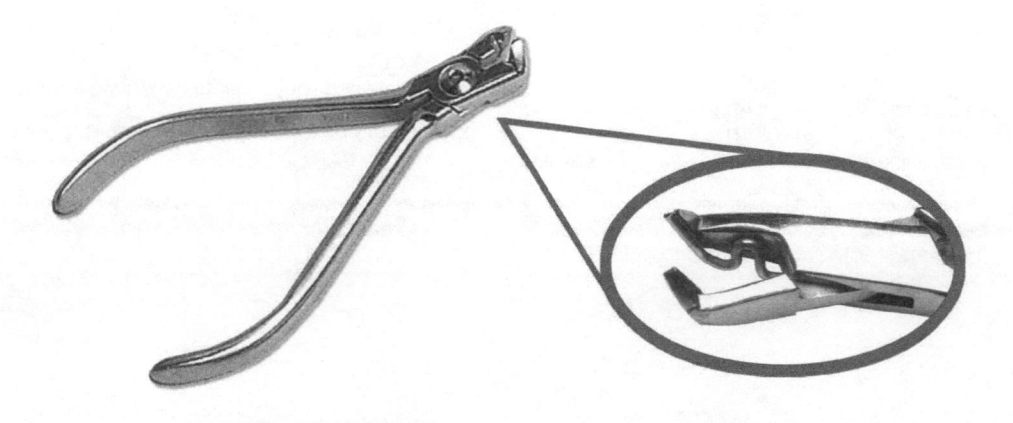

Use
- To cut the distal ends of the arch wire after the wire has been placed and secured in the brackets and the buccal tubes
- Designed to grasp the cut end of the wire

Composition A hinged instrument that has two beaks, one for cutting and the other for grasping the cut wire.

Notes
- The pliers are designed to fit at the distal of the most posterior tooth at a right angle.
- The pliers have a sharp edge to cut the excess arch wire.
- They are sterilizable.

Bracket Removers and Adhesive-Removing Pliers

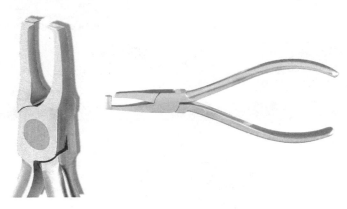

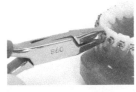

Use	• Bracket remover: To remove brackets from the teeth
	• Adhesive-removing pliers: To remove excess adhesive from the tooth after the brackets have been removed
Composition	• Bracket removers are hinged instruments with two beaks that have sharp right-angle edges.
	• The bracket remover has beaks that come together in a flat pointed edge to fit under the bracket and pry it loose.
	• Bracket removers are available in anterior, where the tips are straight, and posterior, where the tips are at a right angle.
	• Adhesive-removing pliers are hinged instruments; one end has a plastic cap on it and the other working end is a flat surface.
	• Adhesive-removing pliers have two ends. One end of the pliers has a plastic pad that can be changed; the other end of the pliers has a short, straight beak to scrape off the adhesive.
	• They are sterilizable.

Tray Setup for Placement and Removal of Elastic Separators

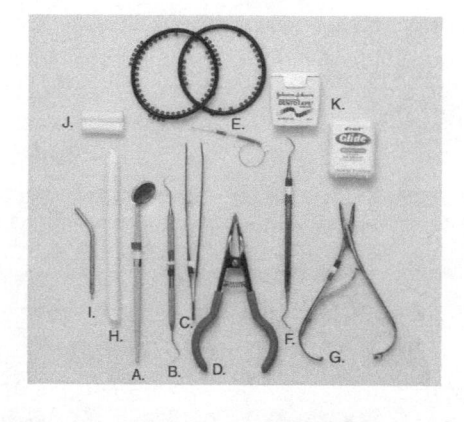

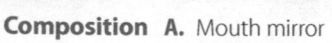

Composition
A. Mouth mirror
B. Explorer
C. Cotton pliers
D. Separating pliers
E. Separators (elastic or metal separating materials)
F. Orthodontic scaler

G. Mathieu pliers
H. High-volume evacuator (HVE) tip
I. Air-water syringe tip
J. Cotton rolls
K. Dental floss or tape

Tray Setup for Cementation of Orthodontic Bands

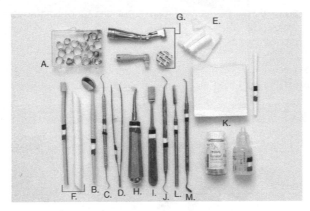

Composition
A. Selection of bands
B. Mouth mirror
C. Explorer
D. Cotton pliers
E. Cotton rolls and 2 × 2 gauze
F. Saliva ejector and HVE
G. Slow-speed handpiece with rubber cup and prophy paste

H. Band pusher
I. Bite stick/band seater
J. Scaler
K. Cement of choice, dispenser for powder, and paper pad
L. Cement spatula
M. Plastic filling instrument

Tray Setup for Direct Bonding of Brackets

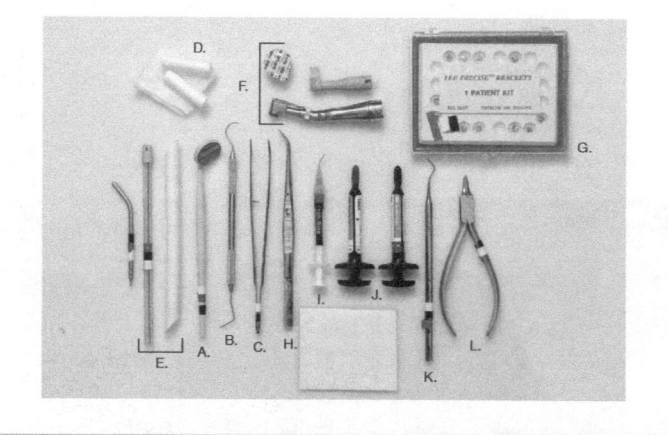

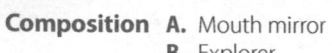

Composition

A. Mouth mirror
B. Explorer
C. Cotton pliers
D. Cotton rolls and 2 × 2 gauze
E. Air-water syringe tip, saliva ejector, and HVE
F. Contra-angle attachment or disposable prophy cup and prophy paste

G. Bracket kit
H. Locking cotton pliers
I. Etchant
J. Bonding agent
K. Scaler
L. Bird-beak pliers

Tray Setup for Placement of Arch Wire and Ligature Ties

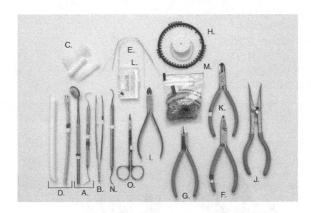

Composition

A. Mouth mirror, explorer
B. Cotton pliers
C. Cotton rolls and 2 × 2 gauze
D. HVE and saliva ejector
E. Selected arch wire
F. Weingart pliers
G. Bird-beak pliers
H. Elastics or ligature wire

I. Ligature-wire-cutting pliers
J. Ligature-tying pliers
K. Distal end-cutting pliers
L. Orthodontic wax
M. Rubber bands
N. Orthodontic scaler
O. Scissors

Tray Setup for Appliance Removal Appointment

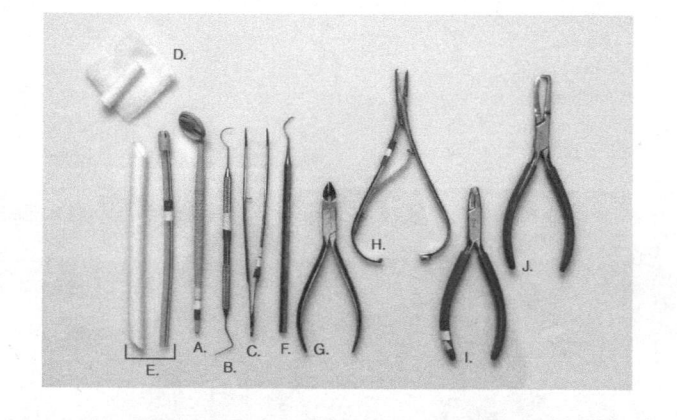

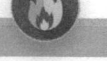

Composition
A. Mouth mirror
B. Explorer
C. Cotton pliers
D. Cotton rolls and 2 × 2 gauze
E. HVE and saliva ejector

F. Orthodontic scaler
G. Ligature-wire-cutting pliers
H. Mathieu pliers
I. Bracket remover and adhesive-removing pliers
J. Posterior band remover

Orthodontic Impression Materials: Jeltrate® Alginate

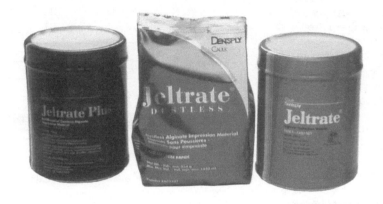

Use   Making dental impressions used for the fabrication of casts for:
- Study models.
- Orthodontic models.
- Opposing models.
- Removable splints.
- Removable retainers.
- Provisional restorations.
- Additional applications in the dental office.

Composition
- Crystalline silica
- Amorphous silica
- Calcium sulfate
- Tetrasodium pyrophosphate
- Potassium alginate
- Magnesium oxide
- Organic glycol
- D&C red dye 30 (fast set)
- Yellow iron oxide (regular set)

Properties
- Supplied in airtight pouches or can (canister), water measure, and a scoop
- Material is supplied with a scoop and measuring device
- Appears to be a creamy color when mixed
- Comes in regular and fast set

Orthodontic Impression Materials: Jeltrate® Alginate *Continued*

Precautions
- Always read the Material Safety Data Sheet (MSDS) for the product.
- Avoid contact with eyes.
- Avoid inhalation.
- Do not ingest.
- Do not use in patients who have history of severe allergic reactions to the components.

Mixing and Setting Time

	Regular Set	Fast Set
Mixing time	1 min	45 sec
Total working time	2 min 15 sec	1 min 30 sec
Initial setting time	2 min 30 sec	1 min 45 sec
Setting time	3 min 30 sec	2 min 30 sec

The temperature of the water will vary the working and setting time. Cooler water increases time; warmer water decreases time.

Directions   After the tray is selected, personal protective equipment (PPE) is in place, and the patient is prepared for the procedure:
1. Cut the pouch and place into a canister with a tight-fitting lid.
2. Fluff powder with lid in place.

3. Dispense material by dipping supplied scoop into powder (do not pack) and tap it lightly against the rim to ensure that the scoop is filled. Use spatula by laying it level across the scoop to scrape excess material from the scoop.

4. Place scoops into dry mixing bowl (rubber or disposable) or into alginate mixer. Place additional scoops into bowl. Normally, two scoops are needed for the mandibular and three scoops for the maxillary arch.

5. Add water from the measuring device. Each line indicates enough water for one scoop. If three scoops are used, the entire water measuring device can be filled. Water should be distilled and the water temperature should be approximately 73°F (23°C).

6. Use a wide-blade spatula to mix water and powder carefully at first to incorporate it together. Then spatulate against the bowl sides to reduce incorporation of air. Do not whip the material. Rotate the bowl and gather the material and then spatulate again against the sides of the bowl. Follow the mixing times for the material.

7. Once the material is mixed to a creamy texture without air bubbles, it can be gathered and loaded into the impression tray for insertion into the mouth.

Coe Alginate™

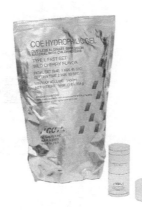

Use

Making dental impressions used for the fabrication of casts for:
- Study models.
- Orthodontic models.
- Opposing models.
- Removable splints.
- Removable retainers.
- Provisional restorations.
- Additional applications in the dental office.

Properties

- Supplied in airtight Ziploc® pouches with a water measure and a scoop
- Use scoop and water measure that is supplied with the material.
- Low flow minimizes gagging
- High compressive strength
- High tear strength
- Regular and fast set in both mint and cherry flavors

Coe Alginate™ *Continued*

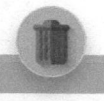

Precautions
- Always read the MSDS for the product.
- Avoid contact with eyes.
- Avoid inhalation.
- Do not ingest.
- Do not use in patients who have history of severe allergic reactions to the components.

Mixing and Setting Time

	Regular Set	Fast Set
Mixing time	45 sec	45 sec
Total working time	2 min 35 sec	1 min 35 sec
Initial setting time	2 min 50 sec	1 min 50 sec
Setting time	3 min 45 sec	2 min 45 sec

*The temperature of the water will vary the working and setting time. Cooler water increases time; warmer water decreases time.

Directions After the tray is selected, the PPE is in place, and the patient is prepared for the procedure:

1. Dispense material by dipping supplied scoop into powder and packing it into the scoop. Use spatula by laying it level across the scoop to further pack the material and scrape excess material from the scoop.

2. Place scoops into dry mixing bowl (rubber or disposable) or into alginate mixer. Place additional scoops into bowl. Normally, two scoops are needed for the mandibular and three scoops for the maxillary arch.

3. Add water from the measuring device. Each line indicates enough water for one scoop. If three scoops are used, the entire water measuring device can be filled. Water should be distilled and at approximately 73°F (23°C).

4. Use a wide-blade spatula to mix water and powder carefully at first to incorporate it together. Then spatulate against the bowl sides to reduce incorporation of air. Do not whip the material. Rotate the bowl and gather the material and then spatulate again against the sides of the bowl. Follow the mixing times for the material.

5. Once the material is mixed to a creamy texture without air bubbles, it can be gathered and loaded into the impression tray for insertion into the mouth.

KromaFaze Alginate

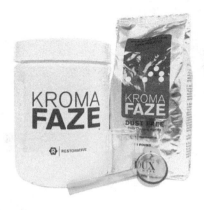

Use

Making dental impressions used for the fabrication of casts for:
- Study models.
- Orthodontic models.
- Opposing models.
- Removable splints.
- Removable retainers.
- Provisional restorations.
- Additional applications in the dental office.

Properties
- Supplied in airtight pouches, with a water measure and a scoop
- Use scoop and water measure that is supplied with material
- High compressive strength
- High tear strength
- Stone models can be separated after 30 minutes
- Dust free
- Color-changing guide for consistency
- Comes in regular and fast set

KromaFaze Alginate *Continued*

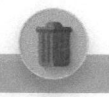

Precautions
- Avoid contact with eyes.
- Avoid inhalation.
- Do not ingest.
- Do not use in patients who have history of severe allergic reactions to the components.

Mixing and Setting Time
Visual color changing guide for consistency

	Regular	Fast
Mix	Purple	Purple
Load	Pink	Pink
Seat	White	White
Set		30–45 seconds

The temperature of the water will vary the working and setting time. Cooler water increases time; warmer water decreases time.

Directions   After the tray is selected, PPE is in place, and the patient is prepared for the procedure:

1. Dispense material by dipping supplied scoop into powder and packing it into the scoop. Use spatula by laying it level across the scoop to further pack the material and scrape excess material from the scoop.

2. Place scoops into dry mixing bowl (rubber or disposable) or into alginate mixer. Place additional scoops into bowl. Normally, two scoops are needed for the mandibular and three scoops for the maxillary arch.

3. Add water from the measuring device. Each line indicates enough water for one scoop. If three scoops are used, the entire water measuring device can be filled.

4. Use a wide-blade spatula to mix water and powder carefully at first to incorporate it together. Then spatulate against the bowl sides to reduce incorporation of air. Do not whip the material. Spatulate until the material turns to a pink color. Rotate the bowl and gather the material and then spatulate again against the sides of the bowl. Mix to a creamy consistency, with all the powder incorporated. Load the pink material into the tray.

5. When the material turns from pink to white, seat the tray in the patient's mouth and wait until the material is firm to remove.

Kromopan® 100 Alginate

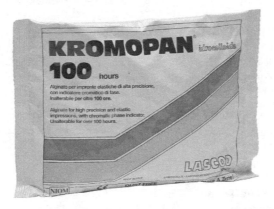

Use

Making dental impressions used for the fabrication of casts for:
- Study models.
- Orthodontic models.
- Opposing models.
- Removable splints.
- Removable retainers.
- Provisional restorations.
- When impression cannot be poured immediately.
- Additional applications in the dental office.

Properties
- Supplied in airtight pouches, with a water measure and a scoop
- Use scoop and water measure that is supplied with material
- Great elasticity
- High compression resistance
- Can be kept for up to 100 hours before pouring without distortion or shrinkage
- Color-changing guide for consistency

Kromopan® 100 Alginate *Continued*

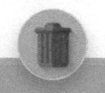

Precautions • Always read the MSDS for the product.
• Avoid contact with eyes.
• Avoid inhalation.
• Do not ingest.
• Do not use in patients who have history of severe allergic reactions to the components.

Mixing and Setting Time
Visual color changing guide for consistency

Spatulate	Purple
Load tray	Pink
Insert into mouth	White

Time from start to finish is just over 1 minute. The temperature of the water will vary the working and setting time. Cooler water increases time; warmer water decreases time.

Directions After the tray is selected, PPE is in place, and the patient is prepared for the procedure:

1. Dispense material by dipping supplied scoop into powder and packing it into the scoop. Use spatula by laying it level across the scoop to further pack the material and scrape excess material from the scoop.

2. Place scoops into dry mixing bowl (rubber or disposable bowl) or into alginate mixer. Place additional scoops into the bowl. Normally, two scoops are needed for the mandibular and three scoops for the maxillary arch.

3. Add water from the measuring device. Each line indicates enough water for one scoop. If three scoops are used, the entire water measuring device can be filled.

4. Use a wide-blade spatula to mix water and powder carefully at first to incorporate it together. Then spatulate against the bowl sides to reduce incorporation of air. Do not whip the material. Spatulate until the material turns to a pink color. Rotate the bowl and gather the material and then spatulate again against the sides of the bowl. Mix to a creamy consistency with all the powder incorporated. Load the pink material into the tray.

5. When the material turns from pink to white, seat the tray in the patient's mouth and wait until the material is firm to remove. After removal, the impression can be rinsed and enclosed in a plastic bag and kept for up to 100 hours without distortion.

Alginate Flavoring

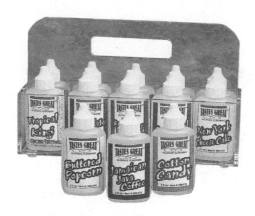

Use	To add a pleasing flavor to alginate products
Properties	• Supplied in 2-oz dropper bottles
	• 10 to 14 sugar-free flavors
	• Alginate Flavoring Carrier is available for use and has 10 different flavors
	• Flavors available:

• Very Strawberry
• Marvelous Mint
• Chillin' Cherry
• Groovy Grape
• Wild Watermelon
• Bubble Gum
• Cotton Candy
• French Vanilla
• Cola
• Jamaican Java Coffee

Precautions Do not use in patients who have history of severe allergic reactions to the components.

Alginate Flavoring *Continued*

Directions

1. Patients identify alginate flavoring preference.
2. Plastic barrier is placed around dropper bottle.
3. Operator adds two to five drops in water before mixing it with the alginate powder.

AlgiNot™

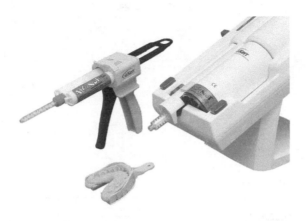

Use

An alternative alginate impression material for use in preparation of:

- Dental impressions.
- Case study models.
- Orthodontic models.
- Opposing models.
- Simple removable dentures.
- Removable retainers and splints.
- Provisional crown and bridge.

Composition A silicone impression material intended as an alternative to traditional alginate materials

Properties

- Extruder operation with mixing tip and cartridge—no hand mixing.
- Impressions remain stable for months.
- Tolerates disinfectants.

Precautions

- Skin, eyes: may cause mild irritation
- Inhalation: may cause mild irritation
- May be harmful if swallowed

AlgiNot™ *Continued*

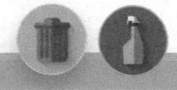

Mixing and Setting Time

	Minimum Working Time from Start of Mix	Removal Time
Cartridge:	45 sec	2 min 30 sec
Volume™	1 min	2 min 45 sec

Directions   After the tray is selected, PPE is in place, and the patient is prepared for the procedure:

1. Insert cartridge into the extruder.
2. Attach mixing tip to cartridge.
3. Squeeze trigger to mix and dispense material.
4. Material will stop flowing when trigger is released.

StatusBlue® Mix Star Material (Alginate Substitute Material)

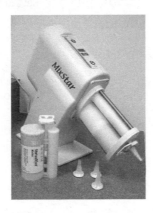

Use

An alternative alginate impression material for use in preparation of:
- Study models.
- Orthodontic models.
- Opposing models.
- Impressions for temporaries.
- Model-cast dentures.
- Additional applications in the dental office.

Composition
- Addition curing polysiloxanes

- Silicon dioxide
- Food pigments
- Additives
- Platinum catalyst

Properties
- Designed as a high-efficiency alternative to traditional alginates
- Supplied Automix cartridges for use with a Zenith/DMG MixStar machine
- Automix Gun Tips are used with the Automix cartridges

StatusBlue® Mix Star Material (Alginate Substitute Material) *Continued*

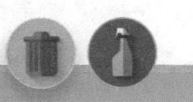

- StatusBlue® also supplied in 50-ml cartridges for Automix guns and tips
- 100% dust free
- Mixing takes place in the MixStar machine if using the MixStar cartridges
- Extremely flowable under pressure
- Low shore hardness
- Dimensionally stable
- Repourable and reusable
- StatusBlue is an additional curing silicone impression material

Precautions
- Always read the MSDS information for the product.
- On MSDS: under Hazards Identification it reads: "None if handled according to directions." "No labeling of hazardous ingredients required."
- Do not use in patients who have history of severe allergic reactions to the components.

Mixing and Setting Time
- Tray is loaded and inserted into mouth no later than 1 minute 15 seconds after mixing.
- Recommended time in mouth is 1 minute 45 seconds.
- Wait a minimum of 10 minutes before pouring impression.

Directions

1. Slide the locking mechanism into open position on the MixStar Cartridge.
2. Remove and discard the cap on the openings of the base and catalyst outlets on the MixStar Cartridge.
3. Seat the mixing tip completely into the open holes on the MixStar Cartridge.
4. Secure the mixing tip by sliding the locking mechanism into the locked position over the mixing tip.
5. Insert the cartridge into the mixing unit.
6. Turn on the mixing unit; as the material is dispensed, flow the material into the tray, keeping the tip in the material and not trapping air into the material.
7. Insert the tray into the patient's mouth and hold for 1 minute 45 seconds.
8. Remove from the patient's mouth, rinse, and disinfect.
9. Wait 10 minutes, then pour the impression.

Flex Mixing Bowls

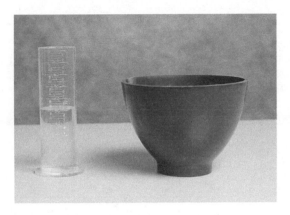

Use	• To mix materials such as alginate and/or gypsum products • To provide flexibility when mixing materials
Composition	Various sizes of rubber, flexible bowls with a firm bottom

Notes
• These bowls are available in various colors.
• They are easy to hold and turn in hand while mixing.
• Some bowls come with disposable liners.
• They are easy to clean after use.

Laboratory Spatula

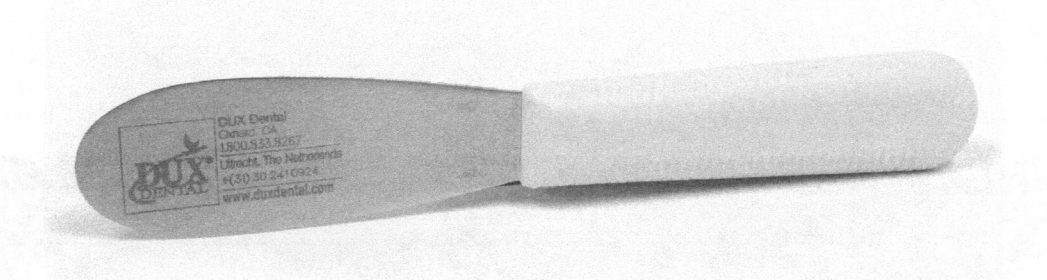

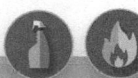

Use
- To mix materials in a flexible bowl
- To mix materials such as a periodontal dressing and/or impression materials on a paper pad

Composition
- Blade with handle.
- Blades are plastic or stainless steel.
- Handles are plastic, wood, or metal.

Notes
- These come in various sizes and styles.
- They are usually 7½ inches long.
- They are available in a variety of colors.
- Some are sterilized.

Disposable Anterior, Posterior, Quadrant, and Full-Arch Trays

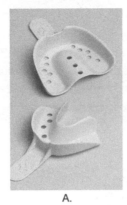

A.

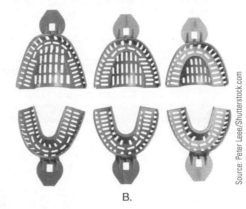

B.

Source: Peter Leee/Shutterstock.com

Use	• To hold various types of impression materials • To carry impression material into the patient's mouth to obtain an accurate impression
Composition	• Plastic perforated trays with handles • Anterior, full maxillary and mandibular, and quadrant styles

A. Disposable Impression Trays
B. Variety of sizes of Impression Trays

Notes
• Various sizes that are color-coded.
• They may be disposable or cold sterilized.
• They can be molded and trimmed if necessary.
• Holes and perforations aid in locking/holding of materials.

Metal Perforated Trays

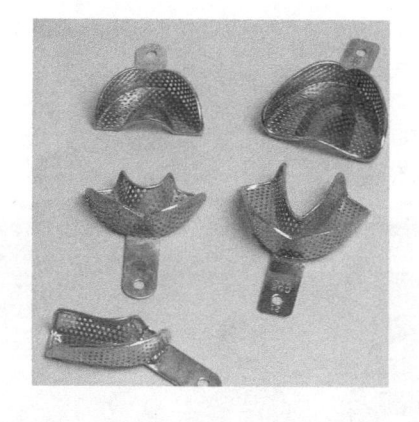

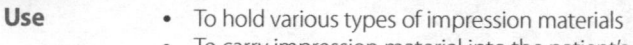

Use	• To hold various types of impression materials
	• To carry impression material into the patient's mouth to obtain an accurate impression
Composition	• Metal perforated trays with handles
	• Anterior, full maxillary and mandibular, and quadrant styles
Notes	• These can be sterilized.

Fuji Ortho LC CEMENT

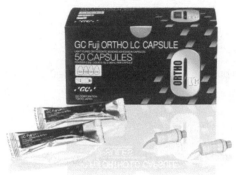

Source: https://www.gcamerica.com/products/ortho/Fuji_ORTHO_LC/

Use	Orthodontic light-cured adhesive that bonds to metal and porcelain brackets and metal bands
Composition	Polybasic carbolic acid, hydroxyethyl methacrylate, and aluminosilicate glass

Properties
- Low sensitivity to moisture
- Used with etching
- Significant fluoride release and recharge
- Available in both powder/liquid and automix
- Prevents caries—no decalcification
- High success rate
- Easy to use and clean up

Precautions
- Eyes: May be irritating to the eyes, rinse for 15 minutes.
- Skin: May be irritating to the skin, wash for 15 minutes.
- Ingestion: Do not induce vomiting. Drink large volumes of water.
- Inhalation of powder: Move to fresh air. Drink water to clear throat and blow nose to remove dust particles.
- If irritation develops, seek medical attention with all of the above.

Fuji Ortho LC CEMENT *Continued*

Mixing and Setting Time
- Total mixing time is 20 to 25 seconds.
- Working time is 3 minutes from start of mix.

Directions

1. Clean the surface with nonfluoridated prophy paste and water.
2. Rinse thoroughly with water.
3. Dispense a few drops of GC Fuji Ortho Conditioner/Etch into a well. Dip a gauze or sponge into the conditioner and apply to the bonding surfaces of the teeth for 20 seconds. Rinse.
4. Enamel bonding surfaces must be moist.
5. Insert the automix cartridge into the dispensing gun.
6. Dispense material and mix for 15 seconds.
7. Place onto orthodontic appliance and position in place. Light-cure into place according to manufacturer's instructions.

Heliosit Orthodontic

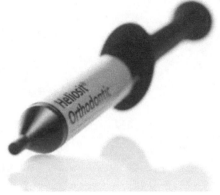

Use	To permanently cement metal or ceramic orthodontic brackets
Composition	Paste of dimethacrylate, bisphenol A–glycidyl methacrylate (bis-GMA), silicone dioxide, catalyst, and stabilizers
Properties	• Light-curing material • Highly translucent • No dosing or mixing required • High-strength bond

Precautions
- May be irritating to the eyes. Flush with water.
- May be irritating to the skin. Wash with soap and water.
- Ingestion: No hazard anticipated from swallowing small amounts incidental to normal handling
- Inhalation: Move to fresh air.
- If irritation develops, seek medical attention with all of the above.

Heliosit Orthodontic *Continued*

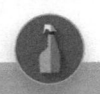

Mixing and
Setting Times
- No mixing required
- Light-cure for 40 seconds

Directions

1. Clean the surface thoroughly.
2. Isolate with cotton rolls and blown air.
3. Apply etchant to the tooth according to manufacturer's instructions. Usually etchant is applied for 30 to 60 seconds.
4. Rinse and dry the area thoroughly. The tooth surface should look chalky.
5. Remove the cap from the Heliosit Orthodontic cement and place a small amount on the bracket according to the bracket manufacturer's instructions. The cement may also be placed on a paper pad and by using an instrument placed on the bracket.
6. Replace the cap.
7. Light-cure the bracket once placed for 20 seconds from the cervical position and 20 seconds from the incisal.

Orthodontic Wax Sticks

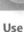

Use	Peripheral lining of impression trays, to increase the tray height, and across the back of the tray as a post dam for impression materials
Composition	• No hazardous components • Less than 10% petroleum hydrocarbons and additives
Properties	• Soft and tacky • Can be adapted to the tray without heating • Come in 6-inch sticks • White in color • Often slightly scented

Precautions Nonhazardous at room temperature

Directions
1. Take one stick of the orthodontic tray wax and place it onto the impression tray.
2. Form the wax on the border of the tray.
3. Form a post dam across the back of the tray.
4. Adjust the wax as necessary.

Orthodontic Wax

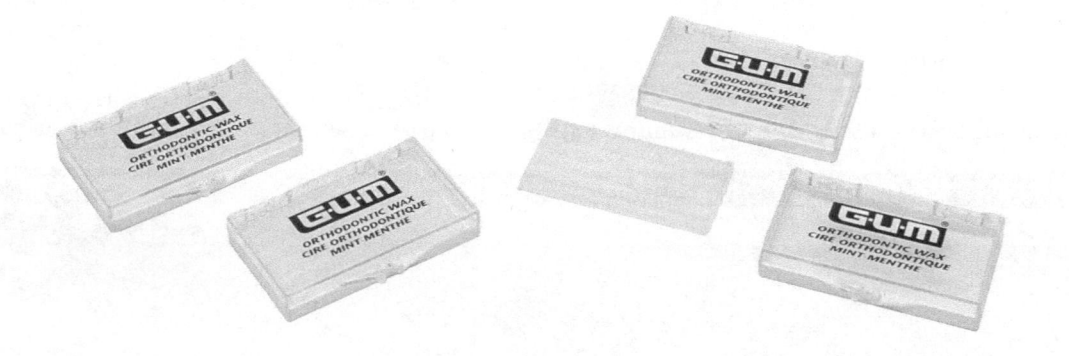

Use   To mold around orthodontic brackets to help relieve irritation and discomfort

Composition
- No hazardous components
- Less than 10% petroleum hydrocarbons and additives

Properties
- Normally comes in a plastic carrying case for patient use
- Comes in mint or regular flavoring
- Soft and pliable
- Does not need to be heated to be adapted to brackets

Precautions   Nonhazardous at room temperature

Directions
1. Plastic case can be opened easily.
2. Take a small amount from the sticks in the case.
3. Adapt the wax around the brackets.
4. Rub it until it is smooth to the touch.
5. Add more as necessary in areas where the brackets are causing irritation.

CHAPTER 15

Pedodontic Instruments, Preventive Dentistry, and Whitening Products

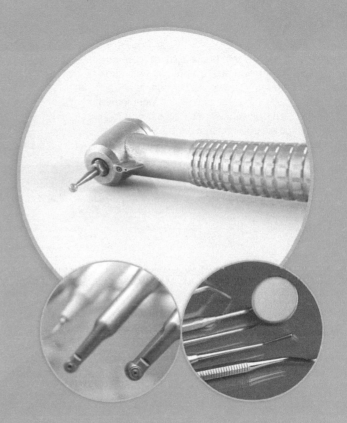

T-Band Matrix

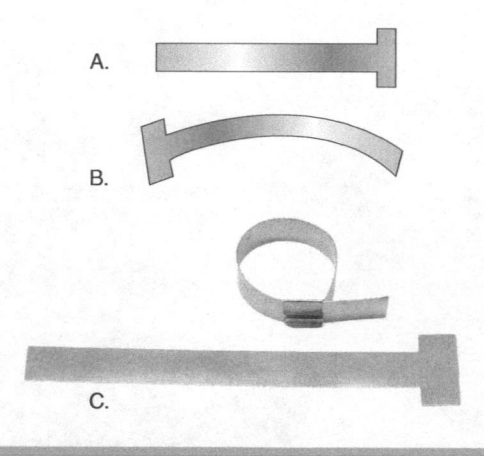

A.

B.

C.

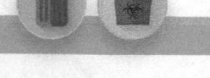

Use On primary teeth, to establish the normal contour of the prepared tooth while the tooth is being filled with the restorative material

Composition Brass strips that are "crossed" at one end

A. Straight.
B. Curved.
C. Straight T-band shown, also as made into a ring, ready to apply.

Notes
- These are available in various designs and sizes.
- They do not require retainers and are adjustable.
- They may replaces a missing wall of the cavity preparation.
- Can be secured on the tooth by bending the "T" extensions at a right angle to the strip and by sliding the strip through it to make a ring that can be pulled tighter on the tooth.

Stainless Steel Crown Kit

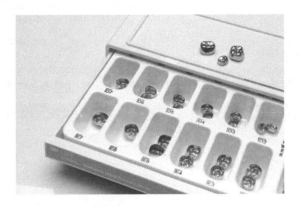

Use

- To replace tooth structure when there have been extensive carious lesions
- To replace tooth structure when there are hypoplastic or hypocalcified teeth
- To replace tooth structure following a pulpotomy or pulpectomy
- To be used as an abutment tooth for a space maintainer
- To be used as a temporary restoration for a fractured tooth

Composition Anatomical stainless-steel crowns in various sizes

Notes These are available in a variety of sizes and can be purchased individually or in a kit.

Crown and Collar Scissors

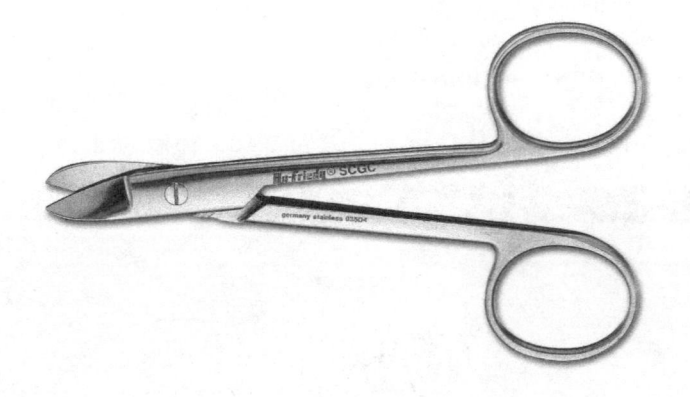

Use
- To trim aluminum temporary crowns on the gingival area
- To trim stainless steel crowns on the gingival area
- To cut gingival retraction cord
- To trim custom provisional restorations
- To trim matrix bands

Composition
- Hinged scissors with enclosed-circle handles that can be manipulated with one hand
- Cutting beaks available in straight or curved tips

Notes
- These scissors are available in narrow or wide cutting edges.
- They are available in a variety of sizes.

Contouring and Crimping Pliers

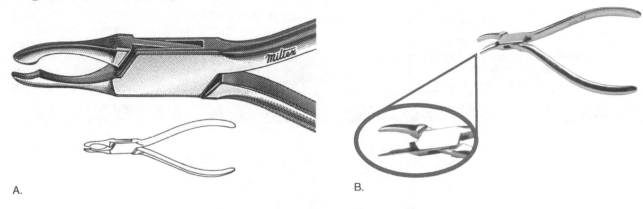

A.

B.

Use	To crimp and contour the marginal edge of the aluminum or stainless-steel crown
Composition	Hinged instruments
	A. Contouring pliers: One beak has a convex surface and the other a concave surface that fits over the convex one.
	B. Contouring pliers: Both ends of the beaks are curved.

Notes
- These are available in a range of sizes and shapes.
- The Johnson contouring plier is a commonly used type of contouring pliers.

Tray Setup for Pediatric Stainless-Steel Crown Placement

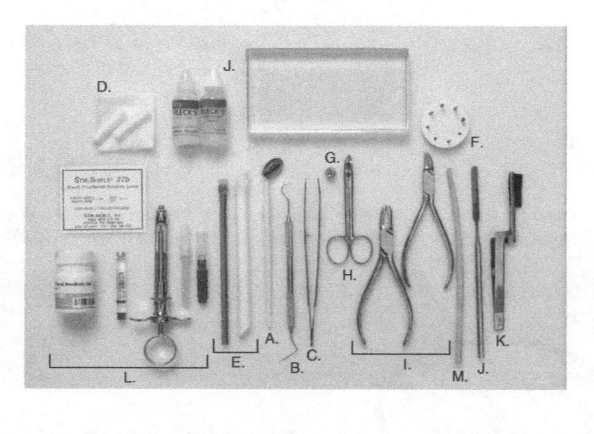

Composition
A. Mouth mirror
B. Expro
C. Cotton pliers
D. Cotton rolls and gauze
E. High-volume evacuator (HVE) and saliva ejector
F. High-speed handpiece (not shown) and selected burs
G. Stainless steel crown
H. Crown and collar scissors
I. Contouring and crimping pliers

J. Mixing spatula, paper pad, permanent cement
K. Articulating forceps and paper
L. Topical anesthetic, syringe, carpules, needles, stick shield
M. Orangewood stick

Not Shown
• Low-speed handpiece with green stone and rubber abrasive wheel
• Spoon excavator
• Dental floss

Tray Setup for Dental Sealant

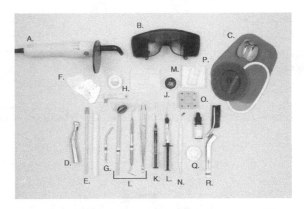

Composition
A. Curing light
B. Protective glasses
C. Dental dam setup
D. Low-speed handpiece
E. Saliva ejector and HVE tip
F. Dry angle
G. Air-water syringe tip
H. Prophy angle with prophy paste without fluoride
I. Basic setup: mirror, explorer, and cotton pliers

J. Dispensing tray
K. Etchant
L. Sealant
M. Dental floss
N. Applicator brush
O. Bur block with assorted burs and/or stones
P. Cotton rolls and gauze
Q. Dappen dish and bonding agent
R. Articulating forceps with paper

Preventive Materials: Pit and Fissure Sealants, Prophy Paste, Fluoride, Whitening Agents, and Clinpro Sealant

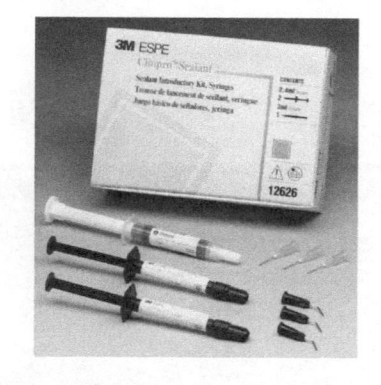

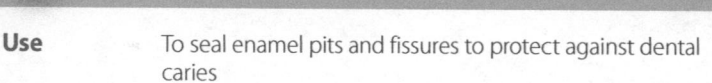

Use
To seal enamel pits and fissures to protect against dental caries

Composition
- Triethylene glycol dimethacrylate
- Bisphenol A diglycidyl ether dimethacrylate
- Tetrabutylammonium, tetrafluoroborate
- Silane-treated silica

Properties
- Low viscosity
- Bonds to enamel
- Fluoride-releasing

- Flows easily into pits and fissures
- Comes with ultrafine tips for easy placement
- Smart color-change technology

Precautions
- May cause mild eye irritation
- May cause allergic reaction on skin or moderate skin irritation
- Prolonged or repeated exposure may cause upper respiratory irritation
- May cause gastrointestinal irritation

Clinpro Sealant

Mixing and Setting Time
- No mixing is required.
- Sealant is light-cured for 20 seconds to set.

Directions

1. Prepare delivery system. Remove cap from the syringe and save.
2. Twist disposable cap onto the syringe until secure.
3. Dispense a small amount of material on a paper pad to ensure the tip is not clogged.
4. Etch each tooth according to the manufacturer's directions, then rinse thoroughly and air dry. The tooth should be a matte frosty white color on the etched area.
5. Do not allow the etched surface to be contaminated.

6. Using the syringe tip, slowly introduce the pit and fissure sealant to the etched surface of the tooth.
7. Stirring the sealant during and after placement with the syringe tip or an explorer will help to eliminate air bubbles and enhance flow of the sealant into the pits and fissures.
8. Hold the tip of the curing light close to the surface and cure for 20 seconds.
9. When set, the sealant forms a hard, opaque film that is light yellow in color with a slight imbibition.
10. Repeat this on each etched tooth.

Delton FS+

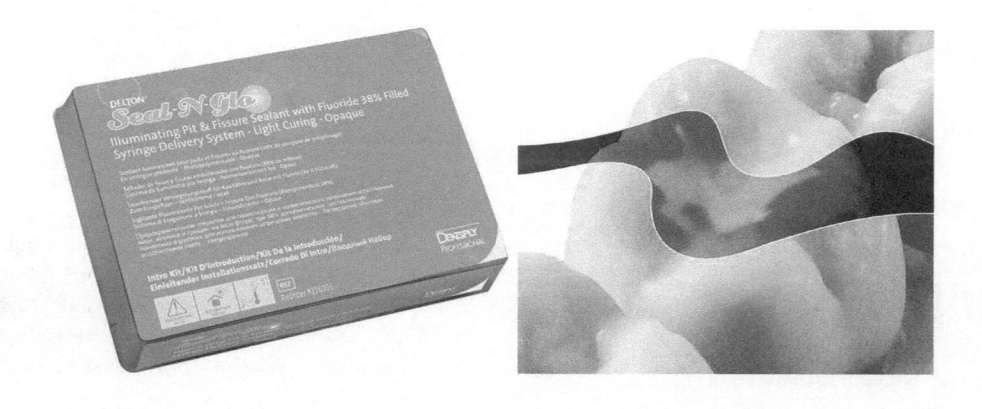

Use
Preventive sealing of pits and fissures in the primary and secondary dentition in combination with the acid-etch techniques

Composition
- Low-viscosity monomers
- Triethylene glycol dimethacrylate
- Bis-GMA
- Barium aluminofluoroborosilicate glass
- Titanium dioxide
- Silicon dioxide
- Sodium fluoride
- Initiators
- Stabilizers
- Fluorescent dye—55% filled

Properties
- Provides visual verification of sealant margins at time of placement
- Easy way to verify retention and integrity of margins at recall appointments
- Contains fluoride

Delton FS+ *Continued*

- Effective sealing properties
- Illuminating dye does not color or change the look of the opaque sealant
- Easy to place

Precautions
- May cause eye irritation.
- Individuals sensitive to acrylics may develop an allergic response.
- Possible nausea on prolonged exposure.
- Possible irritation to the skin.

Mixing and Setting Time
- No mixing is required
- Light-cure to set

Directions

1. Tooth must be cleaned with an air polishing device or prophylaxis treatment with no fluoride.
2. Rinse well with water and isolate the teeth to be sealed.
3. Air dry each tooth with air free of oil or water contamination.
4. Etch the pits and fissures of the teeth to be sealed for 15 to 60 seconds according to the manufacturer's directions.
5. Rinse thoroughly for at least 30 seconds, then dry area.
6. Teeth will have a dull frosty white appearance; if they do not look like this, re-etch for another 20 seconds.
7. Remove cap from the syringe. Attach a disposable applicator tip to end of the syringe. Turn the tip clockwise to secure the applicator tip to the end of the syringe.
8. Express a small amount onto a pad to ensure free flow of material.
9. Apply the sealant into the pits and fissures.
10. Cure each surface for at least 20 seconds, keeping the curing light tip as close as possible to the tooth surface without touching it.
11. Remove the soft (oxygen-inhibited) surface layer after light-curing with cotton pellets or cotton rolls.

FluroShield VLC Pit & Fissure Sealant

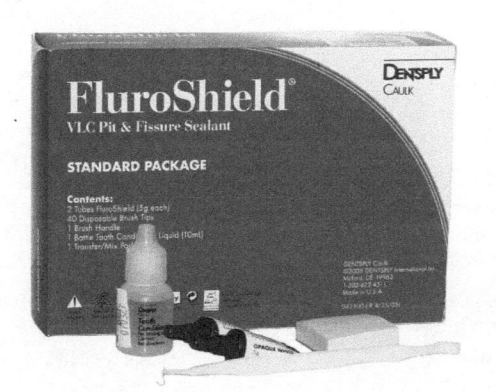

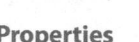

Use
- Preventive sealing in pits and fissures in primary and secondary dentition to protect against dental caries
- Fluoride release that is intended to act as a fluoride supplement

Composition
- Urethane-modified bis-GMA dimethacrylate
- Barium aluminofluoroborosilicate glass
- Polymerizable dimethacrylate resins
- Bis-GMA
- Sodium fluoride
- Photoinitiator

- Photoaccelerator
- Silicon dioxide
- 50% inorganic filler

Properties
- Visible light-cured pit and fissure sealant
- Releasable fluoride that is intended to act as a fluoride supplement
- Decreases the chance of microleakage
- Bonds chemically and mechanically to the enamel
- Low water absorption increases resistance to washout

FluroShield VLC Pit & Fissure Sealant *Continued*

Precautions
- Material may cause irritation to the eyes.
- Material may be a skin irritant.
- Material is probably not harmful if swallowed.

Mixing and Setting Time
- No mixing is required.
- Material is light-cured for 20 seconds per surface.

Directions

1. Prophy the pits and fissures of the teeth with fluoride-free paste to be sealed, then rinse thoroughly and air dry.
2. Isolate the teeth with cotton rolls or a rubber dam.
3. Apply Caulk 50% Tooth Conditioner Liquid with the cotton-tipped applicator for 60 seconds to permanent teeth and 90 seconds for primary teeth then rinse thoroughly and air dry.

4. Tooth should look frosty.
5. Remove the cap and place material on a paper pad. Cover to protect from the overhead light.
6. Pick up a liberal amount of material using the disposable brush and place on the tooth into the pits and fissures.
7. Light-cure all surfaces, keeping the tip of the light about 1 to 2 mm away from the surface for 20 seconds (curing time depends on the light source).

Helioseal Sealant

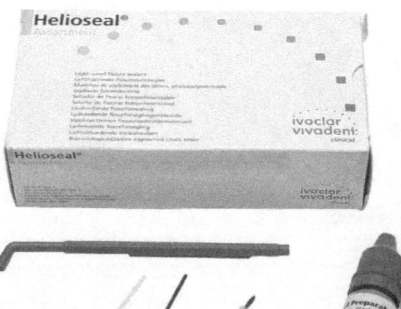

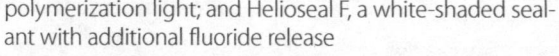

Use	To provide excellent long-term cavity protection in occlusal areas
Composition	Mixture of bis-GMA, dimethacrylate, titanium dioxide, initiators, and stabilizers, 40% fillers
Properties	• Offered in dispensing bottle or syringe • Long-term caries protection • Fast and easy to apply • Available in two formulas: Helioseal Clear, a transparent sealer with reversible color changes using a halogen

polymerization light; and Helioseal F, a white-shaded sealant with additional fluoride release

Precautions	• May be irritating to the eyes—flush with water. • Skin contact—wash thoroughly with soap and water. • Inhalation—move to fresh air. • No hazards anticipated with swallowing a small amount of material with normal handling.
Mixing and Setting Time	• No mixing is required. • Setting time is 35 seconds total, including waiting time and light-curing.

Helioseal Sealant *Continued*

Directions

1. Thoroughly clean the tooth to be sealed.
2. Isolate the area, preferably with a rubber dam.
3. Place the disposable tip on Syringe Total Etch and apply the etching gel for 30 to 60 seconds, then thoroughly rinse and dry with oil-free air. Tooth should have a matte appearance.
4. Shake the Helioseal bottle well and open immediately before use to prevent any premature polymerization by light.

5. Remove the cap and place a cannula on the bottle to apply directly or place Helioseal in well, on paper pad, or directly from bottle and apply with the brush handle and tip supplied in the kit.
6. Wait for 15 seconds and then light-cure with a suitable light source for 20 seconds.
7. Check seal and occlusion.

Procedure for Placing Pit and Fissure Sealants

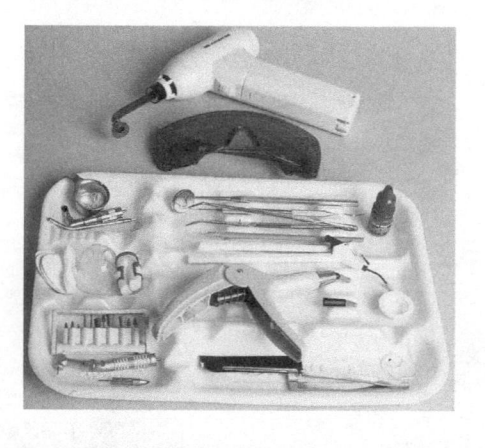

This procedure is performed by the dentist and/or the dental assistant at chairside.

Equipment and Supplies
- Basic setup
- Air-water syringe tip, HVE, and saliva ejector
- Cotton rolls and 2 × 2 gauze sponges, applicator tips
- Rubber cup or brush
- Dri-Angles
- Rubber dam setup, cotton rolls, or Garmer cotton roll holders and short and long cotton rolls

- Low-speed dental handpiece with right-angle (prophy-angle) attachment
- Flour of pumice or prophy paste without fluoride, or air polisher, or dry toothbrush or fissurotomy burs
- Applicators (microbrush, small cotton-tipped applicator, or syringe for etchant)
- Etchant and bonding agent or all-in-one etchant and bonding agent
- Pit and fissure sealant material
- Curing light

Procedure for Placing Pit and Fissure Sealants *Continued*

- Articulating paper and forceps
- Assorted burs, discs, and stones for reducing high spots
- PPE worn by the dental team

Directions

1. Check tooth or teeth with explorer. Polish the occlusal surface of the teeth to receive sealants. The dentist may want x-rays of the teeth to be sealed before beginning the procedure.

2. Polish the teeth using flour of pumice or a nonfluoride prophy paste with a rubber cup to clean the occlusal surfaces. (Some sealants can be used with fluoride prophy materials, check with the manufacturer before using.) An air polisher, dry toothbrush, or fissurotomy burs may also be used.

3. Once the teeth are polished, rinse and dry the teeth thoroughly. If the pits and fissures are deep, check them with an explorer and then rinse and dry again, if necessary.

4. Place the chosen method of isolation—dental dam, cotton rolls, or Garmer clamps.

5. Place a Dri-Angle on buccal mucosa and dry the tooth.

6. Apply the etchant using an applicator or syringe with a disposable tip to the occlusal surface, into the pits and fissures and two-thirds up the cuspid incline.

7. Etch for 15 to 60 seconds according to the manufacturer's directions.

8. Rinse the tooth with water and use the evacuator tip to remove the remaining etchant and water.

9. Dry the tooth; it should have a dull chalky white appearance. If the tooth does not have this appearance, re-etch for 15 to 30 seconds.

10. Follow the manufacturer's directions to prepare and apply the sealant material.

11. With applicator selected, place the sealant so that it flows into the pits and fissures.

12. Light-cure the sealants, holding the curing light 2 mm directly above the occlusal surface and expose for 20 seconds on each surface.

13. Evaluate sealant with an explorer to check for voids and irregularities; repeat the process, if necessary.

Procedure for Placing Pit and Fissure Sealants *Continued*

14. After the sealant has set, rinse or wipe the surface with a moist cotton roll to remove the air-inhibited layer.

15. Remove the dental dam or cotton rolls.

16. Dry the teeth and place articulating paper in forceps to check the bite.

17. Reduce any high spots with slow-speed handpiece and burs or discs.

18. Apply fluoride to the sealed teeth.

19. Record procedure on the patient's chart.

Perfect Choice Prophy Gems Prophy Paste

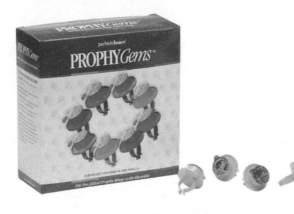

Use	As a cleaning paste to remove deposits and stains from the teeth
Composition	• Blend of cleaning and polishing agents • Sodium fluoride and sodium saccharine
Properties	• Removes tough stains. • Low splatter paste. • Variety of grits. • Contains fluoride. • Rinses easily.

• Variety of flavors.
• Rings are color-coded by flavor.
• Lip for thumb-hold ring in place.
• Ring is comfortable and secure on finger.

Precautions
• Eyes: Direct contact will cause irritation.
• Skin: Prolonged contact will cause irritation.
• Ingestion: Contains sodium fluoride, do not swallow.

Mixing and Setting Time
No mixing or setting time is required.

Perfect Choice Prophy Gems Prophy Paste *Continued*

Directions

1. Determine the grit to use by evaluating the amount of hard and soft deposits.
2. Select the grit and flavor.
3. Remove the foil seal from the Prophy Gems.
4. Remove the prophy paste with a prophy angle and cup to begin the polish.

Nupro Prophy Paste Cups Variety Pak with Fluoride (Dentsply Professional)

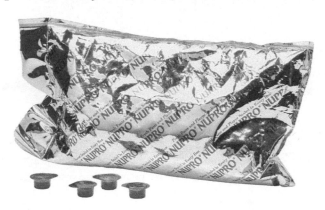

Use	To remove soft and hard deposits from the teeth
Composition	• Blend of polishing and cleaning agents • 1.23% fluoride ion
Properties	• Excellent stain removing and polishing • Variety of grits and flavors • Spatter-free formula • Rinses easily and completely • Always consistent • Comes in unidose cups, jars, and variety packs

- Available with and without fluoride

Precautions
- Skin: Not applicable.
- Eyes: Flush with water. If irritation persists, contact a physician.
- Ingestion: Give copious amounts of water or milk and call a physician.
- Inhalation: Not applicable.

Mixing and Setting Time
- Not mixing or setting time required.

Nupro Prophy Paste Cups Variety Pak with Fluoride (Dentsply Professional) *Continued*

Directions

1. Each cup contains enough prophy paste to complete a procedure on one patient.
2. Remove foil from prophy cup.
3. If finger grip is used, place prophy cup in finger grip and secure.
4. Attach rubber cup to prophy angle.
5. Place the rubber cup into the prophy paste while running the angle at low speed.
6. To avoid overheating the tooth, always keep enough prophy paste in the rubber cup to be used on the teeth.

Preppies Pumice

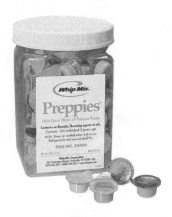

Use   To polish a tooth prior to sealant placement

Composition   Volcanic silica manufactured as a loose abrasive. Flour of pumice is extremely fine.

Properties   Available in grades:
- Pumice, flour
- Pumice, fine
- Pumice, medium
- Pumice, coarse
- Pumice, extra-coarse

Mixing and Setting Times
- No mixing or setting time is required.

Directions

1. Each cup contains enough prophy paste to complete a procedure on one patient.
2. Remove foil from prophy cup.
3. If finger grip is used, place prophy cup in finger grip and secure.
4. Attach rubber cup to prophy angle.
5. Place the rubber cup into the prophy paste while running the angle at low speed.
6. To avoid overheating the tooth, always keep enough prophy paste in the rubber cup to be used on the teeth.

Minute-Foam

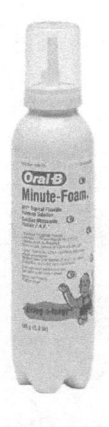

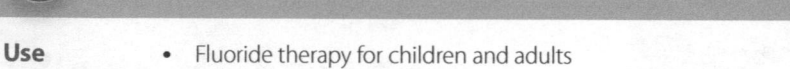

Use
- Fluoride therapy for children and adults
- Protects against dental caries

Composition Sodium fluoride, hydrofluoric acid (equivalent to 1.23% w/w fluoride ion [0.79%t from sodium fluoride and 0.44% from hydrogen fluoride])

Properties
- Pleasant flavor with no aftertaste
- Seven creative flavors
- Fast and effective fluoride uptake—provides 12,000 ppm in just 1 minute

- Low pH—3.5
- Excellent coverage, including the interproximal areas
- Reduces gagging and ingestion because the material stays in the tray
- Light airy consistency
- Foam clears easily from mouth and will not clog suction

Precautions Ingestion may cause abdominal pain, vomiting, diarrhea, and weakness.

Mixing and Setting Time
- No mixing is required.
- Setting time is 1 minute of exposure.

Minute-Foam *Continued*

Directions

1. The first time you dispense from a new bottle, gently lift upward on the nozzle to break the protective shipping tab.

2. Shake the bottle vigorously for 3 to 4 seconds prior to filling each tray.

3. Invert the bottle 180 degrees with nozzle pointing downward.

4. Place the nozzle tip close to the bottom of the tray at one end of the arch. Slowly press down on trigger.

5. Dispense the foam into the fluoride tray. Move from one end of the tray to the other in one motion to evenly fill about a third of the tray.

6. Place the tray in the patient's mouth and have the patient bite down lightly for 1 minute.

7. Instruct the patient not to eat, drink, or rinse for at least 30 minutes.

Topex 2 percent Neutral Foam

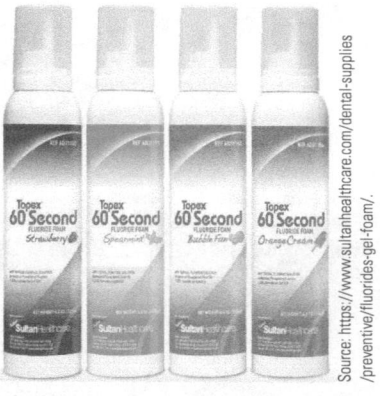

Source: https://www.sultanhealthcare.com/dental-supplies/preventive/fluorides-gel-foam/.

Use
- Fluoride protection
- For patients with reduced salivary flow (xerostomia)
- For patients with resin sealants
- For patients with intolerance to acidic fluoride

Composition 2% sodium fluoride (0.9% fluoride ion)

Properties
- Several flavors
- Available in gel and in foam
- Clearly Strawberry has no dyes, so it is ideal to use after whitening procedures or for patients who are sensitive to acidic fluoride

- Will not harm cosmetic restorations
- Effective caries prevention
- Excellent interproximal coverage

Precautions Primary routes of entry: No acute or chronic health hazards.

Mixing and Setting Time
- No mixing is required.
- Up to 4-minute application time.

Topex 2 percent Neutral Foam *Continued*

Directions

1. After initial use, shake for 10 seconds before each subsequent use.
2. Turn can completely upside down to dispense.
3. Point can downward toward fluoride tray and press the nozzle to fill the tray.
4. Use one press per arch, as foam will expand slightly to fill the tray.
5. Dry the teeth and insert the tray.
6. Have the patient bite down for 4 minutes.
7. Remove the tray and have the patient expectorate excess.
8. Instruct patient not to eat, drink, or rinse for 30 minutes.

Zooby Perfect Choice 1.25% APF Gel

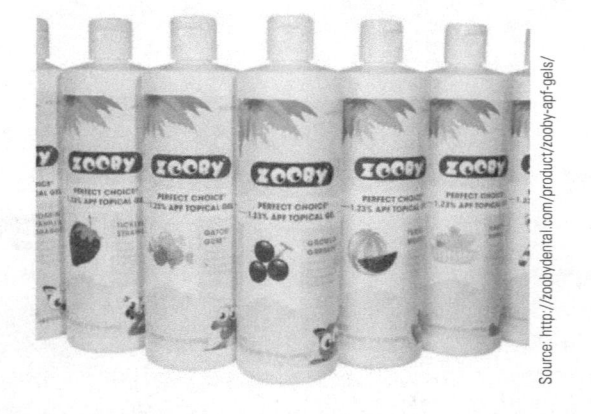

Source: http://zoobydental.com/product/zooby-apf-gels/

Use	Fluoride treatment to prevent dental caries
Composition	• 1.23% acidulated phosphate fluoride • Dyes and flavorings
Properties	• Available in gel, foam, and paint-on techniques • Great tasting • 80% effective at 1 minute and 100% effective at 4 minutes

• Assorted flavors
• Effect fluoride application

Precautions
• May be irritating to the eyes
• May be irritating to the skin if contact is prolonged
• May cause nausea and vomiting if ingested

Mixing and Setting Time
• No mixing time.
• Setting time is 1 to 4 minutes.

Zooby Perfect Choice 1.25% APF Gel *Continued*

Directions

1. After prophylaxis, flip the top open and place gel in fluoride tray (not more than one-third full).
2. Thoroughly air dry the teeth and insert trays into the mouth.
3. Gel may also be applied with a cotton-tipped swab.
4. Instruct the patient to bite down slightly but firmly for 1 to 4 minutes.
5. A slight chewing motion enhances coverage interproximally.
6. Remove trays and have the patient expectorate excess gel.
7. Instruct the patient not to eat, drink, or rinse for 30 minutes.

Duraflor Ultra 5% Cavity Varnish

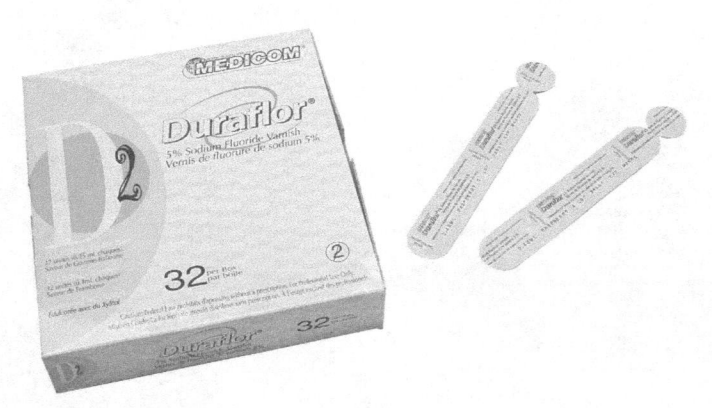

Use	• Relief of hypersensitivity for up to 6 months
	• Reduce postoperative sensitivity
	• Dental caries protection
Composition	• 5% sodium fluoride
	• Nonmedical ingredients: denatured ethyl alcohol, flavor, purified water, rosin, sucralose, xylitol, and yellow beeswax
Properties	• Quickly releases fluoride within 2 to 4 hours
	• Strong desensitizing action when applied to the teeth
	• Water-tolerant

• Adheres well to the tooth surface
• Slight tint for easy visual control and placement verification
• Proven effective up to 6 months
• May be placed on a moist tooth surface

Precautions	• May cause irritation to the skin
	• May cause irritation to the eyes
	• May cause nausea with extensive application
Mixing and Setting Time	• No mixing is required.
	• Hardens rapidly when in contact with saliva.

Duraflor Ultra 5% Cavity Varnish *Continued*

Directions

1. Wash and dry the tooth surface.
2. Remove the top of the container.
3. Apply Duraflor over the surfaces of the teeth with the supplied brush.
4. Gently thin the excess varnish in the surfaces of the tooth until the varnish surface is dry.
5. Duraflor covers even moist teeth with a coating of varnish film for several hours, which occludes the openings of the dentinal tubules.

6. Duraflor hardens on contact with saliva and the patient may leave immediately following the application.
7. Instruct the patient to eat only soft foods for 2 hours following treatment.
8. Clean instruments with alcohol before sterilizing.

DuraShield 5% Sodium Fluoride Varnish

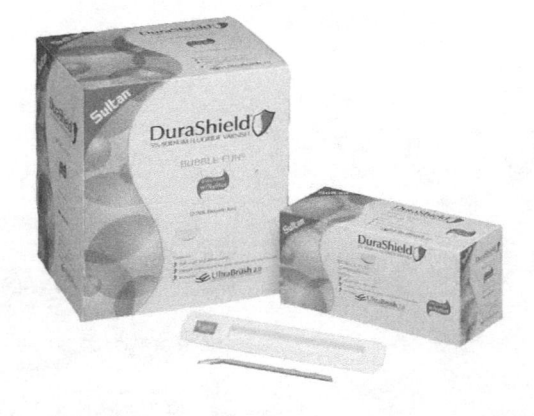

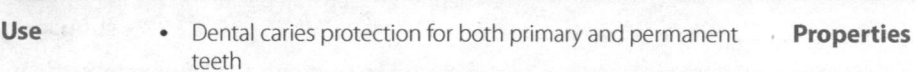

Use
- Dental caries protection for both primary and permanent teeth
- Cavity varnish and desensitizing agent
- Reduces hypersensitivity for high-risk caries patients with root caries or xerostomia where dentin and cementum are exposed

Composition
- Sodium fluoride, 5%
- Colophony resin, synthetic inert polymer, alcohol, silica, and flavoring
- Sweetened with xylitol and contains no dyes

Properties
- Effective in reduction of caries and sensitivity.
- Fast to apply and a wide range of applications.
- No need to prophy before application.
- Sets on contact with saliva and releases fluoride for 4 to 6 hours after application.
- Can be used with small children (infants and toddlers), disabled patients, and patients with active gag reflex.
- Comes in single-use hygienically sealed doses; aids in asepsis and cross-contamination.
- Cleanup is easy and fast.

DuraShield 5% Sodium Fluoride Varnish *Continued*

Precautions	• Inhalation—may be irritating to the throat; may cause headaches, drowsiness, lassitude, loss of appetite, and inability to concentrate • May be irritating to the eyes and skin—seek medical attention • Ingestion—may cause nausea, diarrhea, vomiting, and depression to the central nervous system
Mixing and Setting Time	• No mixing • Hardens rapidly when in contact with saliva
Directions	1. Remove any calculus or plaque. 2. Remove any excess saliva or moisture in area where varnish is going to be applied.

3. Remove the Ultra Brush 2.0 from the sealed packet.
4. Use the brush to mix the contents of the packet and then bend the applicator brush to the angle needed for application.
5. Uniformly brush the varnish over the entire surface to be covered, reinserting the brush into the packet as needed.
6. Allow the area to become wet by rinsing or saliva contact.
7. Instruct the patient to eat soft foods for the remainder of the day; to avoid rinses containing fluoride or alcohol; and to avoid brushing and flossing treated area for 4 to 6 hours after application.

Fluor Protector Assortment Fluoride Varnish

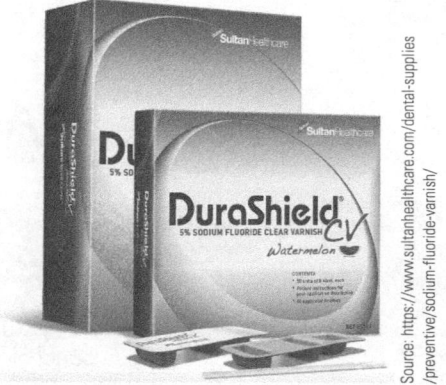

Source: https://www.sultanhealthcare.com/dental-supplies
/preventive/sodium-fluoride-varnish/

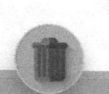

Use
- Professional protection against dental caries and erosion
- Prevents hypersensitivity
- Protective varnish and dentin sealant
- Remineralization of incipient caries
- Used on children, adolescents, and adults

Composition
- Fluoride
- Ethyl acetate, isoamyl propioniate, polyisocyanate, and fluorosilane

Properties
- Excellent seal of enamel.
- Reduces microleakage.
- Hydrogen fluoride varnish penetrating the enamel.
- Simple unit-dose delivery.
- Low fluoride concentration.
- Colorless and fast setting.
- One ampule is sufficient for two to three sets of teeth.
- Single dose is sufficient for one set of teeth.

Fluor Protector Assortment Fluoride Varnish *Continued*

Precautions
- May be irritating to the eyes: Rinse thoroughly.
- May be irritating to the skin: Wash with soap and water.
- No hazards indicated from swallowing small amount.

Mixing and Setting Time
- No mixing is required.
- Apply varnish and wait for 1 minute.

Directions
1. Thoroughly clean the tooth.
2. Dry the tooth with air and isolate area with cotton rolls.
3. Place the bottle or ampule in the plastic base.
4. Ampule opens with enclosed breaker.
5. Apply a thin layer using the enclosed brush (for single use).
6. Use dental floss to apply the material to the proximal surface.
7. Evenly disperse the varnish and then air dry.
8. Keep the area isolated with cotton rolls for 1 minute.
9. Instruct the patient not to rinse, eat, or brush for 45 minutes after placement of the fluoride varnish.

Topex Take Home Care 0.4% Stannous Fluoride Gel

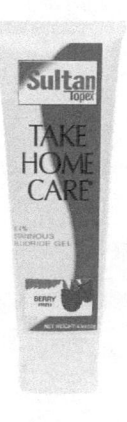

Use
- Reduces sensitivity and plaque biofilm
- Inhibits cariogenic microbial process

Composition
- Glycerin, cellulous derivative, and 0.4% stannous fluoride
- Inorganic halide, saccharide, and polyol

Properties
- Thick, clear gel
- Easy to apply to toothbrush or tray
- No food or drink restrictions after treatment
- Alcohol-free, with no color additives
- Reduced allergenic reactions

Precautions
- Inhalation of vapors may cause breathing difficulty and coughing.
- Contact with skin or eyes may cause dermatitis.
- Ingestion may cause headache, nausea, vomiting, gastrointestinal irritation, convulsions, and unconsciousness.

Mixing and Setting Time
- No mixing is required, but the fluoride gel should be in contact with the teeth for 1 minute.

Topex Take Home Care 0.4% Stannous Fluoride Gel *Continued*

Directions

1. Adults and children 6 years or older use once a day at bedtime.
2. Brush and floss and then remove excess water from toothbrush.
3. Liberally cover bristles of toothbrush with Topex Take Home Care Gel 0.4% Stannous Fluoride.
4. Brush onto all tooth surfaces for 1 minute.
5. Push gel in between the tooth surfaces with the tongue and cheek muscles for 1 minute and then spit gel out.
6. Do not swallow any material, and do not rinse.
7. Adults: Expectorate thoroughly, do not rinse, eat, or drink for 30 minutes.
8. Children 6 years or older: Expectorate and rinse thoroughly.

Rembrandt Whitening Strips

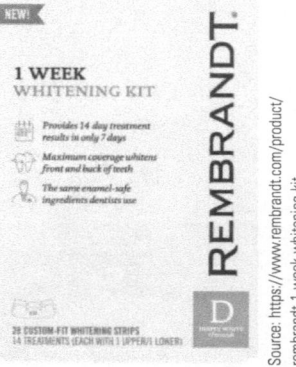

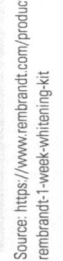

NEW!

1 WEEK
WHITENING KIT

Provides 14 day treatment
results in only 7 days

Maximum coverage whitens
front and back of teeth

The same enamel-safe
ingredients dentists use

REMBRANDT.

D

28 CUSTOM-FIT WHITENING STRIPS
14 TREATMENTS (EACH WITH 1 UPPER/1 LOWER)

Source: https://www.rembrandt.com/product/
rembrandt-1-week-whitening-kit

Use	• To whiten teeth
	• To restore the original brightness of professional whitening
Composition	Polyvinylpyrrolidone (PVP), polyoxyethylene oxide (PEG 78), water, acrylate copolymer, hydrogen peroxide, disodium pyrophosphate, sodium stannate, and disodium ethelyenedi-aminetetraacetic acid (EDTA)
Properties	• 3-day and 7-day options available
	• Apply once to twice a day
	• Form-fit strips

• Economical yet effective whitening
• Quick results and easy application
• Adheres well to the tooth

Precautions
• May cause irritation to the eyes.
• May cause skin irritation and blanching.
• If swallowed, contact doctor or Poison Control Center immediately.

Mixing and Setting Times
• No mixing is required.

Rembrandt Whitening Strips *Continued*

Directions

1. Rinse mouth with water for 15 seconds to moisten the teeth.
2. Remove the upper strip from the blister pack.
3. Apply the upper strip by aligning the straight edge with the gum line and pressing down to fit the curves of the teeth.
4. Press the tabs behind the front teeth to secure strip.
5. Remove the lower strip from the blister pack and repeat the same process on the lower teeth.

6. Wear the strips for 30 minutes and avoid eating, drinking, or smoking.
7. After 30 minutes, rinse mouth with water for 15 seconds.
8. Remove the strips from the upper and lower teeth. Discard the used strips.
9. If whiter teeth are desired, continue using the strips for 7 days.

Opalescence Tooth Whitening Systems

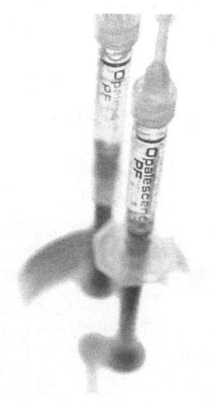

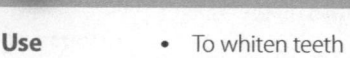

Use
- To whiten teeth
- To remove the colors present on teeth from the time of tooth eruption and/or the stains of aging
- Success with varying degrees of tetracycline and brown fluorosis discoloration
- On nonvital teeth for intracoronal bleaching

Composition
- Carbamide peroxide
- Potassium nitrate
- Fluoride ion

Properties
- Very effective bleaching agent
- Comes in unit-dose syringes and is flavored
- Available in different percentages of carbamide peroxide
- Has sustained release
- Adhesive properties
- Custom designed application tray required
- High viscosity and stickiness

Precautions
- Eye contact: Immediately flush eyes for 15 minutes.
- Skin: Wash thoroughly with soap and water.

Opalescence Tooth Whitening Systems *Continued*

- Ingestion: If swallowed, give the patient a glass of water or milk and call a physician.
- Inhalation: Not defined.

Mixing and Setting Times
- No mixing is required.
- Application time varies depending on the patient's needs, level of sensitivity, and day-to-day activities.

Directions

1. Fabricate the tray according to the manufacturer's instructions.
2. Instruct the patient about the bleaching procedure.
3. Patient should load gel into their custom tray. Use one-half to one full syringe of material to fill the tray.
4. Brush teeth, and then insert the tray. Adjust tray sides to the teeth.
5. Remove excess gel with a clean finger or soft toothbrush. Rinse twice; do not swallow rinses.
6. The dentist will instruct the patient when and how long to bleach. Opalescence carbamide peroxide gel will bleach 8 to 10 hours during the night or 4 to 6 hours during the day. In some treatment sequences, the bleaching procedure is completed by the patient for 30 minutes several times a day.
7. Patient is evaluated every 3 to 5 days of treatment or as needed.

Nu Radiance Duet Tooth Whitening System

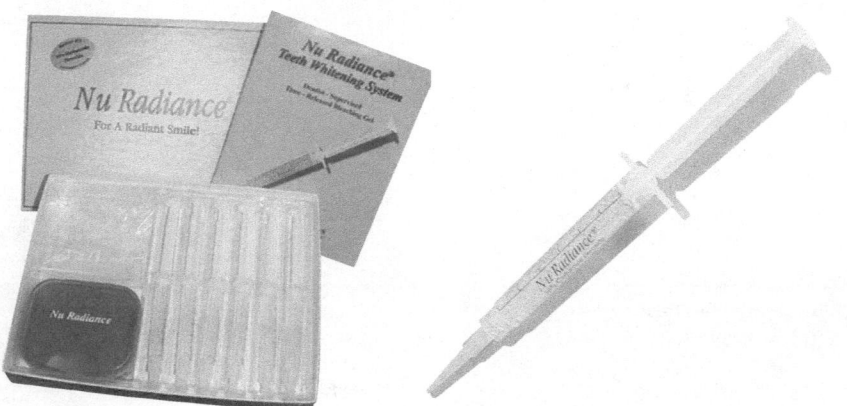

Use   To whiten teeth without sensitivity

Composition   Stabilized carbamide peroxide gel mixed with an accelerator and hydrating agent

Properties
- Easy, comfortable, and effective whitening system
- Takes less time
- Comes in different percentages
- Hydrates the teeth, so it does not cause sensitivity

Precautions
- May cause irritation to the eyes: Flush with copious amount of water.
- May cause skin irritation: Wash with soap and water.
- If swallowed, drink large amounts of water and contact doctor immediately.
- No harm anticipated if inhaled in the amount contained in commercially packaged material.

Mixing and Setting Times
- No mixing is required.
- Application times vary with the percentage of solution.

Nu Radiance Duet Tooth Whitening System *Continued*

Directions

1. Remove and save the small cap from the whitening syringe tip.
2. Express a small dot into the deepest portion of each anterior tooth compartment in custom-made whitening trays.
3. Pat the teeth dry before treatment.
4. Place the tray into the mouth and press the gel against the teeth; remove any excess with a tissue.

5. Follow manufacturer's instruction for time in mouth; remove the tray and rinse.
6. Complete the whitening treatment once a day or as directed by the dentist.
7. Do not eat, drink, or smoke while whitening or for 30 minutes after the treatment.

ZOOM in Office and Home Whitening System

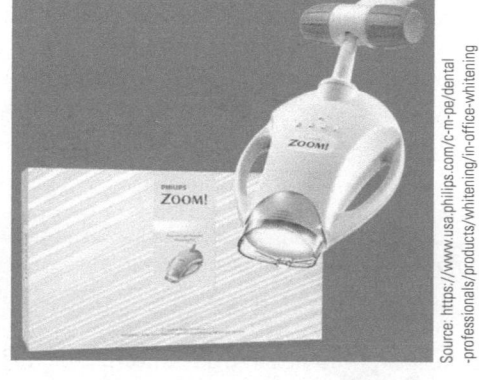

Source: https://www.usa.philips.com/c-m-pe/dental-professionals/products/whitening/in-office-whitening

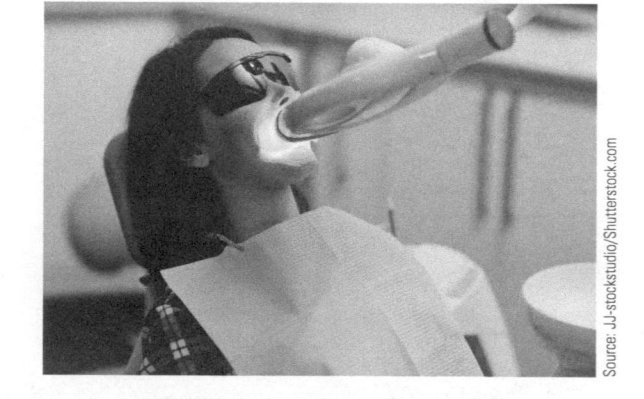

Source: JJ-stockstudio/Shutterstock.com

Use
- To whiten and brighten teeth
- Remove stains

Composition
- 35% hydrogen peroxide in office treatment
- 8%, 9.5%, 14%, and 20% hydrogen peroxide in home treatment
- Ethanol, aminoalkyl methacrylate copolymer, methacrylate acid, polymer with ethyl acrylate, methanol, and proprietary trace elements

Properties
- Achieves the best results in the least amount of time.
- Convenient to use.

- Everything needed is provided in the kit.
- Protectant for gingival tissues provided.

Precautions
- Corrosive to mucous membranes of the skin and eyes
- Eyes: May cause severe damage.
- Skin: May cause irritation and burns.
- Inhalation: Slight nose and throat irritation.
- Ingestion: Corrosive to gastrointestinal tract; may cause irritation and burning.
- Not suitable for persons under 18 years of age.

ZOOM in Office and Home Whitening System *Continued*

Mixing and Setting Time
- One-step gel application.
- Activation time is 15 minutes for each of the three applications.

Directions

1. Determine the existing shade with the teeth moist and no overhead lighting and apply vitamin E on lips.
2. Use prophy paste to polish teeth.
3. Insert cheek retractors provided in the kit and cotton rolls in the upper and lower lip area.
4. Thoroughly dry the teeth and gingiva. Apply LiquiDam along the gingival margin of the teeth and cure for 3 to 5 seconds. Light-cure the material in a slow flowing motion over the teeth. Material should be rubbery and cover all the gingival tissues.
5. Dry teeth and apply vitamin E on LiquiDam and around any exposed tissue near retractors. Do not get on the teeth.
6. Vial 1: Apply whitening varnish evenly using applicator brush. Do not place on tissue. Allow the material to dry (material should not feel sticky). Takes approximately 30 seconds.

7. Apply activator light for 15 minutes.
8. Repeat step 6 for vials 2 and vial 3 for two more rounds of care.
9. Carefully remove LiquiDam without disturbing the whitening varnish.
10. Remove the lip retractors and cotton rolls.
11. Apply vitamin E to the patient's lips.
12. Patient leaves with varnish on their teeth.
13. Give postoperative Instructions.
    a. Apply relief gel into trays as needed for sensitivity for the next 12 hours.
    b. For the next 48 hours, avoid staining foods, such as dark drinks and red sauces, that may compromise results.
    c. Sensitivity is common. If it persists after 1 week, call for a follow-up appointment.
    d. Use at-home whitening as needed to maintain shade. Do not swallow the solution. Leave in for 30 to 60 minutes.
14. Patient can be given take-home whitening treatments.

CHAPTER 16

Periodontic Instruments and Materials

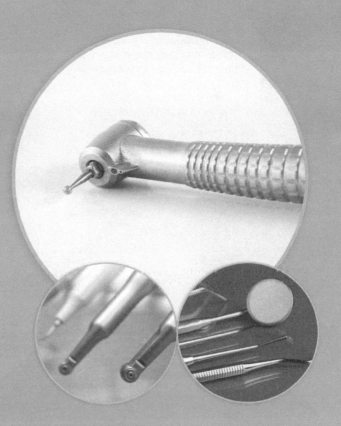

Sharpening Periodontal Instruments

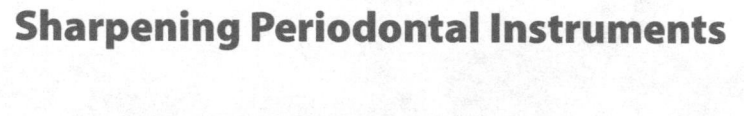

A.

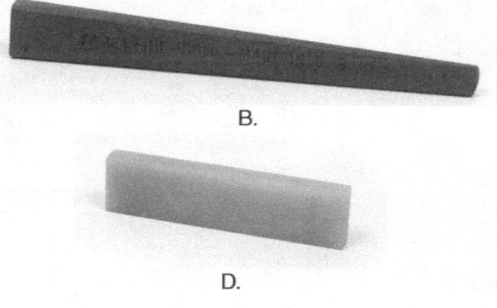

B.

C.

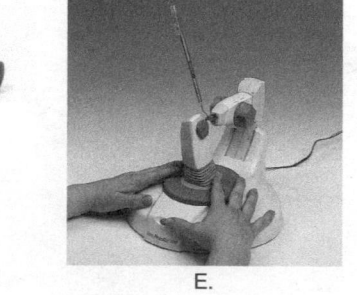

D.

E.

Use
- To sharpen the cutting edges of periodontal instruments
- To improve the effectiveness of the instruments

Composition
- Manual sharpening stones come in several sizes and shapes.
- They are made of various materials, including Arkansas stone, India oilstone, silicon carbide, and ceramic stone.
- The mechanical method for sharpening periodontal instruments is shown here.
  A. Silicon carbide sharpening stone in cone shape
  B. Ceramic sharpening stone in triangle shape
  C. India sharpening stone

D. Arkansas sharpening stone
E. Mechanical sharpening device

Notes
- Mechanical devices provide a consistent and precise sharpening method.
- Sometimes a lubricant is used when sharpening instruments.
- Sharpening periodontal instruments requires training and practice.

Periodontal Probes

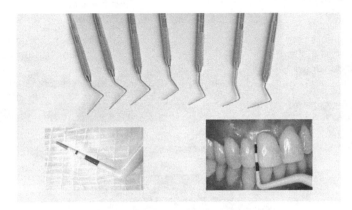

Use	• To measure the depth of periodontal pockets in millimeters • To measure areas of recession, bleeding, or exudate
Composition	Calibrated instrument with a blunted working end
Notes	• The probe may be flat, oval, or round in cross section, but it is thin enough to fit in the gingival sulcus. • Many styles and variations in the millimeter markings are available.

• The calibrations may be indentations or color-coded for easy reading.
• May be double-ended with a probe on one end and an explorer on the other end.
• Computerized probe systems detect and store information on pocket depth, recession, furcation involvement, and mobility.

Florida Periodontal Probe System

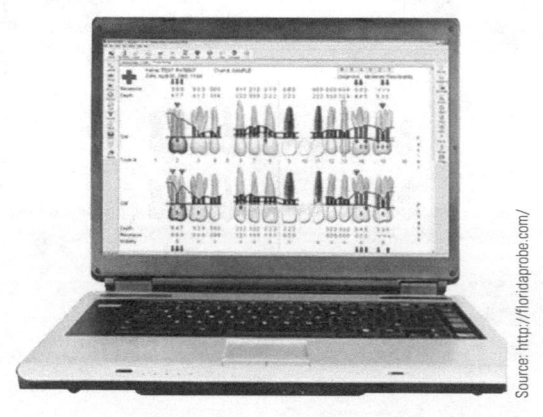

Source: http://floridaprobe.com/

Use
- To measure the depth of periodontal pockets in millimeters
- To measure areas of recession/hyperplasia, bleeding, attached gingiva, minimal attached gingiva suppuration, plaque, furcations, tooth mobility, and missing teeth

Composition
- Calibrated instrument with a blunted working end
- Computerized periodontal pressure-sensitive probing and charting system
- Solo operation: voice call-out system

Notes
- The probe may be flat, oval, or round in cross section, but it is thin enough to fit in the gingival sulcus.
- Patient education handouts and movies are available.
- The calibrations may be indentations or color-coded for easy reading.
- Only need one examiner; may be completed in approximately 10 minutes.
- Computerized probe systems detect and store information on pocket depth, recession, furcation involvement, and mobility.

Furcation Probe

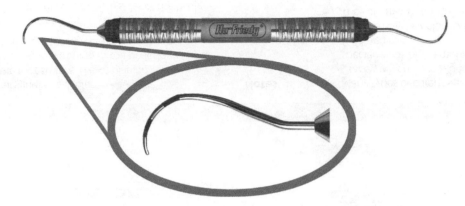

Use	To measure the pocket depth in furcation areas on multirooted teeth
Composition	An instrument with a rounded calibrated working end
Notes	• Furcation probes have blunted or rounded ends. • They can be single- or double-ended.

- The curved working ends have millimeter markings/calibrations.
- Markings may be indented or color-coded.

Periodontal Curettes

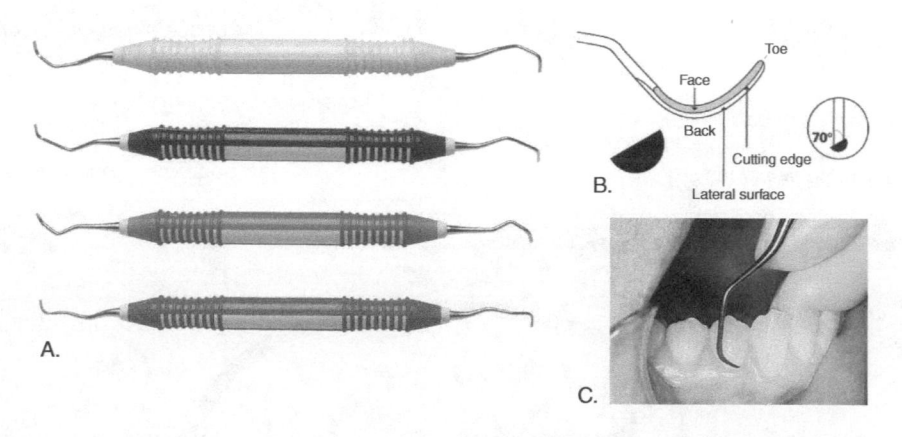

A. Variety of anterior and posterior curettes
B. Drawing of the working end of a curette
C. Curette being used in oral cavity

Use
- To remove subgingival calculus
- To smooth the root surface in root planing
- To remove the soft tissue lining or the periodontal pocket
- Designed to adapt to the curves of the root surface

Composition
- A double-ended instrument in which the working ends have a cutting edge on one or both sides of the blade.
- The end of the instrument is rounded, not pointed like a scaler.
  - **A.** Variety of anterior and posterior curettes
  - **B.** Drawing of the working end of a curette
  - **C.** Curette being used in oral cavity

Notes
- Many types of curettes exist, including the Universal and Gracey, which are designed and angled to be used in specific areas of the mouth, such as the anterior and posterior regions.
- Handles may be color-coded and ergonomically designed.
- They are mainly double-ended.
- They are available in a range of sizes, usually 1/2, 3/4, and so on, with the size label following the manufacturer's name.
- They are often named for the designer, for example, Gracey, McCall, or Langer.

Periodontal Scaler: Sickle and Jacquette

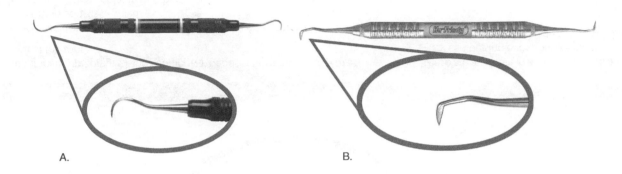

A.

B.

Use   To remove supragingival calculus

Composition
- An instrument with working ends that have two cutting edges along the margins of the curved blade; the end of the instrument is a sharp point.
- There are three angles in the shank of the instrument (Jacquette).
  - **A.** Sickle Scaler.
  - **B.** Jacquette Scaler.

Notes
- The periodontal scaler is also known as the shepherd's hook.
- They can be single- or double-ended.
- The sickle scaler looks like the agricultural tool called a sickle.
- There are a variety of sizes and angles.
- The Jacquette is able to get closer to the root to remove calculus.

Periodontal Chisel Scaler

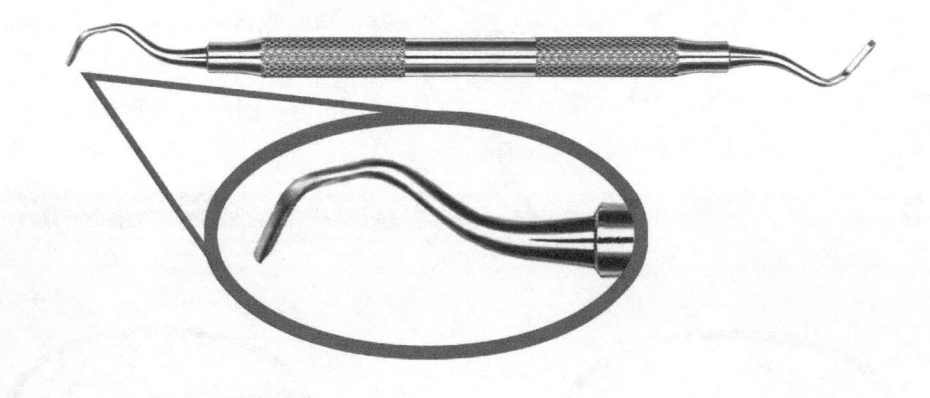

Use   To remove supragingival and subgingival deposits from the root of the tooth

Composition
- The working end is a blade that is slightly curved and the cutting edge is beveled.
- There are two angles in the shank.

Notes
- These are available in a variety of sizes and shapes.
- They can be single- or double-ended.
- Some have a broader blade at the working end.

Periodontal Hoe Scalers

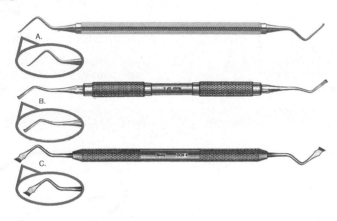

Use
- To remove supragingival and subgingival calculus from around the tooth
- To plane and smooth the root surface

Composition An instrument that resembles the agricultural hoe tool and has a straight cutting edge
- **A.** Mesial/distal hoe
- **B.** Buccal/lingual hoe
- **C.** Back-action hoe

Notes
- Hoes are used in a pulling motion.
- They can be single- or double-ended.
- They come in a variety of sizes and designs.

Periodontal Files

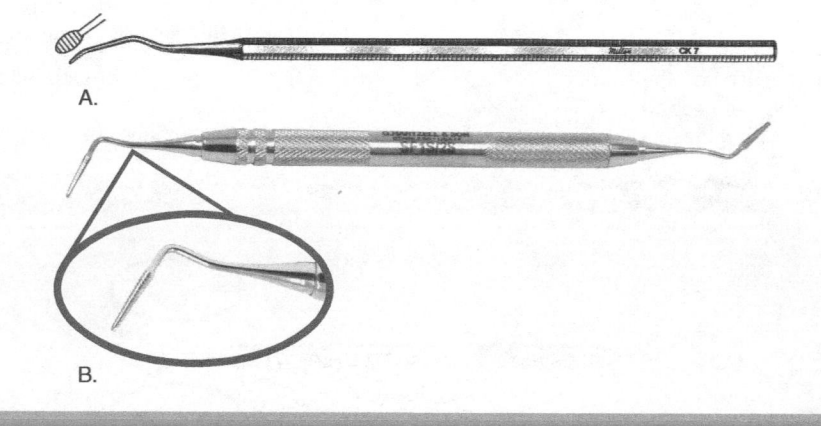

A.

B.

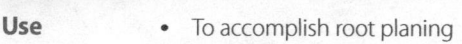

Use
- To accomplish root planing
- To remove supragingival and subgingival calculus from the interproximal surface

Composition An instrument that has a long neck with cutting groves on the working end
A. Single Ended Periodontal File
B. Double-ended interproximal periodontal file

Notes
- There are a variety of blade shapes and shank angulations.
- A pushing and pulling motion is used interproximally.
- Some of these are designed with a long-grooved working end to be used interproximally.
- They come in various sizes and shapes.

Ultrasonic Scaler and Air Polishing Unit (Cavitron®)

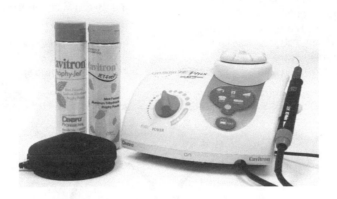

Use
- To remove hard deposits, stains, and debris during scaling, curettage, and root-planing procedures
- To polish surfaces more thoroughly than by conventional means
- To clean tooth surfaces prior to bonding procedures and placing of sealants

Composition A combined ultrasonic scaler and air polishing unit that has a handpiece for use with scaling tips as well as a foot control to regulate the speed of the unit. It has an air polishing insert containing sodium bicarbonate, air, and water.

Notes
- These come with a variety of tips.
- The air polisher delivers a mixture of sodium bicarbonate, air, and water to polish teeth.
- Various sizes and types of ultrasonic and air polishing units are available; they can be purchased as independent units.
- Foot controls can be wireless.
- The ultrasonic unit generates high-power vibrations to a handpiece with a variety of tips.
- Ultrasonic units create heat, so the units have cooling systems that circulate water through the handpieces and out the openings near the tips.

Periodontal Knives and Interdental Knives

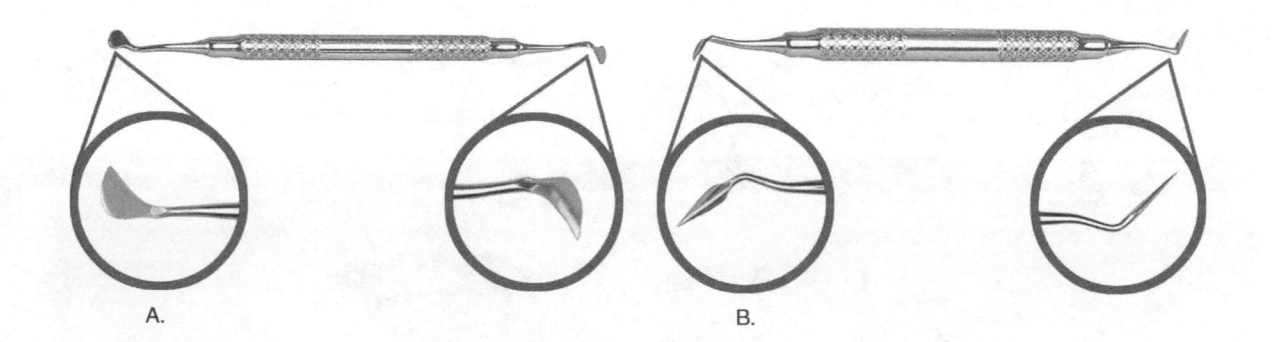

A.

B.

Use
- Periodontal knives remove and contour gingival tissue during periodontal surgery.
- Interdental knives interproximally remove soft tissue.

Composition
- **A.** The periodontal knife is an instrument with a round-bladed working end with cutting edges.
- **B.** The interdental knife is a spear-shaped instrument with long, narrow blades.

Notes
- The most common periodontal knives are kidney-shaped and broad-bladed knives.
- The entire periphery of the blade is sharp.
- They can be single- or double-ended.
- Periodontal knives are also called gingivectomy knives.
- Common periodontal designer names are Kirkland, Buck, and Goldman-Fox.
- Common interdental designer names are Orban and Goldman-Fox.

Electrosurgery Unit

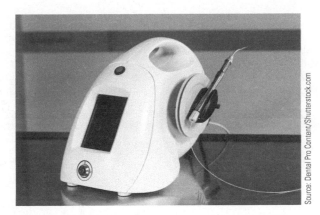

Source: Dental Pro Content/Shutterstock.com

Use
- To incise and contour gingival tissue
- To coagulate the blood during surgical procedures

Composition
- Control box.
- Two terminal plates: One is placed behind the patient's back or shoulders and the other is a probe with various cutting tips that is used during surgery.
- Foot-operated on/off controls.

Notes
- The electrosurgery unit uses timed electrical currents to incise the tissue.
- A dental assistant must keep the high-volume evacuator (HVE) close during the use of the electrosurgery unit to remove debris and odor.
- Many tips are available.

Pocket-Marking Pliers

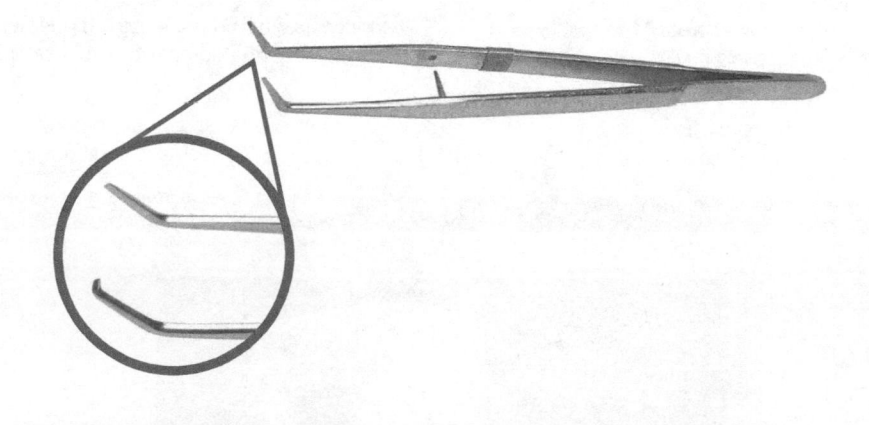

Use   To transfer the measurement of the pocket to the outside of the tissue to indicate the depth of the pocket

Composition Pliers that have one straight thin beak that is placed in the pocket and the other bent at a right angle at the tip.

Notes
- When the beaks are pinched together, the gingival tissue is perforated, which leaves small pinpoint markings.
- It resembles cotton pliers, but the tips are different.

Periodontal Scissors

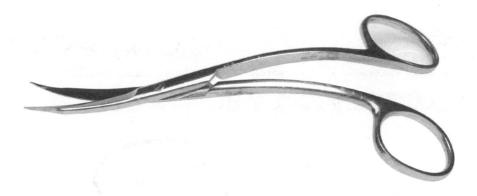

Use	• To remove tags of tissue and to trim margins of tissue • Also used in oral maxillofacial surgeries and periodontic procedures	**Composition** Scissors with long, very thin, and sharp blades **Notes** These come in a variety of shapes and sizes.

Periodontal Rongeurs

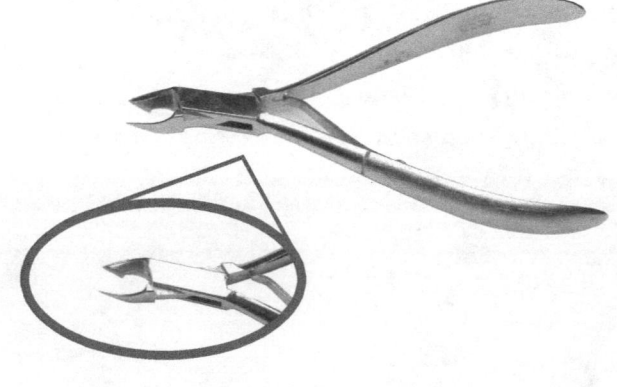

Use To remove excess tissue and to shape the soft tissue

Composition Hinged pliers with sharp cutting edge on one side of the blade of the working end

Notes
- Periodontal rongeurs are smaller than bone rongeurs.
- They are also known as nippers.

Periodontal Retraction Forceps

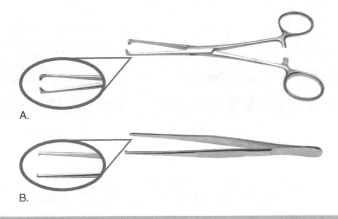

A.

B.

Use
- To retract soft tissue during surgical procedures
- To hold soft tissue in place

Composition This instrument has beaks that are often curved near the end at right angles to each other; the ends are sharp to securely hold the tissue.
A. Hinged locking tissue forceps
B. Cotton-plier-designed tissue forceps with tongue and groove ends

Notes
- These are available in a variety of shapes and designs.
- They are shaped like cotton pliers or hemostats with locking handles.

Periotomes

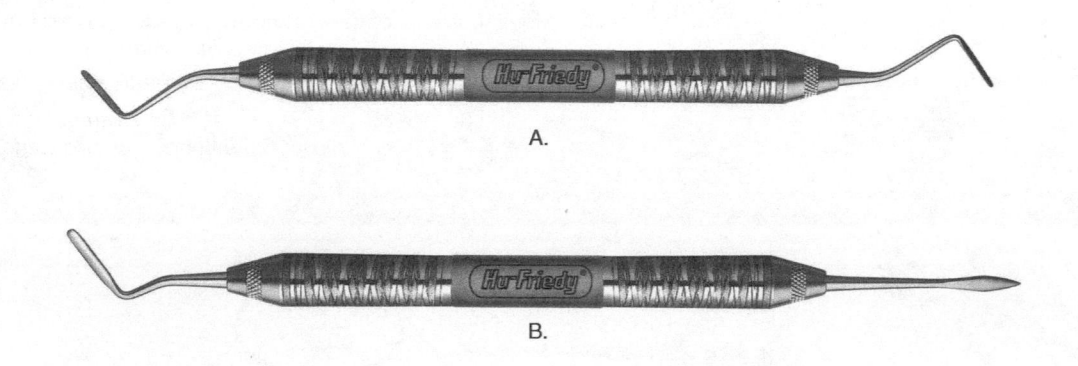

A.

B.

Use
- To sever the periodontal ligament prior to extraction
- To prepare for dental implants

Composition An instrument with flexible fixed blades that are thin, sharp, and designed to cause minimal damage to the periodontal ligament
- **A.** Posterior periotomes
- **B.** Anterior periotomes

Notes
- These may be single- or double-ended.
- An instrument's blade may be straight or angled.
- They are available in a variety of sizes and shapes.
- They are made of stainless steel.
- They are available as a handle with interchangeable blades.
- Wide, narrow, angled, and contra-angled blades are available.

Coe-Pak Automix NDS Periodontal Dressing

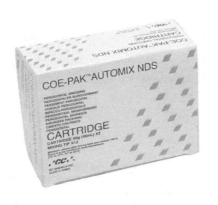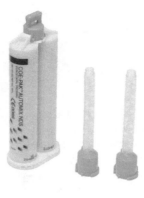

Use   Noneugenol surgical and periodontal dressing

Composition
- Vegetable oil
- Zinc oxide
- Mineral oil
- Magnesium oxide
- Chlorodimethyl phenol ethanol
- Methanol
- Petrolatum

Properties
- No burning sensation.
- No unpleasant taste.
- No strong odor.
- Protection to tissues.
- Promotes cleanliness and healing.
- Resilient hardness to resist fracture or breakage.
- Smooth cohesive mix.
- Automix or two-paste system available.
- Material won't stick to gloves.

Coe-Pak Automix NDS Periodontal Dressing *Continued*

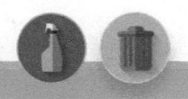

Precautions
- Eyes: May be irritating to the eyes. Flush for 15 minutes.
- Skin: May be irritating to the skin. Wash for 15 minutes with soap and water.
- Ingestion: Drink several glasses of water.
- Inhalation: Remove to fresh air. Drink water to clear throat and blow nose to remove dust particles.
- If irritation develops, seek medical attention with all of the above.

Mixing and Setting Time
- Ready to use in 3 minutes
- Hard- and fast-set ready in 1 minute

Directions

1. Place an Automix cartridge into a GC cartridge dispenser II.
2. Remove the cap from the cartridge and place a mixing tip.
3. Dispense the required amount of material on a paper pad.
4. Using a spatula, form the material into a cylindrical shape.
5. Lightly lubricate your fingers with Vaseline, lanolin, cold cream, or water to test the mix for thickness.
6. Automix material will lose its tackiness in about 30 seconds, whereas the two-paste mix should lose its tackiness in 2 to 3 minutes.
7. Automix will be workable for 8 minutes; two-paste mix can be worked for 10 minutes.
8. Form into ropes. Material is extremely cohesive. Place in patient's mouth.

Barricaid VLC Surgical Periodontal Dressing

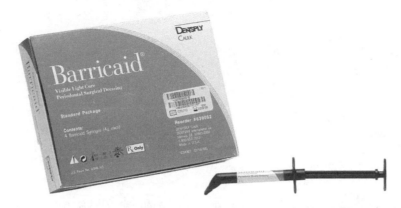

Use	• Light-cured surgical periodontal dressing • Protection for periodontal surgical sites during the healing process
Composition	Dimethacrylate resins
Properties	• Control over the setting time of the material. • Light-cured. • Designed for direct and indirect placement. • Material forms a nonbrittle, elastic protective cover.

• Tasteless.
• Tinted pink with translucent qualities.

Precautions
• Eyes: Rinse with open eyes for several minutes under running water.
• May be irritating to the skin: Immediately wash with soap and water and rinse thoroughly.
• Ingestion: If symptoms persist, contact a physician.
• Inhalation: Move to fresh air.

Barricaid VLC Surgical Periodontal Dressing *Continued*

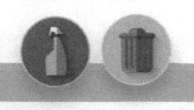

Mixing and Setting Time
- No mixing is required.
- Light-cured for 10 seconds per tooth on both buccal and lingual sides.

Directions
Barricaid Periodontal Dressing can be applied directly or indirectly.

Direct Technique
1. Using sterile gauze, dry the buccal or lingual surfaces adjacent to the surgical site.
2. Remove the cap from the syringe and begin dispensing the material at the juncture of the cervical third of the teeth and the margin of the surgical site.

Indirect Technique
1. Using sterile gauze, dry the buccal or lingual surfaces adjacent to the surgical site.
2. Place a thin layer of lubricant on a paper pad. Remove the cap from the syringe and dispense the amount needed.
3. Place a light layer of lubricant on your gloved hand and roll the material off the pad ready to be placed.
4. Once placement is completed, light-cure the buccal and lingual surfaces of each tooth for 10 seconds.
5. Check for uncured material with a blunt instrument or explorer.

Tray Setup for Scaling, Curettage, and Polish Procedure

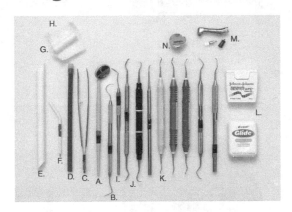

Composition
A. Mouth mirror
B. Explorer
C. Cotton pliers
D. Saliva ejector
E. HVE tip
F. Air-water syringe tip
G. Cotton rolls

H. Gauze sponges
I. Periodontal probe
J. Scalers: Jacquette and shepherd's hook
K. Curettes: universal and Gracey
L. Dental floss and tape
M. Prophy angle: rubber cups and brushes
N. Prophy paste

Tray Setup for Gingivectomy Procedure

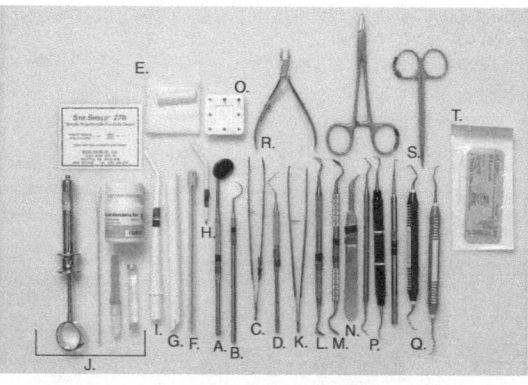

Composition

A. Mouth mirror
B. Explorer
C. Cotton pliers
D. Periodontal probe
E. Cotton rolls and gauze sponges
F. Saliva ejector
G. HVE tip
H. Air-water syringe tip
I. Surgical aspirating tip
J. Anesthetic setup
K. Pocket marker

L. Periodontal knives
M. Interproximal knives
N. Scalpel and blade
O. Diamond burs
P. Scalers
Q. Curettes
R. Soft tissue rongeurs
S. Hemostat and surgical scissors
T. Suture needle and thread

Not shown: Periodontal dressing materials

Tray Setup for Osseous Surgery

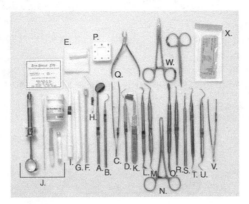

Composition

A. Mouth mirror
B. Explorer
C. Cotton pliers
D. Periodontal probe
E. Cotton rolls and gauze sponges
F. Saliva ejector
G. HVE tip
H. Air-water syringe tip
I. Surgical aspirating tip

J. Anesthetic setup
K. Scalpel and blade
L. Broad-bladed periodontal knife
M. Interproximal periodontal knife
N. Tissue retractor
O. Periosteal elevator
P. Diamond burs and stones
Q. Periodontal rongeurs
R. Chisels
S. Files

T. Scalers
U. Curettes
V. Tissue forceps
W. Scissors
X. Suture setup

Not shown: Periodontal dressing materials

Procedure: Preparation and Placement of Noneugenol Periodontal Dressing

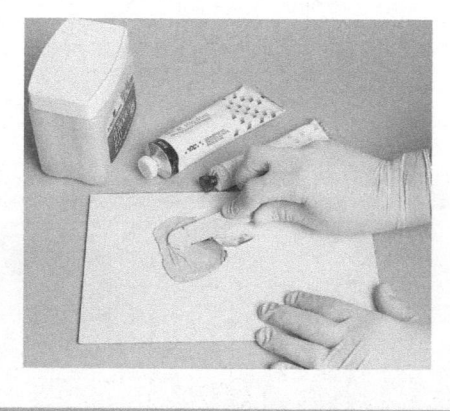

This procedure is performed by the dentist and/or the dental assistant at chairside.

Equipment and Supplies
- Basic setup
- Air/water syringe tip, HVE, and salvia ejector
- Cotton rolls and 2 × 2 gauze sponges
- Periodontal dressing catalyst and base tubes
- Paper pad—large
- Large spatula or tongue depressor
- Lubricant (petroleum jelly, lanolin, cold cream, water)
- Instrument to contour dressing (spoon excavator)
- PPE worn by the dental assistant

Directions After the hemorrhaging is controlled, the patient's lips are coated lightly with a lubricant. Before placement, the dental assistant prepares the periodontal dressing for application as follows:

1. Extrude equal lengths of paste from the catalyst and base tubes onto the paper pad.

2. Spatulate for 30 to 45 seconds until the mix is of uniform color.

Procedure: Preparation and Placement of Noneugenol Periodontal Dressing *Continued*

3. Using the spatula, form the paste into a cylindrical shape.

4. Lightly lubricate gloved fingers with Vaseline, cold cream, lanolin, or water to test the mixed paste for tackiness. It should be ready in 2 to 3 minutes.

5. After 2 to 3 minutes, the dressing paste can be handled. Remove the cylindrical shape from the paper pad and mold into the diameter and length needed to place over surgical site.

6. The dressing paste can be worked for 10 to 15 minutes. This gives the dentist or dental assistant enough time to place and secure the dressing on the buccal and lingual surfaces of the surgical site.

7. The dressing is secured around the most posterior tooth and then pressed interproximally on the buccal surfaces. This procedure is repeated on the lingual surfaces.

8. Once the dressing is placed, it is evaluated for effectiveness and comfort for the patient. Adjust as needed.

9. Give home care instructions to the patient and dismiss.

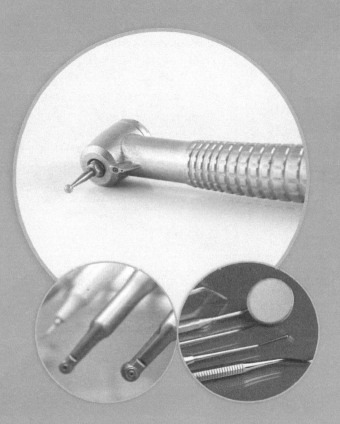

CHAPTER 17

Fixed Prosthodontic Instruments

Impression Wax

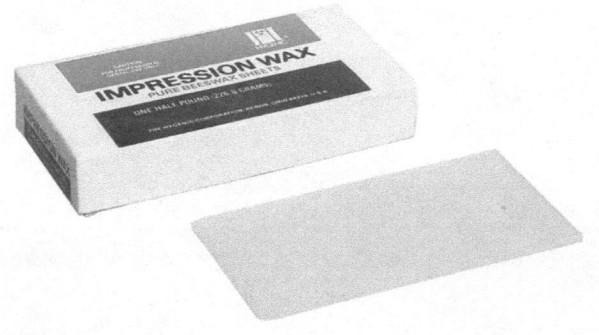

Use	To take an impression of a small area where great detail is not required and to take a bite impression
Composition	• Most often made of pure, natural beeswax with no additives • No hazardous components • Less than 10% petroleum hydrocarbons and additives
Properties	• Softens easily under hot water • Very pliable • Comes in sheets • Often yellow in color

• Softens quickly
• Flows easily
• Sets hard when chilled

Precautions   Nonhazardous at room temperature

Directions

1. Take one sheet from the box.
2. Heat the sheet with warm water.
3. Adapt it to the area where the impression is needed.
4. Let the wax cool and remove it from the area.

Bite Wafers

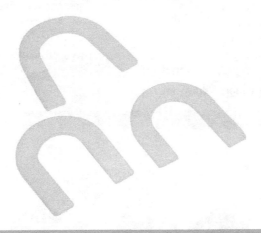

Use
To check occlusal relationships and to take bite registrations

Composition
- No hazardous components
- Less than 10% petroleum hydrocarbons and additives

Properties
- Available in yellow, blue, and green.
- Available in nonlaminated.
- Available in foil laminated: Foil is laminated between two layers of wax to decrease distortion and prevent the patient from biting through the wax bite.
- U-shaped wax.
- Designed to adapt to the dental arch.

Precautions
Nonhazardous at room temperature

Directions

1. Wax bite wafers are heated slightly in warm water.
2. Wafers are placed on the occlusal surface of the maxillary or mandibular arch.
3. The patient is instructed to bite gently in the normal bite pattern.
4. After the patient has bitten into the wax and the wax has cooled, the wax is gently removed and used for bite checks or occlusal transfers.

Coprwax™ Bite Wafers

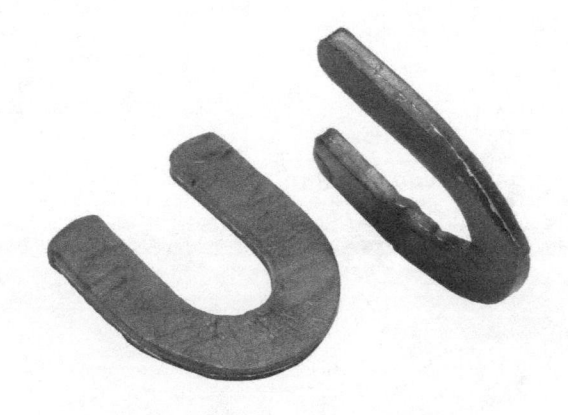

Use To obtain an occlusal registration

Composition
- No hazardous components
- Less than 10% petroleum hydrocarbons and additives
- Copper particles

Properties
- Has a thin foil layer between layers of wax
- Prevents patients from biting through the occlusal registration
- Has copper particles that provide uniform flow of heat and allow the wax to soften quickly
- Sets hard when chilled
- Made in the shape of an arch

Precautions Nonhazardous at room temperature

Directions

1. Coprwax™ bite wafers are heated slightly in warm water.
2. Wafers are placed on the occlusal surface of the maxillary or mandibular arch.
3. The patient is instructed to bite gently in the normal bite pattern.
4. After the patient has bitten into the wax and the wax has cooled, the wax is gently removed and used for bite checks or occlusal registration.

Aluwax™

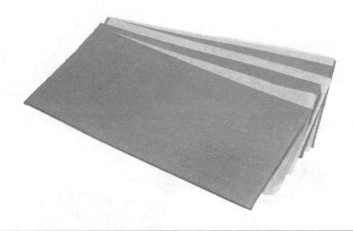

Use For dental bite registration material

Composition
- Contains powdered aluminum
- Trade secret—paraffin and beeswax

Properties
- Comes in a number of shapes
- Contains powdered aluminum to increase the integrity of the compound and provide the heat-retention properties
- Cut to shape for easy use
- Comes in denture forms, denture sheets, scored, and with waxed cloth forms as well as in the shape of an arch
- The waxed cloth forms that contain coarse weave cloth at the center of the wax form to prevent going through the occlusal surface and to prevent tooth skidding

Precautions Nonhazardous at room temperature

Directions

1. Aluwax™ bite wafers are heated slightly in warm water.
2. Wafers are placed on the occlusal surface of the maxillary or mandibular arch.
3. The patient is instructed to bite gently in the normal bite pattern.
4. After the patient has bitten into the wax and the wax has cooled, the wax is gently removed and used for bite checks or occlusal registration.

Occlusal Indicator Wax

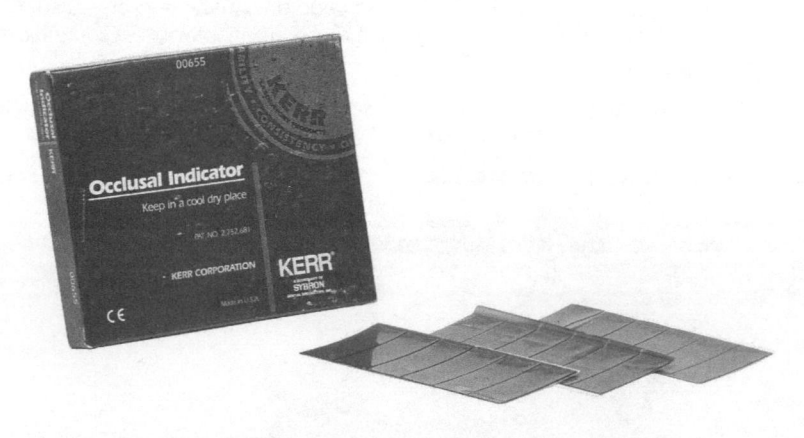

Use To determine whether the occlusal surface of the tooth is high and out of occlusion

Composition No hazardous components

Properties
- Available in a box with 180 strips and a pencil
- Strips can be separated easily
- Green in color

Precautions Nonhazardous at room temperature

Directions

1. Use one wax strip for opposing quadrants.
2. Place on the occlusal surface of one quadrant.
3. Have the patient gently close into the normal bite pattern.
4. Have the patient gently grind from side to side.
5. The green wax will show the biting pattern.
6. Adjust with a bur as necessary.
7. Discard the used wax strip.

Procedure: Taking a Wax Bite Registration with a Bite Wafer

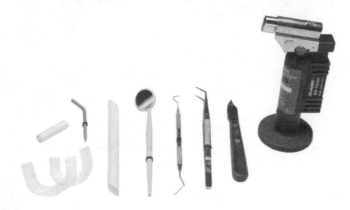

This procedure is performed by the dental assistant in the dental operatory.

Composition
- Basic setup
- Wax wafer
- Laboratory knife
- Heat source (warm water, Bunsen burner, or torch)
- Personal protective equipment (PPE) worn by the dental assistant

Directions

1. Health and medical history is reviewed and the procedure is explained by the dental assistant to the patient.
2. The patient is informed that when the wax is placed into the mouth it will be warm and not to be alarmed.
3. The patient will practice opening and closing the mouth normally. The dental assistant will watch and take note of the correct occlusion positioning.

Procedure: Taking a Wax Bite Registration with a Bite Wafer *Continued*

4. The wax bite wafer is placed over the biting surfaces of the mandibular teeth. The wax bite wafer is checked for length. If the wax extends beyond the occlusal surface of the teeth, the laboratory knife can be used to remove the extra wax.

5. A heat source is used to warm and soften the wax bite wafer. Often the color will change to more clear when the wax is heated.

6. The wax bite wafer is placed on the occlusal surface, and the patient is instructed to bite gently in a normal bite pattern. When the patient closes the teeth, the dental assistant evaluates the position and ensures that the patient is biting properly.

7. The wax is allowed to cool and is removed from the mouth within a minute or two.

8. Carefully remove the wax bite registration to avoid any distortion.

9. The wax bite registration should be disinfected, rinsed, placed in with the impressions or casts related to this patient or labeled, and stored.

Cartridge-Dispensing Guns and Automixer

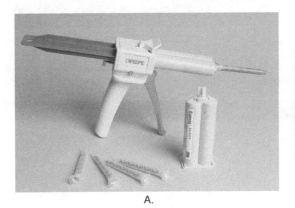

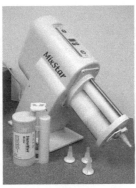

A.

B.

Use	• To dispense a variety of dental materials
	• To mix a variety of dental materials
	• To place mixed dental materials
Properties	• The cartridge-dispensing gun has a pressure rod and an area for the cartridge to be inserted and secured. Pressure is applied to the trigger handle to mix and dispense materials.
	• The Automixer unit has brackets to hold cartridges of catalyst and base material; it also has disposable tips, unit controls with on and off, and a locking area for tips.
	A. Automix Dispensing Syringe.
	B. Automix machine.

Notes

- Automixer is used with cartridges of various impression materials, such as polysulfide, vinyl polysiloxane, and polyether.
- It is used to mix bite registration and temporary/provisional materials.
- Mixing tips are color-coded to indicate various sizes and lengths.
- The tips match the material cartridges they are used with.
- Various styles of Automixers available.
- The Automixer can mix tray material, syringe material, or an alginate substitute material.

Triple Trays/Bite Registration Trays

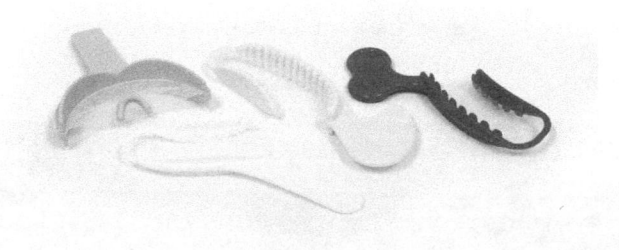
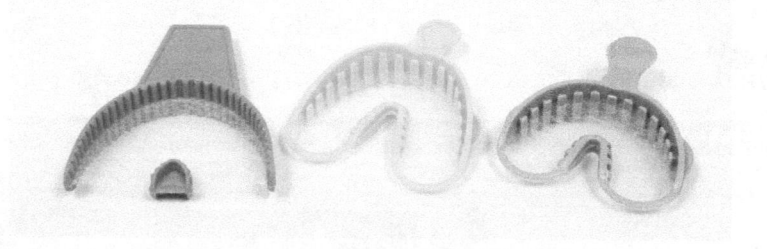

Use
- To take a dual-arch impression at one time (using one tray)
- To take final impressions for crowns and bridges and bite registration
- To take bite registrations for crown and bridge procedures simultaneously while taking the maxillary and mandibular impression (dual-arch–impression technique)

Composition
- Plastic frame with loose webbing to hold impression in tray
- Thin mesh in the middle of the tray
- Plastic handle attached

Notes
- Various sizes and designs are available for anterior, full-arch, or quadrant impression.
- They are disposable.
- They are used with various types of final and bite impression materials.

Blu-Mousse Polyvynylsiloxate Bite Registration

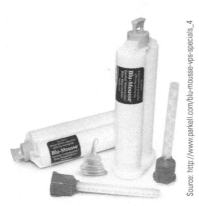

Source: http://www.parkell.com/blu-mousse-vps-specials_4

Use	To take a bite registration for traditional and digital impressions	**Mixing and Setting Time**	• No mixing is required. • Setting time is 30 seconds.
Properties	• Exceptional accuracy • Good tear strength • No slumping • Comes in a variety of flavors • Must have a "standard dispensing gun"	**Directions**	With PPE in place, prepare the patient for the procedure 1. Insert mousse cartridge into impression gun. Twist off and discard the sealing cap. 2. Bleed about ¼ inch of material from both orifices, ensuring that it is extruding evenly from both holes. 3. Wipe the ends clean, avoiding cross-contamination. Attach appropriate mixing tip and tighten one-quarter turn.
Precautions	• Always read the Material Safety Data Sheet (MSDS) information for the product. • Use safety glasses and gloves.		

Blu-Mousse Polyvynylsiloxate Bite Registration *Continued*

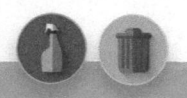

4. Bleed a small amount of mousse through the mixer and immediately dispense the material directly onto the quadrant/full arch as desired.
5. Wait the appropriate time and remove the set impression with a quick, firm motion.
6. Do not reuse the shipping cap. Leave the used mixing tip on the cartridge as the new sealing cap.
7. The cartridge, used mixing tip, and dispensing gun should not be directly sprayed with or soaked in disinfectant.
8. Store the mousse cartridge horizontally until the next use.

Core Post and Retention Pins

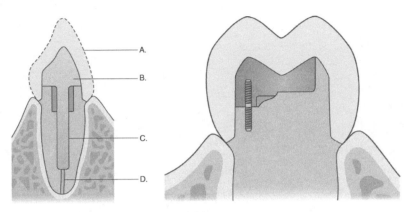

Use

Post
- To support and provide retention for the restoration
- A post-retained core is used when the tooth is nonvital.
- The root canal filling is removed, and the post is fitted in the canal and cemented.

Pins
- For addition or retention of the core buildup material
- For support and retention of a restoration

Composition
- Drill to make the desired preparation.
- Wrenches or keys for hand placement of the core post.
  - **A.** Crown of the tooth
  - **B.** Core buildup
  - **C.** Core post
  - **D.** Apical seal of root canal
- Drills are used in the low-speed handpiece to drill holes for the specific retention pins.
- Hand driver or mechanical placement device.

Core Post and Retention Pins *Continued*

Notes

Pins
- Pins are available in different sizes.
- They are often purchased as a kit.
- After being fitted in the root canal, a pin is cemented in place.
- Made from materials such as titanium, titanium alloy, and stainless steel.

Retraction Cord Placement Instrument

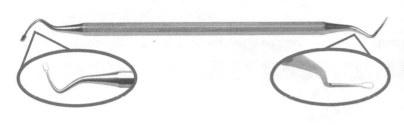

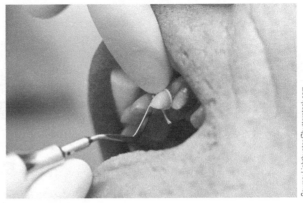

Use	To place retraction cord around a prepared tooth so that the tissue is displaced and ready for an accurate and detailed impression
Composition	• Single- or double-ended instrument • If double-ended, the ends are angled differently and can work differently.

Notes

- Working ends can have smooth or serrated edges.
- This instrument is available in a variety of sizes and shapes.
- Other instruments can be utilized for placing retraction cord, such as explorers, spoon excavators, periodontal probes, and so forth.

Disposable Anterior, Posterior, Quadrant, and Full-Arch Trays

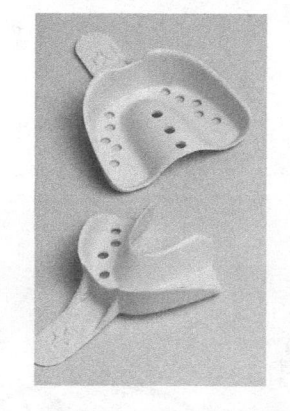

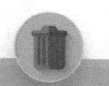

Use	• To hold various types of impression materials • To carry impression material into the patient's mouth to obtain an accurate impression	Notes	• These are available in various color-coded sizes. • They may be disposable or cold sterilizable. • They can be molded and trimmed if necessary. • Holes and perforations aid in locking/holding of materials.
Composition	• Perforated plastic trays with handles • Anterior, full maxillary and mandibular, and quadrant styles		

Metal Perforated Trays

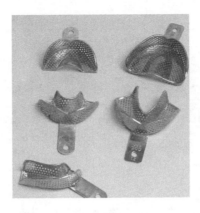

Use	• To hold various types of impression materials
	• To carry impression material into the patient's mouth to obtain an accurate impression
Composition	• Perforated metal trays with handles
	• Anterior, full maxillary and mandibular, and quadrant styles
Notes	They are sterilizable.

COE-FLEX Polysulfide Rubber Base Final Impression Material

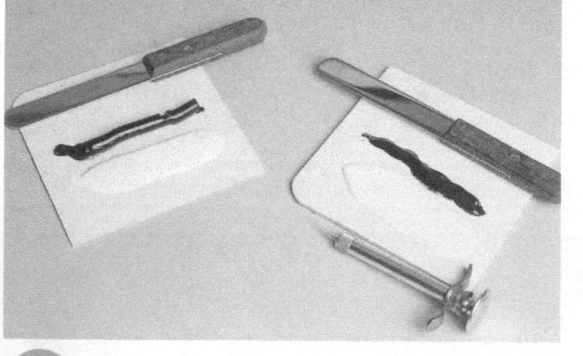

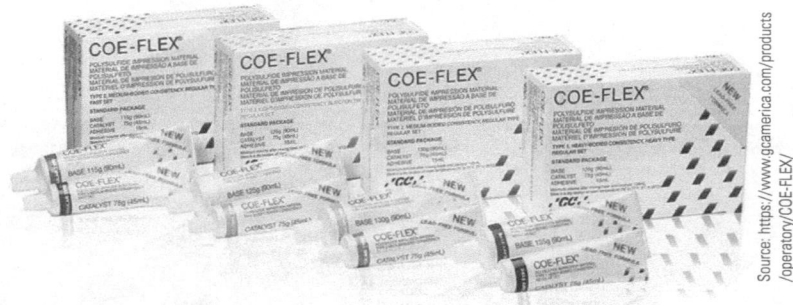

Source: https://www.gcamerica.com/products/operatory/COE-FLEX/

Use	• For taking impressions for the following:
	• Full dentures
	• Partial dentures
	• Inlays
	• Onlays
	• Crowns
	• Bridges
	• Reline and rebase

Properties
• Lead free
• High elasticity

• Excellent tear strength
• Blue-green color, mint flavor
• Available in three viscosities
• Three-year shelf life
• Available in regular body, injection type (light), heavy body, and fast set
• Unmixed catalyst or base may stain clothes

Precautions
• Always read the MSDS information for the product
• MSDS indications refer to the accelerator
• Disposable vinyl gloves recommended

COE-FLEX Polysulfide Rubber Base Final Impression Material *Continued*

- Eye protection
- Respirator protection
- Ventilation

Mixing and Setting Time

	Light-Bodied	Medium-Bodied	Medium-Bodied	Heavy-Bodied
	Type 3	Type 2	Fast Set-Type 2	Type 1
Mixing time	45 sec–1 min	45 sec–1 min	30 sec	45 sec–1 min
Time in mouth	8–10 min	8–10 min	4 min	8–10 min

*To speed up setting time, use more catalyst; to retard setting time, use less catalyst.

Directions   After the tray is selected, the PPE is in place, and the patient is prepared for the procedure:

1. Paint the entire surface of the tray with the tray adhesive. When dry, begin mixing the catalyst and base.
2. The catalyst and base are dispensed by using equal lengths. This is about one part catalyst to two parts base, according to volume.
3. The diameter of the dispensed material should be the same as the orifice of the tubes.
4. Coat the spatula with the blue paste before incorporating the blue and white pastes together. Spatulate with broad strokes until the mixture is free from streaks.
5. Fill an impression syringe with material (injection type—light) to inject onto and around the preparation.
6. Add the material to fill the impression tray that has been painted with adhesive (regular body or heavy body).
7. Firmly place into the oral cavity. Do not apply pressure against the tray while the material is setting. Do not remove impression prematurely. Hold in place for the minimum time indicated. With a blunt instrument, check material for setting prior to removal.
8. Break seal with lateral movement, and remove impression with a straight pull. Rinse off and disinfect or sterilize.
9. Pour model no longer than 8 hours later.

Permalastic Polysulfide Final Impression Material

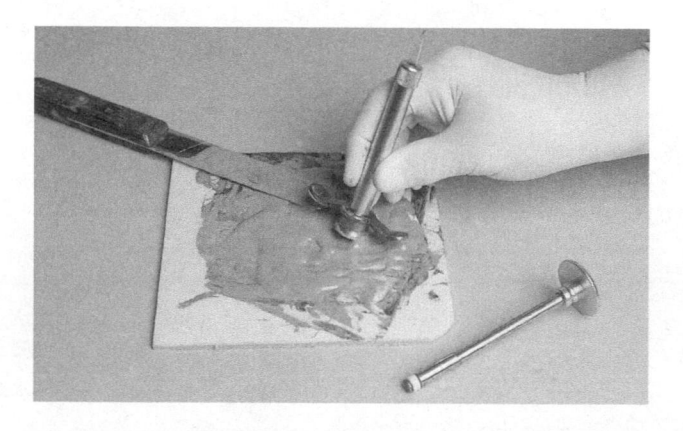

 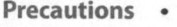

Use
- Regular is recommended for partial or full denture impressions.
- Light is for inlay and fixed bridge impressions.

Properties
- Has a high degree of flow
- Good tear strength
- Comes in regular, light-bodied, and heavy-bodied
- Adhesive available in a 2-oz size

Precautions
- Always read the MSDS information for the product.
- Use safety glasses and gloves.
- Use protective clothing because this product may cause staining.
- This material may cause irritation to skin and eyes.
- If ingested, this material may cause a choking sensation.
- This product contains a lead compound.

Permalastic Polysulfide Final Impression Material *Continued*

Mixing and Setting Time

Mixing time	45 sec–1 min
Tray loading	1.0 min
Syringe filling	10.0 min from start of mix
Mouth removal	6 min in mouth

Directions   After the tray is selected, the PPE is in place, and the patient is prepared for the procedure:

1. Extrude appropriate amounts of base and catalyst pastes onto a mixing pad. Use equal lengths not equal amounts.
2. Using a laboratory spatula, mix materials into each other using a stirring motion.
3. Incorporate thoroughly until a streak-free mixture is obtained.
4. Mixing should be completed within 45 seconds to 1 minute.
5. Immediately fill tray or syringe.
6. The material must stay in the mouth for a minimum of 6 minutes.
7. Remove and disinfect by immersion in a 2% solution of glutaraldehyde.
8. Pouring should occur immediately or within 8 hours.

Coltene Rapid Silicon Final Impression Material

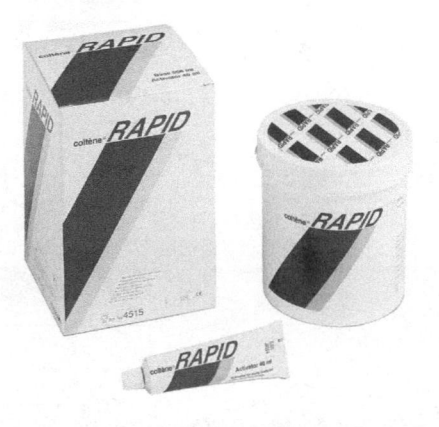

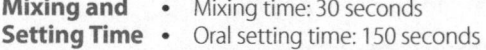

Use	• For inlay and fixed bridge impressions • Partial and full denture impressions
Properties	• Condensation silicone impression material • Seven-day dimensional stability • Material changes color during mixing for easy and reliable handling • Surface-activated hydrophilic to enhance performance when in contact with moist oral tissue • Available in putty, liner with activators, and applicator • Dosing spoon and dosing syringe are available as well.

Mixing and Setting Time
• Mixing time: 30 seconds
• Oral setting time: 150 seconds

Directions

After the tray is selected, the PPE is in place, and the patient is prepared for procedure:

1. Measure the required quantity of rapid line base into the applicator.
2. Add red activator with the precision syringe.
3. Stir briefly. The material turns blue when it's ready for use.
4. Rapid liner is applied from the applicator directly into the primary impression tray or into the syringe.

Impregum Penta Polyether Final Impression Material

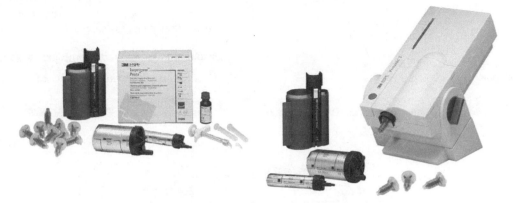

Use	• Impressions of inlays, onlays, veneers, crown, and bridge preparations
	• Fixation and implant impressions
Properties	• Comes in tubes, penta cartridges, syringe in medium and soft medium body.
	• Intrinsic presetting hydrophilicity helps capture and reproduce outstanding detail.
Precautions	• Face and eye protection.
	• Do not ingest.
	• Avoid prolonged or repeated skin contact.

Mixing and Setting Time	• Processing time from start of mixing: 1 minute
	• Time in mouth: 3 minutes
	• Setting time from start of mixing: 4 minutes
Directions	After the tray is selected, the PPE is in place, and the patient is prepared for the procedure:
	1. The dosing and mixing are done automatically in the Pentamix 2.
	2. If using the tubes, dispense in equal lengths and mix until streak free.

Polyjel NF Polyether Final Impression Material

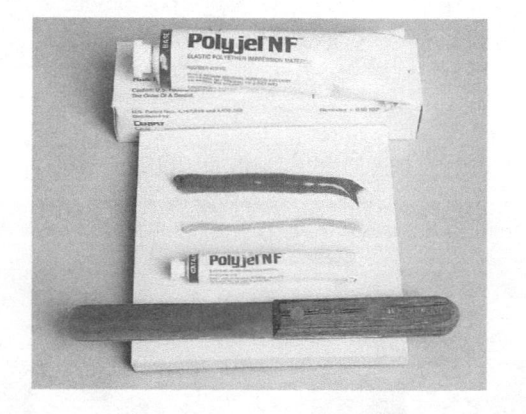

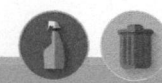

Use	• Reproduction for crown and bridge impressions
Properties	• Easy-to-release polyether-type elastomeric impression material
	• Single viscosity that provides optimal performance
	• Dimensional stability
	• Fast setting time
Precautions	• Always read the MSDS information for the product.
	• Base paste and catalyst paste
	• Flush eyes with plenty of water.

- Wash skin with soap and water.
  - If symptoms persist, seek medical attention.
- Avoid eye and skin contact and ingestion.
- Wear protective eyeglasses.
- Wear protective rubber gloves.
- Use rubber apron to protect clothing.
- Do not eat, drink, or smoke when using product.

Mixing and Setting Time	• Mix material for 30 to 45 seconds.
	• Total working time: 2.5 minutes.

Polyjel NF Polyether Final Impression Material *Continued*

Directions   After the tray is selected, the PPE is in place, and the patient is prepared for the procedure:

1. Measure the required quantity of Polyjel base and catalyst onto mixing pad.

2. The material is dispensed in equal lengths not equal amounts within 45 seconds.

3. Spatulate with broad blade spatula and mix until streak free.

4. Place into the oral cavity and remove when set.

5. Material must be poured within 2 weeks.

Aquasil Smart Wetting Vinyl Polysiloxane Final Impression Material

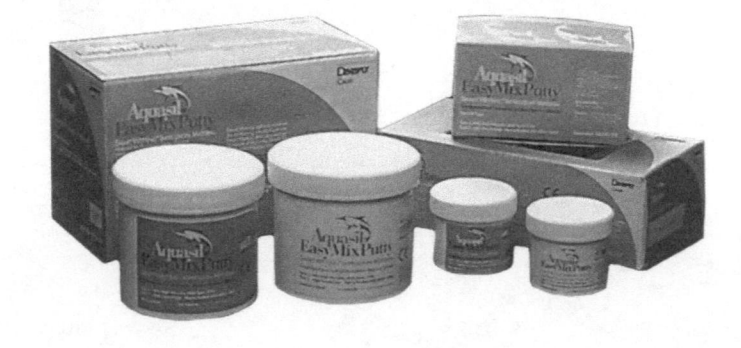

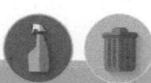

Use
- Suitable for all impression techniques for which high-viscosity materials would be desired by the operator.
- This material can be used for duplication of models.

Composition Aquasil Impression Material is a quadrafunctional hydrophilic addition reaction silicone.

Properties
- Designed to minimize the problems of voids, bubbles, pulls, and drags
- Wettability

- High tear strength
- Available in broad range, many viscosities in regular and fast set
- Mint-flavored

Precautions
- Always read the MSDS information for the product.
- Use safety glasses and gloves.
- Avoid eye and skin contact and ingestion.

Aquasil Smart Wetting Vinyl Polysiloxane Final Impression Material *Continued*

Mixing and Setting Time

	Regular	Fast Set
Working time	2 min 15 sec to 2 min 45 sec	1 min 15 sec to 1 min 45 sec
Setting time from start of mix	5 min	3 min

Directions After the tray is selected, the PPE is in place, and the patient is prepared for the procedure:

1. Insert the cartridge into the extruder.
2. Attach the mixing tip to the cartridge.
3. Squeeze the trigger to mix and dispense material.
4. Material will stop flowing when the trigger is released.

Extrude Vinyl Polysiloxane Final Impression Material

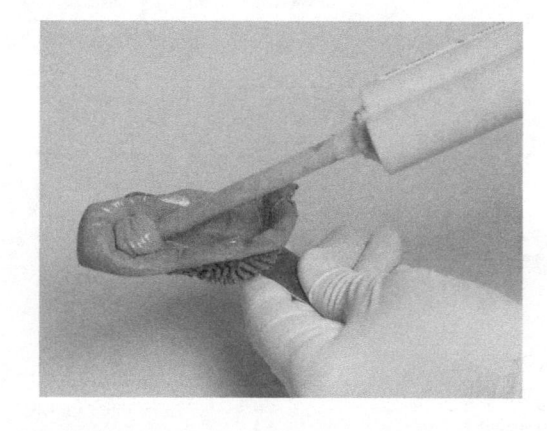

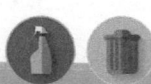

Use
Suitable for all crown and bridge, edentulous, and implant impressions

Properties
- Thixotropic, nonslumping tray material
- Available in cartridge, putty (jars), and tube
- High flow and tear strength
- Putty has 3-year shelf life
- Dimensional stability

- Tasteless
- Odorless

Precautions
- May cause mild skin irritation
- May cause irritation to the eyes
- May be harmful if swallowed
- May cause mild irritation if inhaled

Extrude Vinyl Polysiloxane Final Impression Material *Continued*

Mixing and Setting Time

	Total Working Time from Start of Mix	Minimum Removal Time from Start of Mix
Extrude Wash	3 min	6 min
Extrude Medium	3 min	6 min
Extrude Extra	3 min	6 min
Extrude MPV	2 min 15 sec	5 min 15 sec
Extrude Putty	2 min	6 min

Directions   After the tray is selected, the PPE is in place, and the patient is prepared for the procedure:

1. Insert the cartridge into the extruder.
2. Attach the mixing tip to the cartridge.
3. Squeeze the trigger to mix and dispense material.
4. The material will stop flowing when the trigger is released.

Honigum Hydophilic Final Impression Material

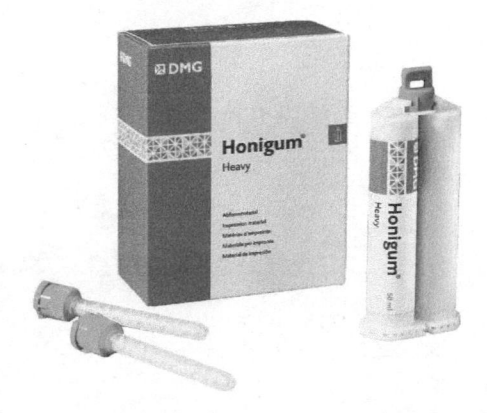

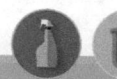

Use	• Crown and bridge impressions • Inlay and onlay impressions • All types of pickup impression—e.g., for implants	**Properties**	• Patented microcrystalline wax matrix chemistry • Pressure-sensitive variable viscosity • Mild honey aroma for great patient acceptance • Available in syringe and MixStar cartridges
Composition	• Addition curing polysiloxanes (an addition of silicone or a viscous liquid that helps in curing into a rubberized material) • Silicone dioxide • Food pigments • Additives • Platinum catalyst	**Precautions**	• Hand and skin protection: Use rubber gloves. • Eye protection: Use goggles. • Consult a physician in case of ingestion.

Honigum Hydophilic Final Impression Material *Continued*

Mixing and Setting Time

	Automix Heavy	Automix Heavy Fast	MixStar Heavy	MixStar Heavy Fast
Working time	2 min	1 min 15 sec	2 min 15 sec	1 min 15 sec
Recommended time in mouth	3 min 15 sec	2 min	3 min 15 sec	2 min

Directions   After the tray is selected, the PPE is in place, and the patient is prepared for the procedure:

1. Insert the cartridge into the extruder.
2. Attach the mixing tip to the cartridge.
3. Squeeze the trigger to mix and dispense material.
4. The material will stop flowing when the trigger is released.
5. Insert the tray into the patient's mouth; hold time varies according to material used.
6. Remove from patient's mouth, rinse, and disinfect.
7. Wait 30 minutes and pour the impression.

Hydrocolloid-Reversible Hydrocolloid Final Impression Material

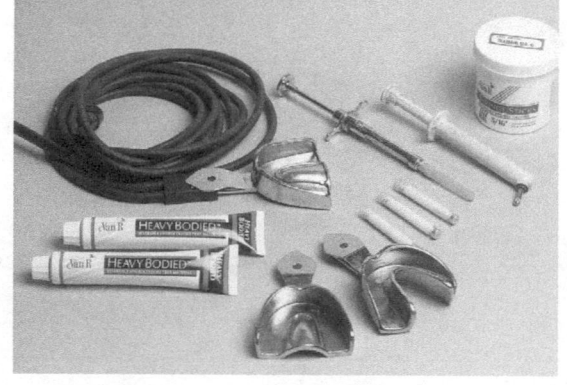

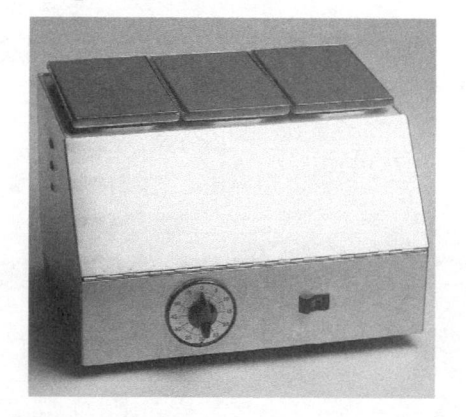

Use	• Crown and bridge impressions • Inlay and onlay impressions
Composition	Made from water and the ocean's agar
Properties	• Wetness. • Small amounts of blood and saliva do not affect the accuracy of the impression. • Available in syringes and tubes. • Must be used with a hydrocolloid machine.

Precautions • No principal hazardous components
• No occupational control measures needed

Mixing and Setting Time

Acculoid, Lavender, Extra Strength
• 5 minutes tempering at 110°F (43°C)
• 7 minutes cooling in the mouth with room temperature water
• Stores 5 days once liquefied

Hydrocolloid-Reversible Hydrocolloid Final Impression Material *Continued*

AgarLoid, Blue, Fast Tempering
- 4 minutes tempering at 110°F (43°C)
- 5 minutes cooling in the mouth with room temperature water
- Stores 5 days once liquefied

Slate, Gray, High Strength
- 5 minutes tempering at 110°F (43°C)
- 5 minutes cooling in the mouth with room temperature water
- Stores 4 days once liquefied

Qwik, Chocolate
- 3 minutes tempering at 110°F (43°C)
- 3 minutes cooling in the mouth with room temperature water
- Stores 3 days once liquefied

Directions   After the tray is selected, the PPE is in place, and the patient is prepared for the procedure:

1. Remove the tube from the storage compartment of the hydrocolloid conditioner. Fill the water-cooled tray and place in the tempering bath.

2. Set the timer to the correct time for tempering according to the material being used.

3. After the time has concluded, remove the syringe material that is in the cartiloid and place it into the syringe. Attach a hydrocolloid syringe tip to the cartiloid and apply pressure to the syringe to expel a small amount of material while taking to the operator to use. This ensures that the material does not set up in the tip.

4. Remove the impression from the tempering bath and place 2 × 2 gauze over the material to dry the top surface. Attach the tubing to the impression and hand it to the operator to place into the mouth. Remove the 2 × 2 prior to placement.

5. After the impression is seated in the mouth, attach the tubing to the water source and start the water flowing. Set the timer.

6. Remove from patient's mouth, rinse, and pour immediately.

Jet Self Cure Temporary Crown Acrylic

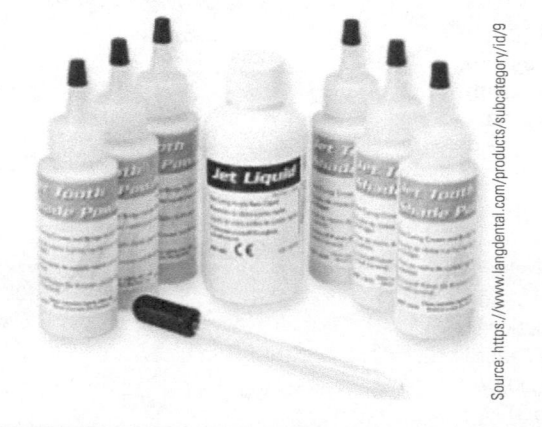

Source: https://www.langdental.com/products/subcategory/id/9

Use	To make a provisional (temporary) restoration	**Jet Liquid**	• Highly flammable.
Composition	• Hazardous ingredient • Methyl methacrylate		• It is irritating to eyes, respiratory system, and skin. It may cause sensitization by skin contact. High atmospheric concentrations may lead to irritation of the respiratory tract and anesthetic effects. Repeated and/or prolonged contact may cause dermatitis.
Properties	• Methyl methacrylate hardness • Easy to polish and trim • Available in a wide range of shades, including dark and light incisal and clear	**Jet Powder**	• Primary routes of entry: Skin or eyes, inhalation of dusts. • Avoid inhalation of dust. Keep dust out of eyes to prevent possible irritation.
Precautions	Use appropriate PPE and follow all Occupational Safety and Health Administration (OSHA) guidelines.		

Jet Self Cure Temporary Crown Acrylic *Continued*

Mixing and Setting Time
- No mixing is required.
- 1 to 2 minutes working time.
- Setting time:
  - 2 minutes intraoral time.
  - 6 to 9 minutes total cure time.

Directions

1. Before preparing the teeth, take a preimpression of the teeth to be restored.
2. Rinse the impression and remove excess water from it.
3. Select the shade of Jet Powder desired.
4. Place a small amount of Jet Liquid in all abutment teeth and pontic areas.
5. Add sufficient Jet Powder to absorb the liquid.
6. Abutment and pontic areas should be slightly overfilled.
7. Coat the prepared teeth and adjacent gingival tissues with a thin film of petroleum jelly.
8. Wait approximately 30 to 60 seconds until the Jet mixture reaches the desired flow.
9. Place the impression in the mouth with pressure.
10. Remove the impression from the mouth before exothermic heat begins, approximately 3 minutes.
11. Reseat impression in mouth and place in and out of patient's mouth until material reaches a rubbery state and cannot be distorted. Place and remove the Jet temporary in the oral cavity.
12. Allow the Jet temporary to cure.
13. Remove the Jet crown or bridge from the impression.
14. Place in the oral cavity to adjust bite.
15. Trim and polish as necessary.
16. Clean patient's teeth of any residual silicone lube. Place provisional into mouth and secure with suitable temporary cement.

Luxatemp

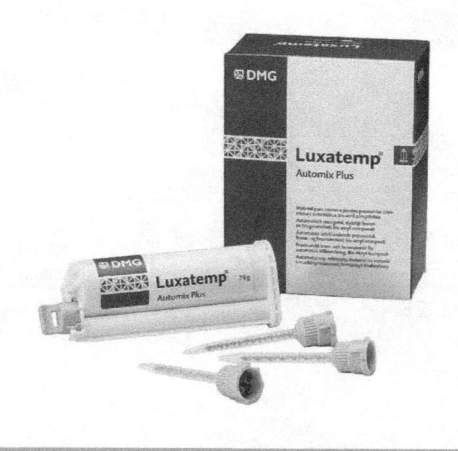

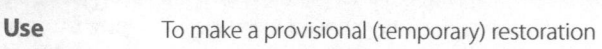

Use	To make a provisional (temporary) restoration
Composition	• Urethane dimethacrylate
	• Aromatic dimethacrylate
	• Glycol methacrylate
Properties	• Excellent marginal adaptation.
	• Provisional restoration is easily removable.
	• No heat damage.
	• Does not contain liquid monomers.

- Does not need to be removed and replaced multiple times during polymerization.
- No hand mixing or reloading syringes.
- No need for mixing pads, spatulas, or application syringes.
- Self-sealing mixing tips allow easy control of the material being used.
- Material available in cartridge gun and tip.
- Luxaglaze is available to provisional restoration for high polish.

Luxatemp *Continued*

- Luxaflow, which is light-cured, is available to repair provisional restoration.
- Luxatemp with Fluorescence is available to make temporaries look as good as final in all lighting conditions.
- Luxatemp Solar Plus is a light-cured format for temporization.

Precautions Use appropriate PPE and follow all OSHA guidelines.
- None, if handled according to directions
- Irritating to eyes, respiratory system, and skin

Mixing and Setting Time
- No mixing is required.
- Setting time:
  - 0 to 45 seconds: insertion in the mouth.
  - 2 to 3 minutes: removal from the mouth.
  - 6 to 7 minutes: end of setting.

Directions

1. Take preimpression or make matrix prior to teeth being prepared.
2. Dry-prepared and lightly lubricate prepared teeth and surrounding tissue with petroleum jelly or a similar separating medium.
3. Match shade and place appropriate Luxatemp cartridge into the application instrument.
4. Dispense Luxatemp into the preimpression or matrix, first on the occlusal surfaces and then bring it gingivally, overbuilding it slightly.
5. Insert the impression or matrix, filled with Luxatemp within 45 seconds with gentle pressure over the prepared teeth and hold firmly in place.
6. Approximately 2 to 3 minutes from start of mix the provisional crown or bridge can easily be removed together with the impression from the prepared teeth.
7. The crown or bridge may be contoured and polished after 4 additional minutes. Remove the soft, sticky inhibition layer on the surface of the Luxatemp restoration by wiping with ethyl alcohol.
8. The temporary can be trimmed.
9. Upon completion, the surface of the temporary can be glazed with Luxaglaze and light-cured.

Protemp™ Crown Temporization Material

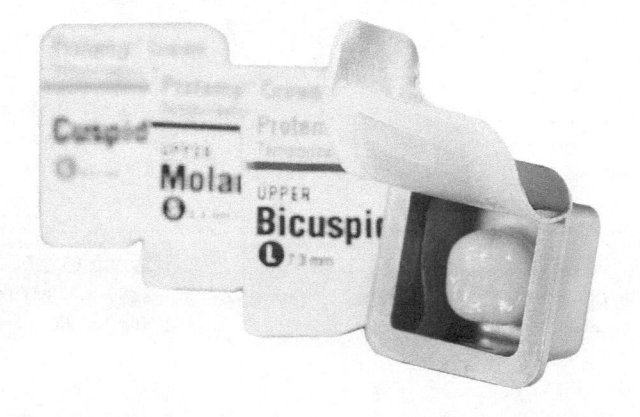

Use

To make short-term temporary restorations

Composition
- Diacetate
- Glass powder
- Substituted pyrimidine

Properties
- No preimpression or matrix
- Easier to obtain good occlusion
- Easier to obtain interproximal contact
- Very low oxygen-inhibited layer
- No odor

- Low exothermic temperatures
- Light-cured on demand
- Anatomical shape similar to natural dentition that you can polish and customize
- Can be repaired using conventional composite or flowable materials

Precautions
- Use appropriate PPE and follow all OSHA guidelines.
- No critical hazards.

Protemp™ Crown Temporization Material *Continued*

Mixing and Setting Time
- No mixing is required.
- Set time: Operator controlled due to light-curing:
  - Tack-cure buccal surface 2 to 3 seconds.
  - Tack-cure lingual surface 2 to 3 seconds.
  - Tack-cure occlusal surface 2 to 3 seconds.
  - Light-cure outside of the mouth for 60 seconds.

Directions

1. Determine the mesial-distal width and temporary crown height using the 3M ESPE crown size tool. Refer to size selection chart to select the appropriate size crown.
2. Remove the crown from sealed crown case.
3. Hold film between the thumb and finger. Carefully remove film from Protemp Crown.
4. Measure the height of the adjacent teeth as a guide to the amount of excess to be trimmed off the crown.
5. Follow the gingival contour when trimming excess material from the crown.
6. Place the crown on the prepared tooth and adapt, shape, and establish interproximal contact for a snug fit onto the moist preparation.
7. Have the patient gently close the mouth to adapt buccal surface and establish occlusion. Adapt buccal margin and adjust occlusion.
8. While patient is in occlusion, check the buccal margin. Tack-cure the buccal surface for 2 to 3 seconds.
9. Have the patient open the mouth for adaptation of the lingual surface.
10. Apply finger pressure to the buccal surface to prevent dislodging of the temporary crown. Adapt the lingual margin.
11. Tack-cure the lingual surface for 2 to 3 seconds.
12. Tack-cure the occlusal surface for 2 to 3 seconds.
13. Gently remove the Protemp Crown from the preparation. Light-cure outside the mouth for 60 seconds.
14. Trial fit the cured crown and adjust occlusion, trim margin, and contour if necessary. Finish using a fine carbide bur and 3M ESPE Sof-Lex™.
15. Polish the ProTemp Crown using a dry muslin rag wheel or polishing brush.

UniFast Light Cure Temporary Crown Acrylic

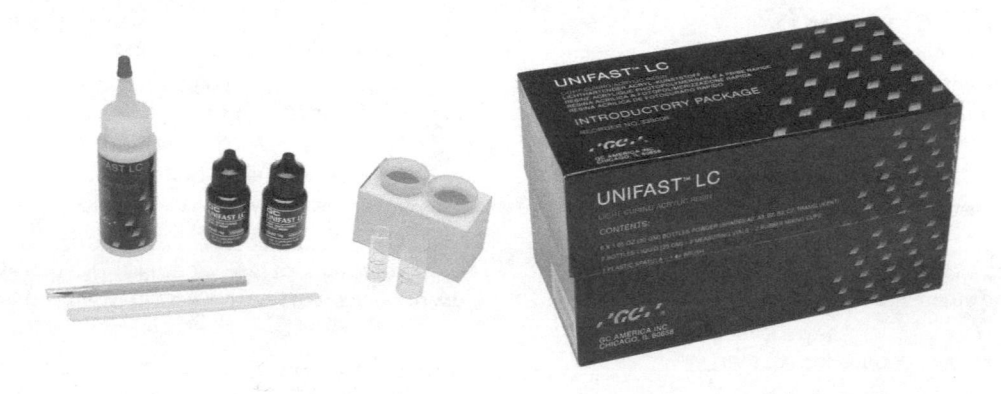

Use
To make a provisional (temporary) restoration

Composition Hazardous ingredients: methylmethacrylate

Properties
- Five shades and translucent.
- Dense, nonporous.
- Light-cured.
- Operator has control over working time.
- Partial cure possible.
- Glaze available.

Precautions
- Use appropriate PPE and follow all OSHA guidelines.
- Inhalation may cause nose and throat irritation. It may cause nervous system depression. Reports have associated repeated and prolonged overexposure with brain damage and nervous system damage. It may cause irritation or burning of eyes, skin, and mucous membranes. Repeated exposure may cause skin burns and allergic reaction. It may cause abnormal liver and kidney function.

UniFast Light Cure Temporary Crown Acrylic *Continued*

Directions

1. Take a preimpression prior to cutting the preparation.
2. Mix powder and liquid quickly for 10 to 15 seconds.
3. Pour Unifast LC mixture into the impression.
4. Seat the impression back into its original position.
5. Hold the impression in place for 2 minutes.
6. Remove the impression from the mouth. Carefully remove the rubber-like Unifast from the impression, trim off the extra, and replace it into the mouth.
7. Partially cure the resin while having the patient bite in occlusion.
8. Remove the partially cured material from the mouth and cure any area that may not have been exposed to the curing light.
9. Adjust occlusion and shape and final trim.

Digital 3D Scanners

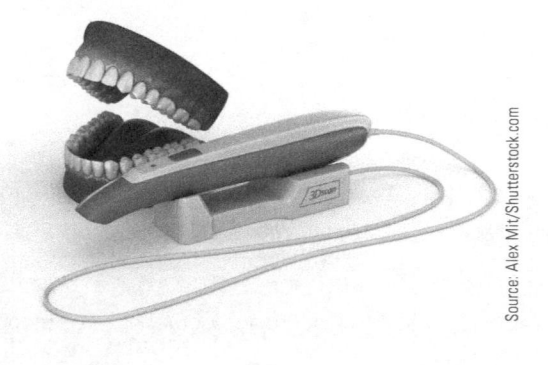

Source: Alex Mit/Shutterstock.com

Use	• To obtain a virtual impression of the teeth • Transmits the obtained information to the in-office or professional dental laboratory for its use (e.g., to construct crowns, etc.)
Composition	• A handheld scanner that is placed into the oral cavity to obtain a digital image. • The image is then saved and used in office to design and fabricate a crown or is sent to a professional lab for design and fabrication of a crown. • Some units require powder on the teeth to obtain the impression.

Notes

Complete System

- The system can scan, design, and fabricate within the dental office.
- The system can scan and then send to a professional lab.

Incomplete system

- The system can scan and then send to a professional lab.

Computer-Aided Design (CAD) and Computer-Aided Manufacturing (CAM) Systems

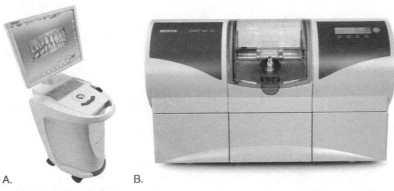

A. B.

Use	• To obtain a virtual impression of the teeth • To design restoration using software • Can be scanned and sent to a dental laboratory for design and fabrication of crown or scanned and designed and fabricated in the office • A specially designed machine to mill the restoration from ceramic blocks	• A computer with a scanner to obtain the impression intraorally. • Uses a specially designed machine to mill the restoration from ceramic blocks. • Software to obtain the image, design the restoration, and send it to the milling unit. • A specially designed milling unit that uses the directions from the software and cuts the ceramic block to the specifications.
Composition	• Considered a "Complete" system owing to the availability to scan, design, and fabricated the crown in the dental office.	

Computer-Aided Design (CAD) and Computer-Aided Manufacturing (CAM) Systems *Continued*

- Ceramic blocks in various shades
  A. Cerec CAD System
  B. Cerec CAM System

Notes
- Powder is normally used to obtain an image.
- The Cerec scanner uses a blue-light LED camera and the E4D scanner uses a red-light laser to obtain the virtual image.
- The restorations can be milled in the office, which saves the patient from wearing a provisional restoration and coming back for another appointment.
- Auxiliary personnel can become proficient in designing the restorations to assist the dentist with the procedure.
- Some systems will mill bridges and others will do only individual crowns.
- The unit can be moved from room to room for easier access to patients.
- The restoration can be designed, milled, polished, glazed, and seated in one appointment.

Cement Mixing Spatula

Use	To mix dental cements and materials
Composition	Single-ended flat spatula and handle
Notes	• The spatula is flexible or rigid and allows proper manipulation of materials.
	• It is made of stainless steel.
	• The spatula is sterilizable.
	• The edge of the spatula can be used to gather the materials for use.
	• It is available in a range of sizes.

Wooden Bite Stick

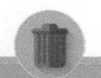

Use	To aid in seating the permanent crown during adaptation and cementation
Composition	Wooden bite stick, also known as an orangewood stick; 6 inches long and 3/16 inch in diameter
Notes	• Sticks come in a range of sizes. • They are made of soft wood.

TempBond, TempBond NE, and TempBond Clear

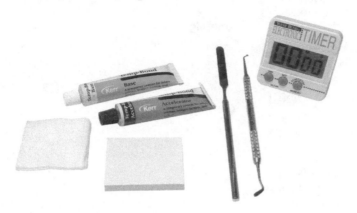

Use	• To cement temporary restorations • To temporarily cement for trial cementations
Composition	• TempBond-Accelerator: eugenol and oil of cloves • Temp Bond-Base: zinc oxide, mineral oil, and cornstarch • TempBond NE-Accelerator: resin, ortho ethoxybenzoic acid, carnauba wax, and octanoic acid • TempBond NE-Base: zinc oxide, mineral oil, and cornstarch • TempBond Clear-Resin-based: uncured urethane diacrylate ester monomer, mineral fillers, activators, and fillers

Properties	• Flows easily. • Strong enough for temporary cementation. • Withstands mastication forces. • Seals the margins and prevents leakage. • Easy to mix and clean up. • Easy to remove. • Matches dentin color. • TempBond NE will not interfere with the polymerization of resin cements and acrylic temporaries. It has the same flow and retentive qualities.

TempBond, TempBond NE, and TempBond Clear *Continued*

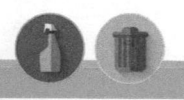

- There are three delivery systems: two-paste, automix syringe, and unidose packets.
- Unidose packets are ideal to give patients who are traveling in case they lose their temporary restoration.
- TempBond Clear has the same properties as TempBond and is also a dual-cure material.

Precautions
- May be irritating to the eyes and skin.
- Irritating to the respiratory system. Move the exposed person to fresh air.
- If ingested, contact a physician.

Mixing and Setting Time
- Mixing time is 30 seconds.
- Working time is 1½ minutes.
- Setting time is 7 minutes for TempBond and TempBond NE, and 5½ minutes for TempBond Clear.

Notes
To accelerate the set with the TempBond Clear, light-cure all surfaces for 20 seconds.

Directions

Tube or Paste

1. Dispense equal lengths of the base and accelerator on the mixing pad that is provided. Length and size is determined by the size of the temporary restoration.

2. Replace the caps tightly.
3. Mix for approximately 30 seconds until the mix is smooth, creamy, and uniform in color.
4. Wipe off the spatula and using a cement spatula or plastic filling instrument (PFI), place TempBond cement into the temporary restoration.
5. Firmly seat the restoration in the mouth and once the material is set, remove the excess cement from the buccal/facial and lingual surfaces with a scaler and floss the interproximal surfaces.

Unidose

1. Using scissors, cut along the dotted line.
2. Squeeze the material on a mixing pad.
3. Mix for 30 seconds.
4. Continue as described with the tube techniques.

Syringe

1. Remove the cap from the syringe and dispense a small amount onto a gauze or paper pad.
2. Place the automix tip on the syringe and turn until locked in place.
3. Material is ready to dispense directly into the temporary or on the tooth.

TempoCem, TempoCem NE, TempoCem NE SmartMix; TempoCem ID

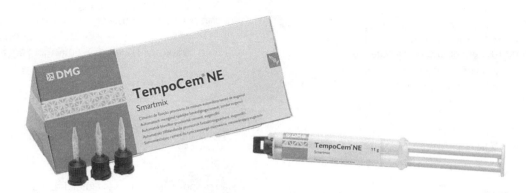

Use

Temporary cement for attaching all kinds of temporaries, such as crowns, bridges, inlays, and onlays

Composition

- TempoCem: Catalyst consists of natural resins, eugenol, and additives.
- TempoCem NE formulas: Catalyst consists of natural resins, fatty acids, and additives.
- Base for both materials is zinc oxide, paraffin, and additives. The noneugenol materials are used with resin and resin-reinforced glass ionomer materials.

- TempoCem ID: "Invisible" cement used for resin temporaries.

Properties

- Comes in eugenol and noneugenol formulas
- Resists forces of mastication
- Securely retains the temporary restoration
- Easy to remove
- Resistant to saliva, and protects the gingival tissues
- Radiopaque on x-rays
- Easy flow, and no heat generated

TempoCem, TempoCem NE, TempoCem NE SmartMix; TempoCem ID *Continued*

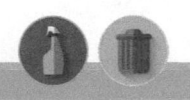

- Protects against thermal sensitivity
- Comes in a variety of forms with automixing and direct dispensing

Precautions
- May be irritating to the eyes and skin.
- Irritating to the respiratory system. Move exposed person to fresh air.
- If ingested, contact a physician.

Mixing and Setting Time
- No mixing is required.
- Working time is 1 minute.
- Setting time is 1 to 3 minutes.

Directions

Smartmix

1. Prepare the tooth and the temporary by rinsing thoroughly and air drying.
2. Remove the cap from the Smartmix syringe and dispense a test amount on a paper or gauze pad.
3. Place a disposable syringe tip on the syringe and twist to secure.
4. Dispense the amount needed onto the tooth or into the temporary restoration.

5. Place the temporary restoration on the tooth and apply pressure until the material has set.
6. Remove any excess material from the margins.

Cartridge

1. Prepare the tooth and temporary by rinsing thoroughly and air drying.
2. Prepare the DMG Type 25 Applicator Gun by releasing the small lever in the back, and make sure the slide is in position.
3. Lift the top level and slide the cartridge into place. The notch on the bottom of the cartridge aligns with the notch in the gun. Push down firmly to lock into place.
4. Remove the cap on the cartridge and dispense a small portion. Place the disposable cannula on the cartridge by lining up the notches. Twist it clockwise 90 degrees to lock into place.
5. Pull the trigger to dispense the material.
6. When finished, remove the cannula and replace the storage cap on the end of the capsule.

Zone Temporary Cement

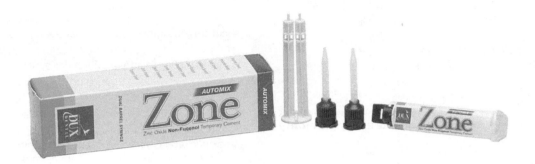

Use
- Temporary cement for all provisional restorations
- Temporary cement for trial cementation of permanent restorations for evaluation purposes

Composition Crystalline zinc oxide preparation

Properties
- Smooth
- Rigid-setting
- Consistent retention
- Easy removal and clean-up
- Compatible with provisional materials

- Does not soften, craze, or discolor polycarbonate or acrylic crown forms
- Kind to the tooth
- Available in tubes, unidose, and syringe
- Noneugenol

Precautions
- May be irritating to the eyes and skin.
- Irritating to the respiratory system. Move exposed person to fresh air.
- If ingested, contact a physician.

Zone Temporary Cement *Continued*

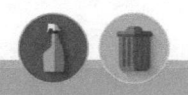

Mixing and Setting Time
- Mixing time is 30 seconds.
- Working time is approximately 1½ minutes.
- Setting time is 5 to 7 minutes.

Directions

Standard Two Tubes

1. Dispense equal lengths of the base and accelerator onto the mixing pad that is provided. Length and size is determined by the size of the temporary restoration.
2. Replace the caps tightly.
3. Mix for approximately 30 seconds until the mix is smooth, creamy, and uniform in color.
4. Wipe off spatula and using a PFI, place Zone cement on the tooth or temporary restoration.
5. Firmly seat the restoration in the mouth; once the material is set, remove the excess cement with a scaler.

Unidose

1. Using scissors, cut along the dotted line.
2. Squeeze the material onto a mixing pad.
3. Mix for 30 seconds.
4. Place in temporary restoration with a PFI. Seat the restoration in the mouth and hold in place until set. Remove excess cement.

Automix Syringe and Autoaspirating Dual-Cartridge, Single-Plunger Syringe

1. Remove the cap from the syringe and dispense a small amount on a gauze or paper pad to be sure the materials are mixing evenly.
2. Place the automix tip on the syringe and turn until locked in place.
3. Material is ready to dispense directly into the temporary restoration or onto the tooth.

Zinc Phosphate Cement-Fleck's Cement

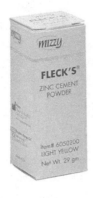
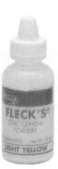
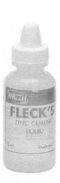
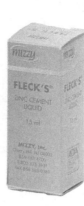

Use	• Permanent cement for indirect restorations including inlays, onlays, crowns, and bridges
	• Orthodontic cement
	• High-strength base

Composition
• Powder: zinc oxide, magnesium oxide, and pigments
• Liquid: phosphoric acid and water

Properties
• High strength
• May be irritating to the pulp, so a liner is used first
• Has an exothermic reaction when mixed

• Specific guidelines for mixing to minimize the temperature rise and slow the reaction process and improve the strength

Precautions
• Eye and skin irritation possible.
• Should not be ingested.
• Avoid cross-contamination.

Mixing and Setting Time
• Mixing time is 2 minutes.
• Working time is 3½ minutes.
• Setting time is 2 to 8 minutes.

Zinc Phosphate Cement-Fleck's Cement *Continued*

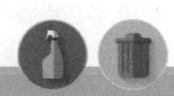

Directions

1. Obtain a clean, cool, dry glass slab and flexible cement spatula.
2. Fluff the powder and dispense appropriate amount for cementation.
3. Divide the powder in half, then into fourths, then divide one of the fourths into two eighths, and then one of the eighths into two sixteenths.
4. Dispense the liquid (6 to 12 drops) holding the dropper vertical to the glass slab.
5. Incorporate one-sixteenth portion of powder into the liquid and mix for 15 seconds. Repeat by adding the second sixteenth and mix for 15 seconds.
6. Add the eighth portion and mix the material using three quarters of the glass slab for 15 seconds.
7. Add one of the quarters and spatulate for 20 seconds; follow by a second quarter, then spatulate again for 20 seconds.
8. Add enough of the last quarter of powder to achieve the consistency the dentist requires. Mix should be completed in 2 minutes.
9. For cementation, the consistency is fluid and should follow the spatula up about an inch from the glass slab.
10. Using the PFI, prepare to pass the cement to the dentist. Have the gauze ready to remove any excess cement from the spatula.
11. Clean the glass slab and spatula immediately.
12. For the base consistency, add more powder to the liquid until you reach a putty-like consistency and the cement can be rolled into a ball.

Polycarboxylate Cement-DurElon

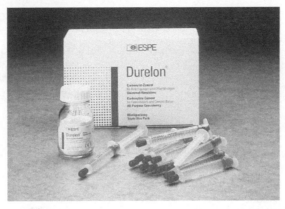

Use
- Permanent cement for crowns, bridges, inlays, and onlays
- Orthodontic cementation
- High-strength base

Composition
- Powder: zinc oxide with small amounts of magnesium oxide
- Stannous fluoride
- Liquid: polyacrylic acid copolymer in water
- Liquid comes in a squeeze bottle or calibrated syringe

Properties
- High strength
- Does not exhibit exothermic heat
- Bonds chemically to the tooth structure and mechanically to the restoration
- More viscous
- Less irritating
- Has a shelf life and should be discarded if the liquid discolors and becomes thick

Polycarboxylate Cement-DurElon *Continued*

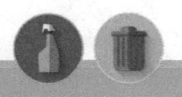

Precautions
- Eye and skin irritation possible.
- Should not be ingested.
- Avoid cross-contamination.

Mixing and Setting Time
- Mixing time is a minimum of 30 seconds.
- Working time is 2 minutes.
- Setting time is 5 to 10 minutes.

Directions

Powder and Squeeze Bottle

1. Gather the paper pad, cement spatula, powder, dosing rod, liquid, and gauze.
2. Fluff the powder and then, using the dosing rod, measure and dispense one scoop of powder onto the paper pad. Press the dosing rod into the powder and then, using the spatula, remove excess powder before placing on the paper pad.
3. Holding the squeeze bottle vertically, dispense two drops onto the paper pad next to the powder.
4. Mix all the powder into the liquid in one move and mix until a uniform, homogeneous consistency is attained—approximately 30 seconds.
5. Gather the cement and prepare to pass to the dentist. Use wet gauze to remove excess material before it sets on the spatula and placement instrument.

Powder and Calibrated Syringe

1. Prepare the powder as described above.
2. Dispense the liquid from the syringe using the calibrations. For one scoop of powder, use two scale units of liquid.
3. Mix all the powder into the liquid in one move until a uniform, homogeneous consistency is attained—approximately 30 seconds.

Glass Ionomer Cement Type I-Rely X

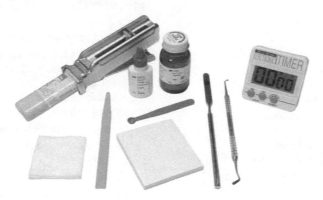

Use	• Cementing porcelain fused to metal crowns and bridges, amalgam composite, or glass ionomer core buildups
	• Metal inlays, onlays, and crowns
	• Prefabricated and cast postcementation
	• Cementation of orthodontic appliances
Composition	• Powder is a radiopaque fluoroaluminosilicate glass.
	• Liquid is an aqueous solution of modified polyalkenoic acid.
Properties	• High strength
	• Chemically adheres to tooth structure and restoration

- Releases fluoride
- Low solubility
- Low viscosity, nonstringy, slump-resistant mix
- Nonirritating
- Easy to mix and clean up

Precautions
- Eye and skin irritation possible
- Should not be ingested
- May cause mild respiratory irritation
- Contains hydroxyethyl methacrylate (HEMA)—a known allergen

Glass Ionomer Cement Type I-Rely X *Continued*

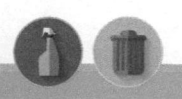

Mixing and Setting Time	• Mixing time is 30 seconds.
	• Working time is 2½ minutes from the start of the mix at room temperature.
	• Setting time is within 10 minutes.

Directions Comes in a powder/liquid system and a clicker dispenser system

Powder/Liquid System

1. Gather a paper pad, cement spatula, and gauze.
2. Keep the caps on the powder and liquid when not in use.
3. Fluff the powder. Using the specific scoop that is supplied with Rely X, dispense three scoops of powder onto the paper pad. Three scoops of powder and three drops of liquid is adequate to seat one typical crown. Use an equal number of powder scoops and liquid drops.
4. Holding the squeeze bottle vertically, dispense three uniform-sized drops.
5. Bring all the powder into the liquid and mix in a small area to minimize water evaporation and maximize working time. Complete the mix in 30 seconds.
6. The mix should be smooth and uniform.
7. Prepare to pass the cement to the dentist. Use a gauze pad to wipe the excess from the spatula and PFI.

Clicker Dispenser System

1. Dispense one portion to ensure that the dispenser is working correctly.
2. Dispose of the test material and onto new paper squeeze the dispenser until you hear a clicking, continue to dispense one to three clicks depending on the restoration(s) to be cemented.
3. Mix the material into a homogeneous mix within 30 seconds. It is then ready for cementation.

Fuji-Glass Ionomer Type I Luting Cement

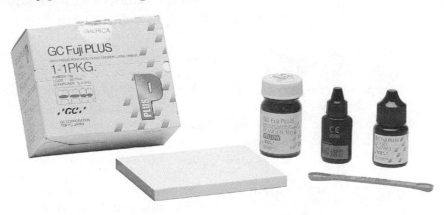

Use	• For final cementation of crown and bridge restorations • Metal inlays, onlays, posts • Orthodontic appliances	• Does not require a dry field • Low film thickness and low solubility • Easy to mix and clean up
Composition	• Powder: radiopaque fluoroaluminosilicate glass • Liquid: polyacrylic acid and water	**Precautions** • Eye and skin irritation possible • Should not be ingested • May cause mild respiratory irritation
Properties	• Strong direct bond • Marginal integrity for long-term restorations • Minimizes microleakage • Releases fluoride	**Mixing and** • Mixing time is 20 to 30 seconds, depending on the size of **Setting Time** the mix. • Setting time is approximately 5 minutes.

Fuji-Glass Ionomer Type I Luting Cement *Continued*

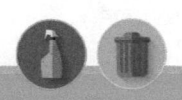

Directions

Powder/Liquid System

1. Gather the paper pad, cement spatula, and gauze.
2. Keep the caps on the powder and liquid when not in use.
3. Fluff the powder. Using the specific scoop that is supplied with Fuji, dispense one scoop of powder onto the paper pad. Divide the powder into two equal parts.
4. Holding the squeeze bottle vertically, dispense two uniform-sized drops.
5. Mix the first portion for 10 to 15 seconds with the liquid. Add the second portion and mix for 15 to 20 seconds.
6. Mix in a small area to minimize water evaporation and maximize working time. Complete the mix in 20 to 30 seconds.
7. The mix should be smooth and uniform.
8. Prepare to pass the cement to the dentist. Use a gauze pad to wipe the excess from the spatula and PFI.

Premeasured Capsules

1. Tap the capsule on a flat surface to fluff the powder.
2. Depress the button on the bottom of the capsule to activate.
3. Place the capsule in a high-speed amalgamator and triturate for 10 seconds.
4. Place in designated dispenser. It is ready to use.

Ketac-Cem Radiopaque, Ketac-Cem Aplicap, and Ketac-Cem Maxicap Type I Glass Ionomer

Use	All of these materials are used for permanent cementation of inlays, crowns, bridges, and orthodontic bands/brackets.
Composition	• Powder: calcium–aluminofluorosilicate glass • Liquid: polyacrylic acid and water
Properties	• High compressive strength • Adheres chemically to tooth structure • Very low solubility • Adheres to slightly moist tooth structure • Minimal film thickness

• Releases fluoride ions to tooth structure
• Comes in various forms for easy use and cleanup
• Nonirritating to the pulp

Precautions	• Eye and skin irritation possible • Should not be ingested • May cause mild respiratory irritation
Mixing and Setting Time	• Powder/liquid mix: Mixing time is 60 seconds. • Aplicap and MAXICAP: 10 seconds. • Setting time for all is 7 minutes.

Ketac-Cem Radiopaque, Ketac-Cem Aplicap, and Ketac-Cem Maxicap Type I Glass Ionomer *Continued*

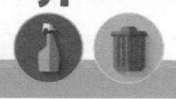

Directions

Powder/Liquid Mix

1. Gather a paper pad, cement spatula, and gauze.
2. Keep the caps on the powder and liquid when not in use.
3. Fluff the powder. Using the specific scoop that is supplied with Ketac-Cem, dispense one scoop of powder onto the paper pad.
4. Holding the squeeze bottle vertically, dispense two uniform-sized drops.
5. Mix the powder into the liquid in one portion. Mix for 60 seconds until the mix is smooth and has a glossy appearance. If the surface becomes dull, the setting reaction has started and the mix should be discarded.
6. Prepare to pass the cement to the dentist. Use a gauze pad to wipe the excess from the spatula and PFI.

Aplicap and MAXICAP

1. Both of these systems are prepared in the same manner; the difference is in the amount of cement. The MAXICAP capsules contain a larger mix than the Aplicaps.
2. Shake the capsule to fluff the powder and then place in the designated activator to release the liquid into the powder in the capsule.
3. Place the capsule in the amalgamator and triturate for 10 seconds.
4. Remove the capsule from the amalgamator and place in the designated applier.
5. Materials are ready to dispense at this point.

Tray Setup for the Crown Preparation Appointment

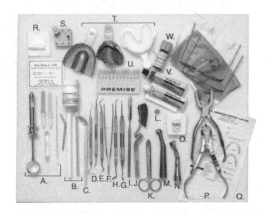

Use

This tray is set up when the patient comes into the office for the tooth to be prepared for the restoration. A preliminary (temporary) crown or bridge is normally placed over the prepared tooth until the final restoration can be fabricated unless a CAD/CAM system will be used.

Composition

A. Anesthetic syringe, carpule, needles, cotton swab, topical anesthetic, and Stik-Shield
B. Three-way syringe tip, high-volume evacuator (HVE) tip, and saliva ejector

C. Mouth mirror and explorer
D. Spoon excavator
E. Curette
F. Cotton pliers
G. Plastic instrument
H. Retraction cord placement instrument
I. Mixing spatula
J. Articulating paper and holder
K. Crown and collar scissors
L. Temporary crown

Tray Setup for the Crown Preparation Appointment *Continued*

M. High-speed handpiece
N. Latch-type contra-angle
O. Dental floss
P. Rubber dam placement instruments: punch, forceps, material, face mask, clamp with ligature, and frames
Q. Laboratory prescription

R. Cotton rolls and gauze
S. Miscellaneous burs
T. Alginate and final impression trays
U. Shade guide
V. Temporary bonding material
W. Retraction cord

Tray Setup for the Crown Cementation Appointment

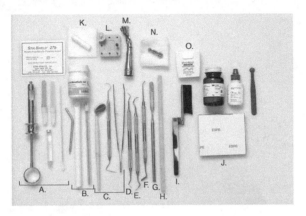

Use

This tray is set up when the patient comes into the office for the final crown or bridge to be cemented over the prepared tooth.

Composition

A. Anesthetic syringe, needles, carpule, cotton-tip applicator, topical -anesthetic, and Stik-Shield
B. Three-way syringe tip, HVE tip, saliva ejector
C. Basic setup: mouth mirror, expro (explorer and periodontal probe -combination), and cotton pliers
D. Spoon excavator

E. Curette
F. Plastic instrument
G. Mixing spatula
H. Wood bite stick
I. Articulation paper and holder
J. Final cementation materials
K. Cotton roll and gauze
L. Miscellaneous burs
M. Latch-type contra-angle
N. Bridge ready for cementation
O. Dental floss

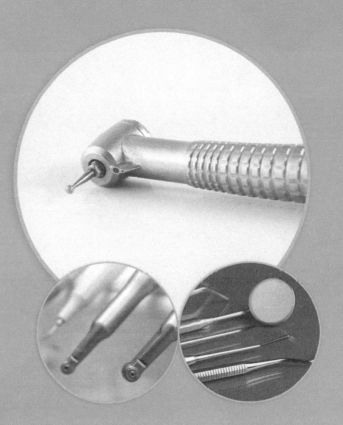

CHAPTER 18

Implant Instruments and Systems

Sterile Water With Tubing

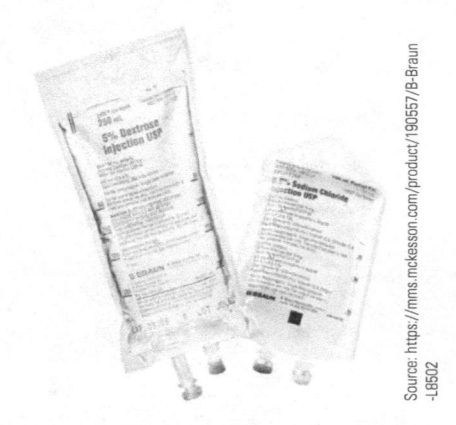

Source: https://mms.mckesson.com/product/190557/B-Braun -L8502

Use	Water used with implant handpieces for sterile field
Composition	Sterile, hypotonic nonpyrogenic water
Properties	• Clear, colorless, and odorless liquid
	• Contains no latex, polyvinyl chloride (PVC) or di-ethylhexyl phthalate (DEHP), bacteriostat or antimicrobial agents
	• In Excel 250 ml flexible plastic bag

Tissue Punch

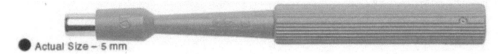

● Actual Size – 5 mm

Source: https://www.salvin.com/5-0mm-Sterile-Tissue-Punch-pluPUNCH-5.0.html

Use	To surgically remove tissue in order to expose underlying bone for implant placement	**Notes**	• A tissue punch is used when there is an excellent ridge. • It is used when there is good access to place the punch. • It can be disposable or sterilizable.
Composition	• Stainless steel edge • Tissue punch at one end of the single-handled instrument		

Electric Implant Drill System

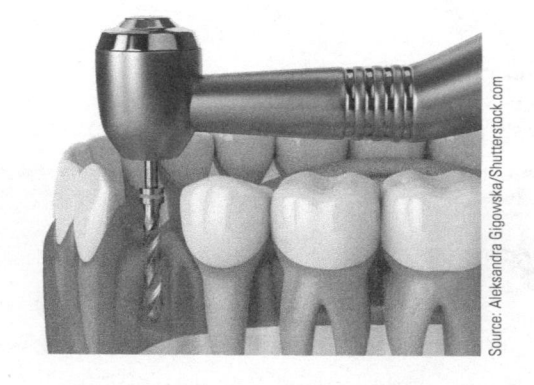

Source: Aleksandra Gigowska/Shutterstock.com

Use
- To create a hole in the bone with the precise apical diameter of the dental implant
- To place the implant once desired diameter and length is reached

Composition
- Electric handpiece unit has:
  - A rheostat.
  - A specialized handpiece.

- An attachment on handpiece connects to irrigation tubing.
- Adjustable speeds and water drip.

Notes
The black attachment for the irrigation drip system on the handpiece is sterilizable.

Implant Drill Kit

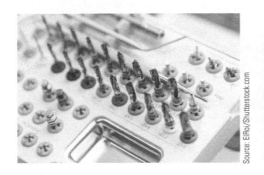

Source: ElRoi/Shutterstock.com

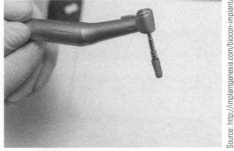

Source: http://implantgenesis.com/biocon-implant/

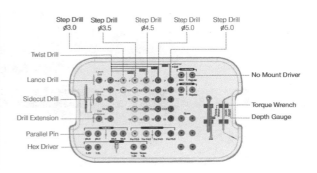

Step Drill ⌀3.0 · Step Drill ⌀3.5 · Step Drill ⌀4.5 · Step Drill ⌀5.0 · Step Drill ⌀5.0

Twist Drill
Lance Drill
Sidecut Drill
Drill Extension
Parallel Pin
Hex Driver

No Mount Driver
Torque Wrench
Depth Gauge

Use

An implant system can include the following:
- Pilot drills
- Implant drill stops
- Dental handpiece with no torque and latch-type contra-angle
- Seating tips
- Sulcus reamers
- Latch reamers
- Depth gauge/bone depth plugger
- Surgical mallet
- Paralleling pins
- Guide pin

Notes

- These drills come in various shapes and sizes that fit into a dental handpiece with a latch attachment that operates without torque.
- The procedure begins with the smallest drill, and the size of the drill gradually increases.
- Many different systems are available.

Implant Surgical Placement Guide

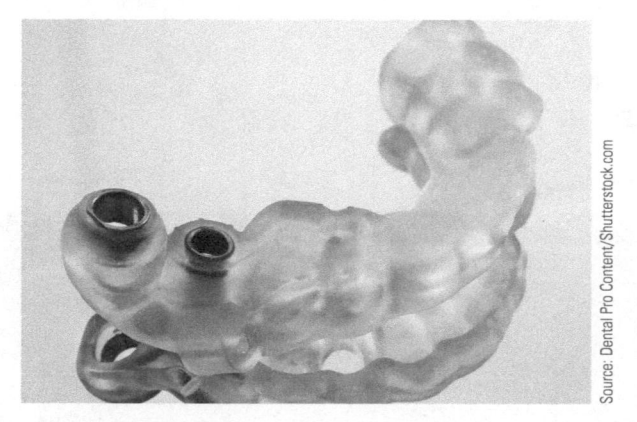

Source: Dental Pro Content/Shutterstock.com

Use	An implant system can include a customized template to align the implant at optimal angle for patient anatomy.
Notes	An impression is taken, and an acrylic guide can be fabricated in the dental office or in a lab.

Endosteal Implant

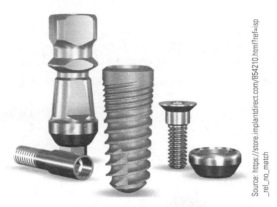

Source: https://store.implantdirect.com/854210.html?ref=isp_rel_no_match

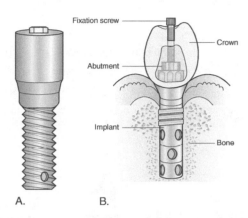

Fixation screw

Crown

Abutment

Implant

Bone

A.   B.

Use	To replace a single tooth
Composition	**A.** Endosteal implants with abutment and impression coping.
	B. Drawing of an osseointegrated implant in the bone after the healing stage. The abutment of the implant is covered with a crown that is held in place by a screw.

Notes

- Implants are available in a variety of styles and sizes.
- Implants are available in a variety of diameters and lengths.
- Many implant systems are available.
- Implant systems may be purchased in a single unit, sterile package.

Implant Healing Cap and Collars

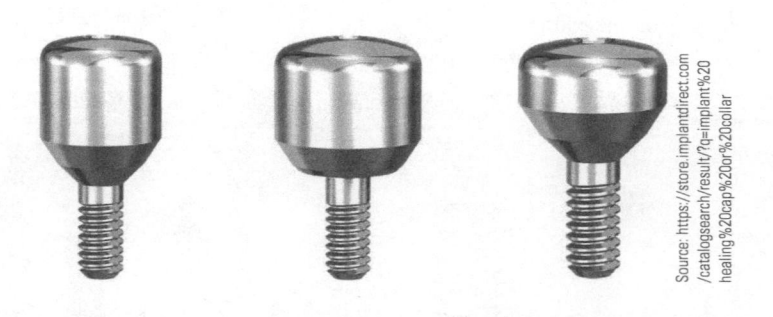

Source: https://store.implantdirect.com /catalogsearch/result/?q=implant%20 healing%20cap%20or%20collar

Use	Attached to implant directly after implant placement; to be worn during healing time
Properties	• Diameter of healing cap or collar must match the implant inserted
	• Height of the healing collar or cap is determined by operator preference and by height of surrounding teeth.
	• Removed after osseointegration is complete and patient is ready for restoration.

Implant Torque Wrench

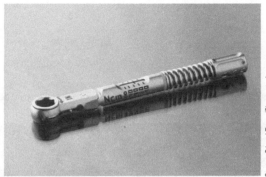

Source: Eduard Tanga/Shutterstock.com

Use	To tighten abutment of healing cap/collar to the implant
Properties	• Each brand of implant has its own specialized torque wrench.
	• Adjustable in Ncm (newton centimeters).
	• Some torque wrenches will "break," indicating that it is at the set NCM.

Implant Driver

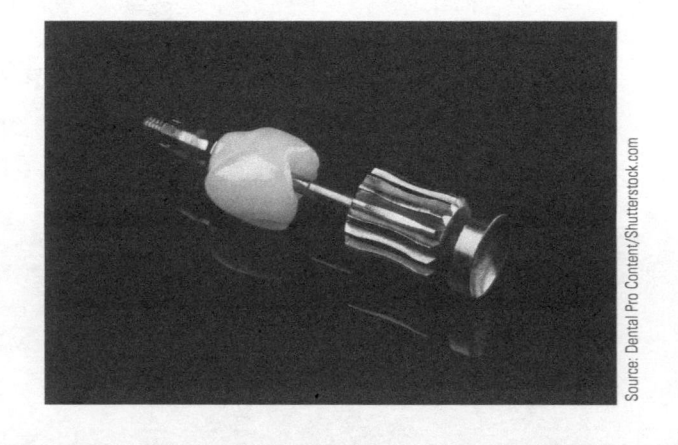

Source: Dental Pro Content/Shutterstock.com

Use	To tighten abutment of healing cap/collar to the implant by hand
Properties	Each brand of implant has its own specialized implant driver.

Implant Scaler

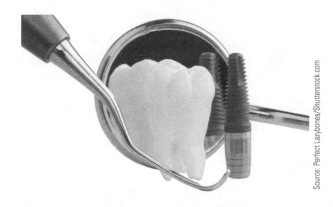

Source: Perfect Lazybones/Shutterstock.com

Use	To remove deposits from the dental implants
Parts	Shown is an implant scaler positioned around a dental implant.
Notes	• Various designs are available to reach around implants.
	• These are made of materials that will not scratch the titanium implant.

Screw-Retained Implant Prosthesis

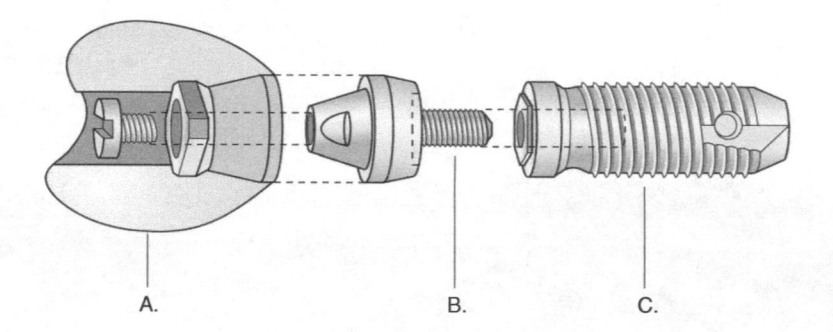

A.   B.   C.

Use	• To replace a single tooth
	• To replace a tooth and become an abutment for a bridge
Composition	**A.** Crown covering that screws in to attach the abutment to the prosthesis
	B. Screw to attach the abutment to the implant
	C. Implant that is placed into the bone
Notes	Most often, a composite restoration is placed over the screw that attaches the abutment to the prosthesis.

Cement-Retained Implant Prosthesis

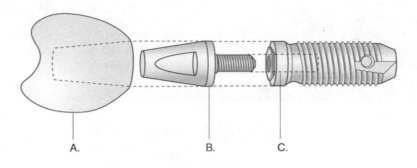

A.   B.   C.

Use	• To replace a single tooth • To replace a tooth and become an abutment for a bridge
Composition	**A.** Crown cemented onto the abutment **B.** Abutment post that is screwed into the implant **C.** Implant that screws into the bone
Notes	• Use transitional cement to attach the prosthesis to the abutment. • Use in case of problems with the implant.

Tray Setup for Dental Implant Surgery

A. Oral rinse with cup
B. Betadine with cup
C. Irrigation syringe
D. Low-speed handpiece
E. Sterile surgical drilling unit/implant kit
F. Sterile saline solution
G. Surgical high-volume evacuator (HVE) tip on 4 × 4 gauze
H. Bite block
I. Anesthetic setup

J. Mouth mirror
K. Sterile template
L. Scalpel and blade
M. Periosteal elevators
N. Rongeurs
O. Hemostat
P. Tissue forceps
Q. Cheek and tongue retractor
R. Surgical curette
S. Tissue scissors

T. Needle holder
U. Suture scissors
V. Sutures

Subperiosteal implants are used on patients whose dentures have failed because the alveolar bone has atrophied (commonly placed on the mandible).

Endosteal implants are used to replace a single tooth (placed into the bone and are most commonly used).

CHAPTER 19

Sterilization Equipment

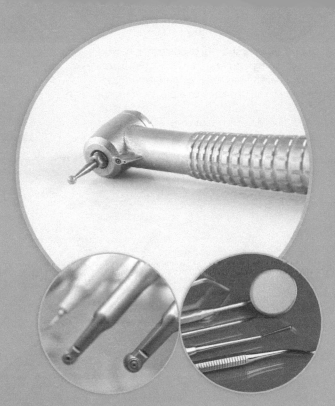

Sterilization Instrument Cassette

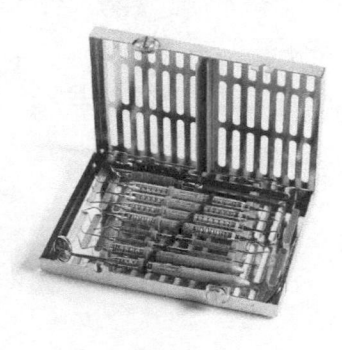
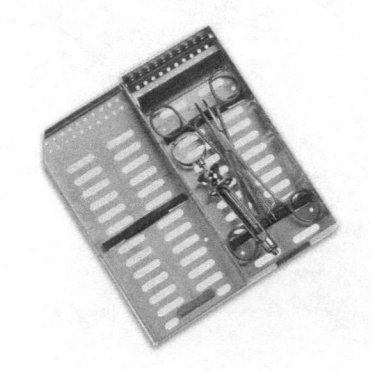

A.

B.

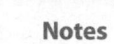

Use
- To contain instruments while being sterilized and/or stored
- To use for tray setup and organization

Composition
- Available in metal or plastic
- Available in various sizes
- Many different types of closing devices, but normally hinged on one side

Notes
- Often instruments are color-coded to make it easy to identify which instruments go in which sterilization cassette.
- Instruments in the cassette can be cleaned in the ultrasonic unit, rinsed, sterilized, and stored in the cassette.
- Dosage indicator strips may be added into the cassette prior to sterilization to that ensure sterilization has occurred.

Cassette Wrap and Label System

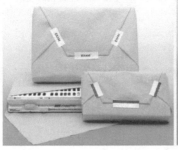
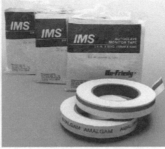
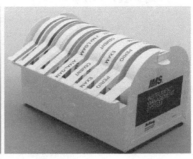

Use	• To wrap cassette during and after sterilization.
	• To use as a tray cover during the procedure.
	• To store the sterilized instruments.
	• The tape is used to secure the wrap and identify contents.
	• Include process indicator dye to verify sterilization.

Composition Wrapping paper, tape, or tape with identification labeling that is used to cover and secure sterilized items or cassettes

Notes
- They are available in a wide range of sizes.
- Tape or labeled tape can be used on sterilization pouches.
- Tape can be color coded.

Sterilization Pouches

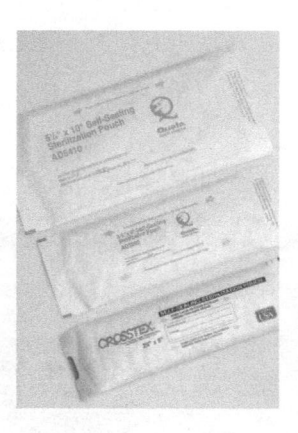

Use
- To hold instruments for sterilization
- Include process indicator dye to verify sterilization

Composition
- Made of clear plastic or paper
- Sealing strip on the open end
- Normally have area for labeling

Notes
- Instruments should be stored in these tightly sealed sterilizing pouches until ready for use.
- They are available in various sizes.
- A dosage indicator strip can be added into the sterilization bag to ensure sterilization.

Sharps Container

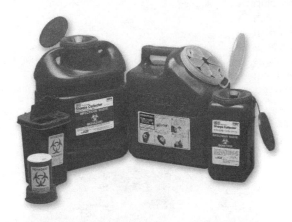

Use	To contain contaminated sharps, blades, wires, and needles
Composition	• Leak-proof container normally red in color
	• Puncture-resistant
	• Labeled
Notes	• Broken glass, anesthetic capsules, and orthodontic wires can also be placed in the sharps container.
	• When sharps disposal containers are full, they are sealed, sterilized using an autoclave if possible, and sent to an outside biohazard agency for safe disposal.

- Must be labeled according to Occupational Safety and Health Administration (OSHA) standards (biohazard).
- They are available in different shapes and sizes.
- Many states are requiring that sharps containers be in each operatory.

Ultrasonic Unit

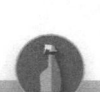

Use
- To clean and remove debris (bioburden) from dental instruments and burs
- To replace hand scrubbing instruments

Composition
- Basket
- Ultrasonic cleaning device
- Lid

Notes
- The ultrasonic cleaning unit significantly reduces the high risk of infection to the dental assistant.
- It uses sound waves that travel through glass and metal and a special solution to clean the debris from

- This process takes 3 to 10 minutes to complete. During this time, the bubbles implode and produce a cleaning effect on anything within the solution.
- After cleaning is complete, the instruments are rinsed thoroughly and dried and sterilized.
- Can be on top of the counter or seated into the counter.
- Units are available that appear similar to a dishwasher to handle large trays and a number of trays at one time.

Sterilizer: Steam (Flash)

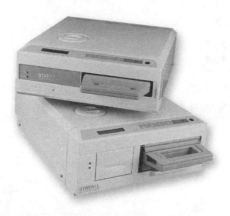

Use	To quickly sterilize instruments with steam under pressure
Composition	• Steam sterilizing unit. • Hinged cassette that is closed and inserted correctly into the sterilizing unit.
Notes	• It sterilizes instruments at 270°F. • The time is 3 minutes for unwrapped instruments and 15 minutes for wrapped instruments.

- It is easily monitored for accuracy.
- Distilled water is required.
- It may corrode instruments.
- It is not for use with many plastics.
- Various styles and sizes are available.

Sterilizer: Steam Autoclave

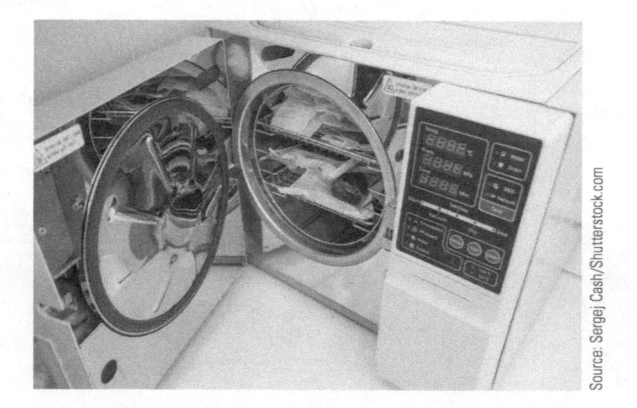

Use	To sterilize instruments using steam under pressure
Composition	Sterilization unit with door
Notes	• It sterilizes instruments at 250°F.
	• The time is 15 minutes for wrapped instruments/cassettes.

- It is easily monitored for accuracy.
- Distilled water is required.
- It may corrode instruments.
- Various styles and sizes are available.

Sterilizer: Chemiclave

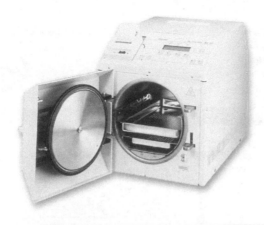

Use	To sterilize instruments using chemical vapor under pressure
Composition	Chemical vapor sterilizing unit with door and pressure chamber

Notes
- It sterilizes instruments at 270°F.
- The time is 20 minutes for wrapped or unwrapped instruments.

- It is easily monitored.
- It requires proper ventilation.
- A special chemical solution is required.
- Various types and sizes are available.

Sterilizer: Dry Heat

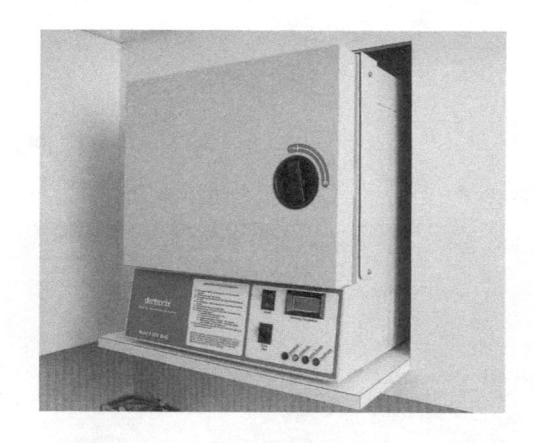

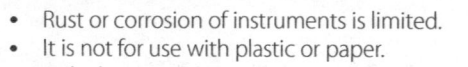

Use   To sterilizes instruments using dry heat

Composition Sterilizing unit with door

Notes
- It sterilizes instruments at 340°F.
- The time is 1 hour for wrapped or unwrapped instruments.
- It is easily monitored.

- Rust or corrosion of instruments is limited.
- It is not for use with plastic or paper.
- A dry heat unit that uses forced air is available; this sterilizes in 6 to 12 minutes.
- Various types and sizes are available.

Biological Monitors

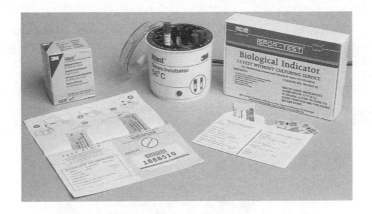

Use   Commercially prepared monitors to assess that sterilization has occurred

Composition   Supplied as paper strips or sealed glass ampules of bacterial endospores

Notes
- These are placed in the sterilizer along with the instrument load.
- When the cycle is complete, the spores are cultured to determine if any have survived.
- The culture can be completed in a dental office if incubators are available for culturing.
- Many are sent out for incubation and a report is returned to the office.
- Machines should be tested weekly.

Process/Dosage Indicators

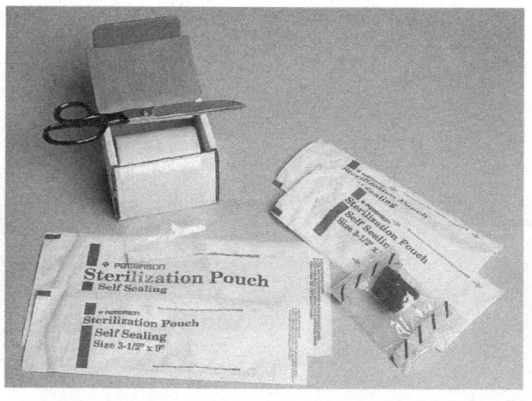

Use
- Process indicators identify whether the packages have been exposed to heat but do not indicate that sterilization has taken place.
- Dosage indicators identify whether the correct conditions were present for sterilization to take place.

- Dosage indicators are dyes placed in the sterilization packing that change color when exposed to dry heat, chemical vapor, or steam for a specific amount of time.
- Heat-sensitive tapes or inks are printed on packaging materials.

Composition
- Process indicators are normally heat-sensitive tapes or inks printed on packaging materials.

Notes
Process and dosage indicators should also be used with biological monitors.

CHAPTER 20

Laboratory Equipment and Materials

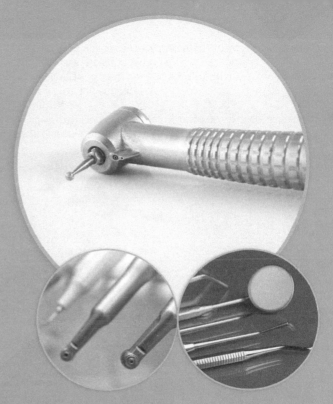

Gypsum Products: General Information Related to Gypsum Materials

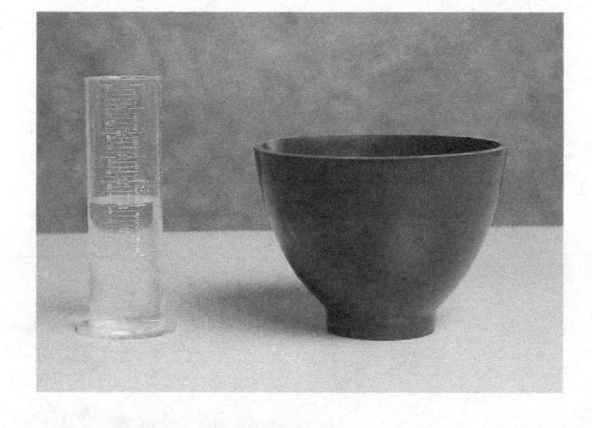

- Setting of gypsum products is chemical and it gives off an exothermic reaction.
- The set can be determined when heat has dissipated the model.
- It is important to have the correct water/powder ratio.
  - Less water—The model can have greater setting expansion, increased strength, and hardness, but mix will become a dry and crumbly mass that will not flow properly.
  - Too much water—The model is weak, is slow to set, and has a greater number of air spaces.
- Temperature of the water is important.
  - Hotter water—The model sets more rapidly (d___ ____ ___ __ __)

- Incorporating the water
  - Overspatulating will cause the breakdown of crystals and soft spots in the model.
- Setting time and enhancers
  - Retarders such as borax and sodium citrate can be added to the material to slow the setting time.
  - Potassium sulfate can be added to the material to accelerate the setting time.

Impression Plaster Type I

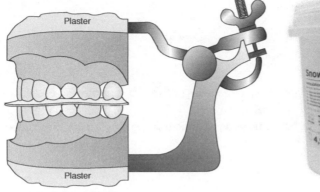

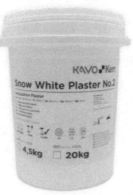

Source: https://www.kerrdental.com/en-dk/dental-laboratory-products/snow-white-plaster-dental-gypsum-products

Use	• To make impressions prior to newer materials being developed • Mounting casts
Composition	Impression plaster type I is produced by heating mineral gypsum in an open kettle at temperatures of 110 to 120°C. This produces crystals that are slender and porous and relatively soft.
Properties	• Beta-hemihydrate. • Reproduction detail poor.

- Formatted for remounting casts.
- Fast-setting plaster.
- Requires more water to wet each surface.
- Calcinated in an open kettle method.
- Takes more water to incorporate the mixture.
- After the mixture dries, the areas where the water was now become air spaces.
- Weaker than stone or type II model or laboratory plaster.
- White color.

Impression Plaster Type I *Continued*

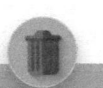

Precautions
- Eye and skin irritation possible
- Should not be ingested
- May cause respiratory tract irritation if inhaled

Mixing and Setting Times
- Ratio: 60 ml of water to 100 g of powder
- Sets in 4 to 5 minutes

Directions

1. Use a rubber bowl and a stiff spatula.
2. Press against the bowl; do not whip (which causes more air to be incorporated into the mixture).
3. Mixing should take about 1 minute.
4. Overspatulating will cause a breakdown of crystals and soft spots in the model.

Type II Plaster

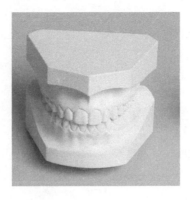

Use
- Versatile formulation for multiple applications
- Study models
- Opposing models
- Repairing casts
- Mounting models and casts

Composition Type II plaster is produced by heating mineral gypsum in an open kettle at temperatures of 110 to 120°C. This produces crystals that are slender and porous and relatively soft.

Properties
- Beta-hemihydrate.
- Requires more water to wet each surface.
- Calcinated in an open kettle method.
- Takes more water to incorporate the mixture.
- After the mixture dries, the areas where the water was now become air spaces.
- Weaker than stone, stronger than type I model or laboratory plaster.
- White color.

Type II Plaster *Continued*

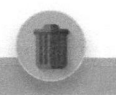

Precautions
- Eye and skin irritation possible
- Should not be ingested
- May cause respiratory tract irritation if inhaled

Mixing and Setting Times
- Ratio: 50 ml of water to 100 g of powder.
- Working time 5 to 7 minutes.
- Initial set loses glossiness and does not flow.
- Final set can no longer be penetrated.
- Sets in 15 to 30 minutes for separation.

Directions

1. Use a rubber or disposable bowl and a stiff spatula.
2. Press against the bowl; do not whip (which causes more air to be incorporated into the mixture).
3. Place the mixture on a vibrator to allow the air bubbles to rise to the surface.
4. Mixing should take about 1 minute.
5. Consistency should be one in which the spatula can cut through the mixture and it stays to the sides without changing position.
6. It will appear like whipped cream, with a smooth, creamy texture.
7. Overspatulating will cause a breakdown of crystals and soft spots in the model.

Orthodontic Plaster/Stone

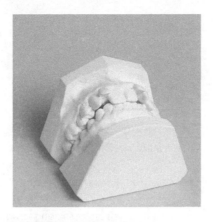

Use	For making orthodontic casts (models)
Composition	Type II plaster and type III laboratory stone mixed together

Properties
- Mixture of type II plaster and type III stone
- Purchased as orthodontic stone, premixed
- Sets harder than models made from type II
- Denser than ordinary plasters
- Easy to trim
- White color

Precautions
- Eye/face protection.
- Skin protection to prevent drying or irritation of hands.
- Respiratory protection—National Institute for Occupational Safety and Health (NIOSH)–approved dust mask or filtering facepiece is recommended in poorly ventilated areas.

Mixing and Setting Times
- Ratio: 40 ml of water to 100 g of powder.
- Working time 5 to 7 minutes.
- Initial set loses glossiness and does not flow.
- Final set can no longer be penetrated.
- Sets in 15 to 30 minutes for separation.

Orthodontic Plaster/Stone *Continued*

Directions

1. Use a rubber or disposable bowl and a stiff spatula.
2. Press against the bowl; do not whip (which causes more air to be incorporated into the mixture).
3. Place the mixture on a vibrator to allow the air bubbles to rise to the surface.
4. Mixing should take about 1 minute.
5. Consistency should be one in which the spatula can cut through the mixture and it stays to the sides without changing position.
6. It will appear like whipped cream, with a smooth, creamy texture.
7. Overspatulating will cause a breakdown of crystals and soft spots in the model.

Type III Laboratory Stone

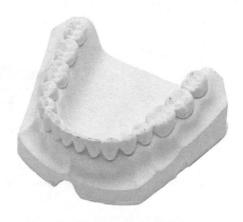

Use	• Diagnostic casts • Working casts • Models for partial and full dentures • Articulating • Flasking	

Composition Produced by driving off water of crystallization under an elevated steam pressure at about 125°C

Properties
• Calcinated by steam under pressure
• More strength than type I and type II
• Usually yellow, green, or blue in color
• Referred to as alpha-hemihydrate

Precautions
• Skin contact: May cause dry skin, discomfort, and irritation
• Inhalation—Breathing dust may be harmful; use mask
• Ingestion: Small quantities not known to be harmful, but large amounts may cause an obstruction

Mixing and Setting Times
• Ratio: 30 ml of water to 100 g of powder.
• Working time 5 to 7 minutes.
• Initial set loses glossiness and does not flow.
• Final set—no longer can be penetrated.
• Sets in 15 to 30 minutes for separation.

Type III Laboratory Stone *Continued*

Directions

1. Use a rubber or disposable bowl and a stiff spatula or a vacuum mixing device.
2. Press against the bowl; do not whip (which causes more air to be incorporated into the mixture).
3. Place the mixture on a vibrator to allow the air bubbles to rise to the surface.
4. Mixing should take about 1 minute.
5. Consistency should be one in which the spatula can cut through the mixture and it stays to the sides without changing position.
6. It will appear like whipped cream, with a smooth, creamy texture.
7. Overspatulating will cause a breakdown of crystals and soft spots in the model.

Type IV Die Stone

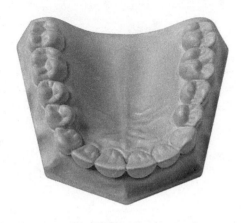

Use	• For making dies (A die is a positive replica of the prepared tooth made from stone.) • In making a cast or model where strength is important • Computer-aided design/computer-aided manufacturing (CAD-CAM) restorations
Composition	Commonly produced by dehydration in an autoclave in the presence of sodium succinate or in a kettle with a 30% calcium chloride solution
Properties	• Extra strong, extra hard • High strength, low expansion

• Hard, smooth surfaces when poured
• Calcinated by autoclaving in the presence of calcium chloride
• Modified alpha-hemihydrate that is referred to as die stone
• Stronger and denser than types I, II, and III
• Normally supplied in colors rose, peach, light blue, or light buff

Precautions	• Skin contact: May cause dry skin, discomfort, and irritation • Inhalation—Breathing dust may be harmful; use mask • Ingestion: Small quantities not known to be harmful, but large amounts may cause an obstruction

Type IV Die Stone *Continued*

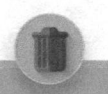

Mixing and Setting Times
- Ratio: 24 ml of water to 100 g of powder (normally supplied in premeasured packets).
- Working time 5 to 7 minutes.
- Initial set loses glossiness and does not flow.
- Final set—No longer can be penetrated.
- Sets in 15 to 30 minutes for separation.

Directions

1. Use a rubber or disposable bowl and a stiff spatula or a vacuum mixing device.
2. Press against the bowl; do not whip (which causes more air to be incorporated into the mixture).
3. Place the mixture on a vibrator to allow the air bubbles to rise to the surface.
4. Mixing should take about 1 minute.
5. Consistency should be one in which the spatula can cut through the mixture and it stays to the sides without changing position.
6. It will appear like whipped cream, with a smooth, creamy texture.
7. Overspatulating will cause a breakdown of crystals and soft spots in the model.

Type V Die Stone

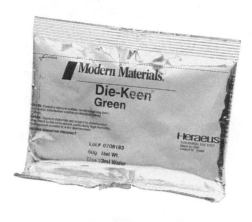

Use	• When a really strong die model is needed • Implants, inlays, crown and bridge dies
Composition	It is commonly produced by dehydration in an autoclave in the presence of sodium succinate or in a kettle with a 30% or more calcium chloride solution. Additional refining and increased pressure of the powder by grinding results in a denser stone.
Properties	• High strength • High expansion

• Approved by the American Dental Association (ADA)
• Optimal expansion for dies and crown and bridge work
• Ultrafine
• Flows easily during vibration

Precautions
• Skin contact: May cause dry skin, discomfort, and irritation
• Inhalation—Breathing dust may be harmful; use mask
• Ingestion: Small quantities not known to be harmful, but large amounts may cause an obstruction

Type V Die Stone *Continued*

Mixing and Setting Times
- Ratio: 21 ml of water to 100 g of powder (normally supplied in premeasured packets)
- Initial set in 10 to 13 minutes
- Final set—no longer can be penetrated

Directions

1. Use a clean, flexible rubber, disposable or plastic bowl.
2. Use the proper ratio of water to powder. Measure room-temperature water into mixing bowl.
3. Add powder to liquid.
4. Use a clean, stiff spatula and spatulate at a rate of 120 RPM for 60 seconds until a smooth and uniform mix is achieved. If using a vacuum mixer, the recommended time is 15 seconds.

Undercut Wax

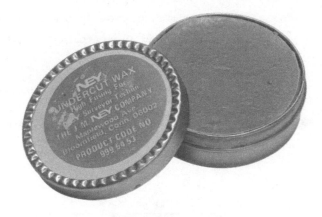

Use   To place into undercuts in models prior to making the final restoration

Composition   No hazardous components

Properties
- Hard wax
- Not sticky
- Available in a small metal container

Precautions
- Nonhazardous at room temperature.
- If a person is exposed to melted wax, fumes may cause irritation.
- Direct contact with molten material may cause injury. Flush area with cold water.

Directions

1. Heat wax spatula under a flame.
2. Insert the hot spatula into the undercut wax.
3. When the undercut wax melts, place it into the undercut on the model.
4. When the undercut is filled and the wax is cooled, remove any extra wax.

Other Laboratory Equipment: Dental Vibrator

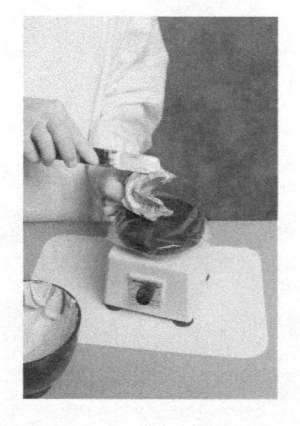

Use	To vibrate materials such as plaster or stone to remove air
Composition	• Small motor topped with a rubber platform work surface. • Three speed controls. • Some come with rubber-cup suction feet to secure the vibrator to the counter.
Notes	The rubber platform surface is often covered with a paper towel or plastic to make cleanup easy.

Flex Mixing Bowls

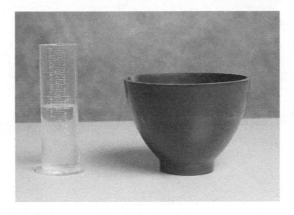

Use
- To mix materials such as alginate and/or gypsum products
- To provide flexibility when mixing materials

Composition Various sizes of rubber, flexible bowls with a firm bottom

Notes
- These are available in various colors.
- They are easy to hold and turn in hand while mixing.
- Some come with disposable liners.
- They are easy to clean after use.

Laboratory Spatula

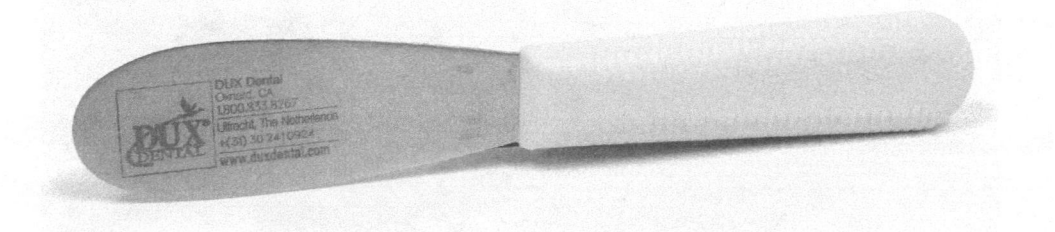

Use
- To mix materials in a flexible bowl
- To mix materials such as a periodontal dressing and/or impression materials on a paper pad
- Sometimes called a beaver tail spatula

Composition
- Blade with handle.
- Blades are plastic or stainless steel.
- Handles are plastic, wood, or metal.

Notes
- These come in various sizes and styles.
- Usually 7½-inch long.
- They are available in a variety of colors.
- Some are sterilized.

Alginator

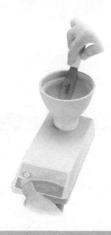

Use To provide a bubble-free, smooth mix of alginate (irreversible hydrocolloid) material

Composition Motorized unit with controls and pad for flexible mixing bowl

Notes

- The design is small and portable, easy to move from room to room.
- Bowl rotates to mix alginate and water together while using a spatula.
- Easy-to-clean bowls come in different sizes.

Procedure: Mixing the Plaster for an Alginate Impression

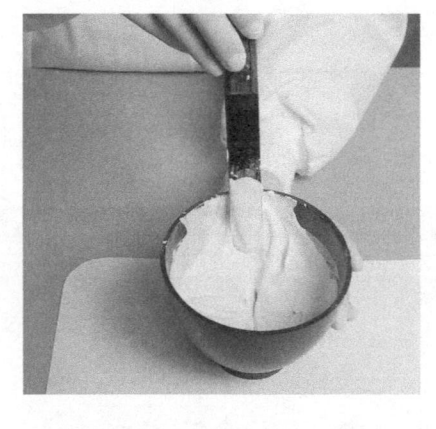

This procedure is performed by the dental assistant in the dental laboratory.

Equipment and Supplies

- Spatula, metal with rounded end and stiff, straight sides
- Two flexible rubber mixing bowls
- Scale
- Type II plaster (100 g)
- Gram-measuring device
- Water-measuring device
- Vibrator with paper or plastic cover on the platform

- Room temperature water
- Alginate impression (disinfected) personal protective equipment (PPE) worn by assistant

Directions

1. Measure 50 ml of room temperature water into one of the flexible mixing bowls.

2. Place the second flexible mixing bowl on the scale and set the dial to zero. This allows the plaster powder to be weighed.

3. Weigh out 100 g of plaster in the second rubber bowl.

Procedure: Mixing the Plaster for an Alginate Impression *Continued*

4. Add the powder from the second bowl to the water in the first bowl. Placing the water in first allows for all the powder to become incorporated into the mixture. Allow several seconds for the powder to dissolve into the water.

5. Use the spatula to slowly mix the particles together. The initial mixing should be completed in 20 seconds. The total mixing procedure should take about 1 minute.

6. Turn on the vibrator to medium or low speed.

7. Place the rubber bowl on the vibrator platform, pressing lightly.

8. Rotate the bowl on the vibrator to allow the air bubbles to rise to the surface. The mixing and vibrating should be completed within a couple of minutes. The mixture is ready if the spatula can cut through it and it stays to the sides without changing positions. It will appear like whipped cream, with a smooth, creamy texture. Another way to check whether the powder and water are in the correct ratio is to place a spoonful on the spatula and turn it upside down—if the material remains in place, the mixture is ready.

Laboratory Knife

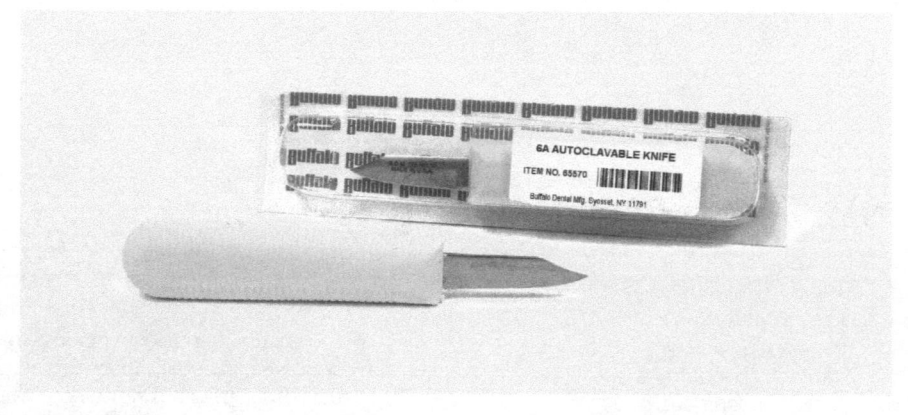

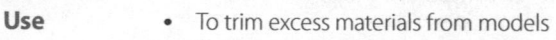

| **Use** | • To trim excess materials from models |
| | • To separate models from impression tray and material |

Composition Wooden handle with stainless steel knife blade or autoclavable handle and stainless-steel knife blade

| **Notes** | • These are available in different styles, with curved or straight blades. |
| | • Various sizes are available. |

Model Trimmer

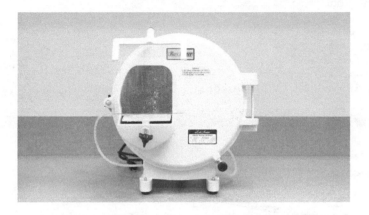

Use
- To trim models of extra plaster or stone
- To remove excess gypsum material and to trim for diagnostic or orthodontic presentation

Composition
- Heavy cast unit with motor
- Cutting or grinding wheel
- Working table
- Water spray and connection
- Splash shield

Notes
- These are available in a variety of styles, including a unit with dual grinding wheels.
- The working table is adjustable to create the angles needed.
- The wheels may be reversible.
- Water sprays on the wheel to reduce heat, keep dust down, and assist in keeping the wheel clean.
- Units are usually secured to a table or counter near a water source.

Dental Waxes: Pattern Inlay Wax

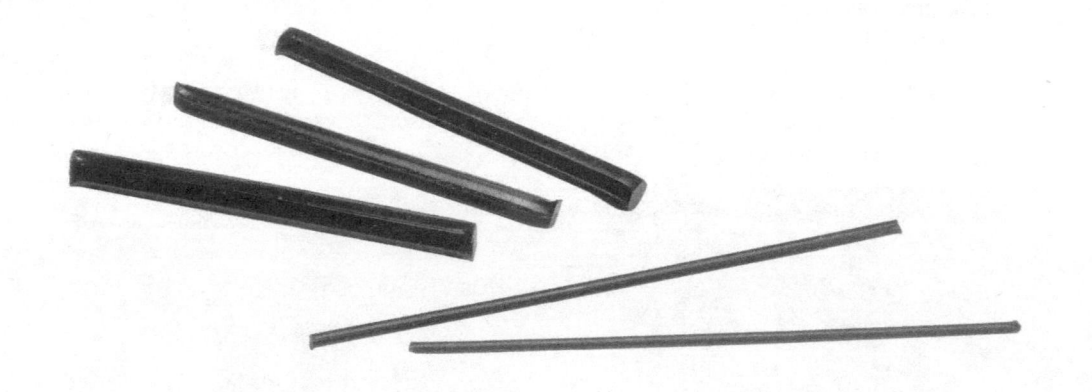

Use To fashion a wax pattern of the restoration (crown or bridge) to be made

Composition
- 40–60% paraffin wax
- 10% gum dammar
- 25% carnauba wax
- 10% ceresin wax
- 5% beeswax

Note: Composition will vary from manufacturer to manufacturer.

Properties
- Hard wax used in crown and bridge construction.
- Dark blue, green, or purple rods or sticks about 7.5 cm long and 6 mm in diameter (3 inches by 0.25 inches diameter).
- Used on a die to make a replica of the final restoration.
- Type I is used for direct techniques (establishing the initial form of the tooth in the oral cavity) and is a little softer.
- Type II, most often used in the dental laboratory, is used for indirect techniques where the wax pattern is carved on the die (stone model).

Dental Waxes: Pattern Inlay Wax *Continued*

Precautions
- This product is nonhazardous at room temperature.
- If a person is exposed to melted wax, fumes may cause irritation.
- Direct contact with molten material may cause injury. Flush area with cold water.

Directions
The wax is melted and applied to the die (a positive replica of the prepared tooth made of stone) layer by layer until the contacts, margins, anatomy, and occlusion are correct. It will resemble the final crown or bridge.

Pattern Wax: Baseplate Wax

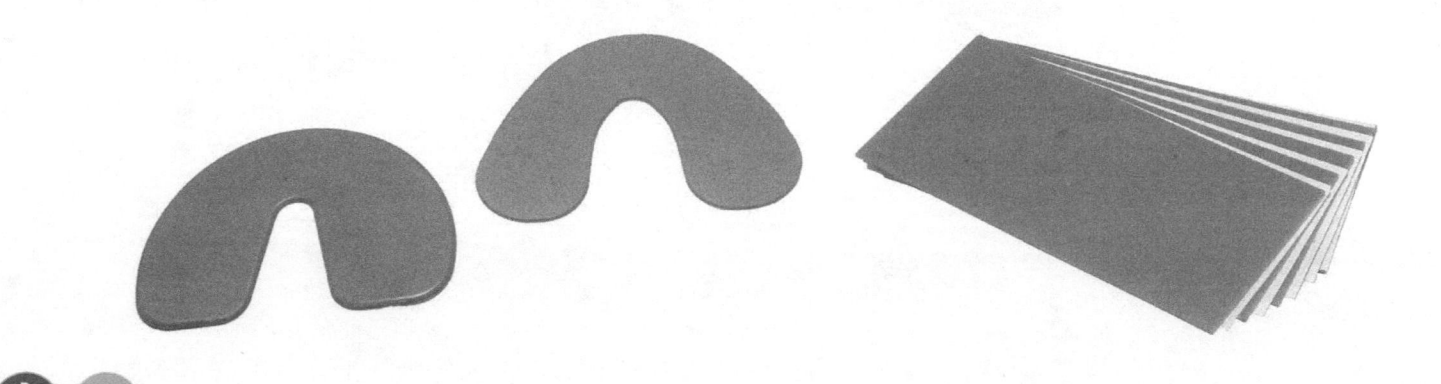

Use

Construction of the baseplate tray to establish the vertical dimension in the initial arch for a denture or partial

Composition

- 80% ceresin
- 12% beeswax
- 2.5% carnauba
- 5% natural or synthetic resins

Note: Composition will vary from manufacturer to manufacturer.

Properties

- Available in three types:
  - Type I—a softer baseplate wax that is used for building contours and veneers
  - Type II—a medium wax used for patterns to be tried into the mouth in temperate climates (most commonly used)
  - Type III—a harder wax to be used in the mouth in tropical weather or when extra hardness is required

Pattern Wax: Baseplate Wax *Continued*

- Carves without chipping.
- Boils out cleanly.
- Pliable.
- Shaded pink to resemble gum tissue.
- Unlimited shelf life.
- Available in shapes that resemble the dental arches.
- Type II can be heated with warm water or a flame and used for taking a bite registration.

Precautions
- This product is nonhazardous at room temperature.
- If a person is exposed to melted wax, fumes may cause irritation.
- Direct contact with molten material may cause injury. Flush area with cold water.

Directions

1. Dental baseplate wax can be heated with a torch and adapted easily to a stone model of the edentulous arch.
2. It should be adapted closely, and the excess should be trimmed with a wax spatula or blade. The softer wax is tough yet pliable all-purpose wax.
3. The margins of the wax should be made smooth to the touch because it is going to be reinserted into the patient's mouth.

Pattern Wax: Occlusal Rims or Bite Blocks

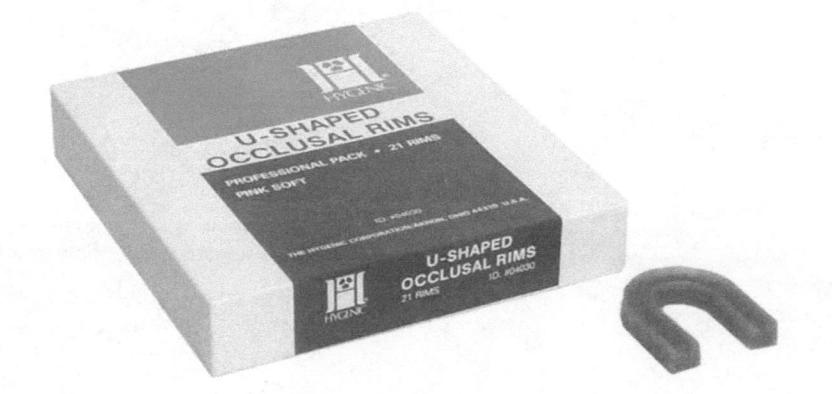

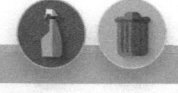

Use

This is a softer wax block that is attached to the baseplate wax that is used in the construction of the tray to establish the vertical dimension in the initial arch for a denture or partial.

Composition
- No hazardous components
- Less than 10% petroleum hydrocarbons and additives

Properties
- Can be shaped at room temperature.
- Some types come with a recessed base to aid in adapting it to the baseplate.

- Can be adapted to fit any arch.
- Can be easily heated to set the denture teeth into it.
- U-shaped.
- Pink in color.
- Soft but not sticky.
- Referred to as either occlusal rim or a bite block.

Precautions
- Nonhazardous at room temperature.
- Above its melting point, wax becomes liquid and flows more readily as its temperature increases. Use special handling with hot liquid wax.

Pattern Wax: Occlusal Rims or Bite Blocks *Continued*

Directions

1. Adapt the U-shaped wax arch to the baseplate on the stone model of the edentulous arch.
2. Heat the recessed base of the arch and stick it to the baseplate.
3. Ensure that the two are adapted securely.
4. Smooth the area where the two waxes (baseplate and bite rim) come together.

Pattern Wax: Casting Wax

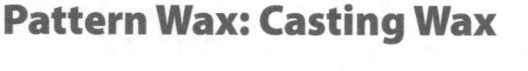

Use	To fabricate the pattern for the metal framework for removable partial dentures and other similar structures.
Composition	The composition is the same as inlay waxes but contains reduced amounts of hard waxes and increased amounts of beeswax.
Properties	• Easily trimmed with sharp knife • Has a smooth, glossy surface after gently flaming

- Sold in:
  - Thin sheets
  - Preshaped like completed metal framework or clasps
  - Square sheets
  - Long thin strips

Precautions
- Nonhazardous at room temperature.
- Above its melting point, wax becomes liquid and flows more readily as its temperature increases. Use special handling with hot liquid wax.

Pattern Wax: Casting Wax *Continued*

Directions

1. Place the wax on the stone model where the metal framework will be after fabrication.
2. Attach all wax on the model and secure it together.
3. Use a flame to smooth areas and obtain the glossy finish needed.

Processing Wax: Sticky Wax

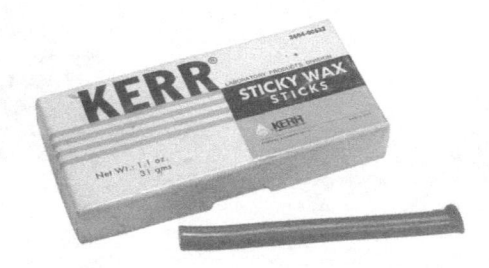

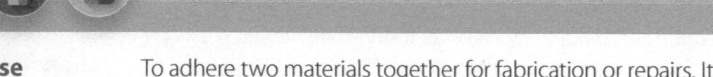

Use
To adhere two materials together for fabrication or repairs. It has many uses.

Composition
- No hazardous components
- Less than 10% petroleum hydrocarbons and additives

Properties
- Brittle at room temperature but sticky when melted with a flame
- Adheres to a number of surfaces such as metal, stone, plaster, tooth structure, etc.

- Will fracture rather than flow if deformed
- Comes in a number of colors—usually orange or dark red
- Normally available in sticks
- Melting temperature 136°F (58°C)

Precautions
- Nonhazardous at room temperature.
- Above its melting point, wax becomes liquid and flows more readily as its temperature increases. Use special handling with hot liquid wax.

Processing Wax: Sticky Wax *Continued*

Directions

1. Place together the two materials that need to be adhered.
2. Heat the tip of the sticky wax stick with a flame.
3. Touch the end that has been heated to the items that need to be attached; the sticky wax will set up rapidly.
4. The wax will change to a milky color when set.

Processing Wax: Boxing Wax

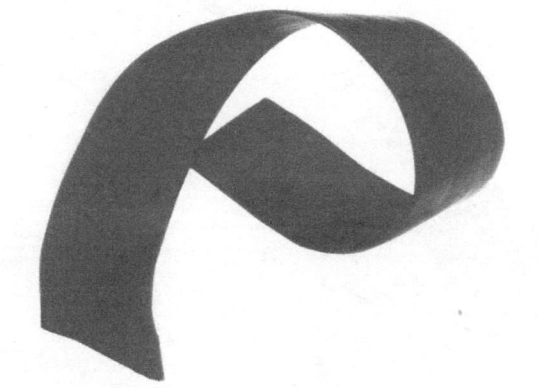

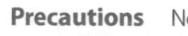

Use   To form a wax box around an impression of an arch into which freshly mixed plaster or stone can be poured.

Composition
- No hazardous components
- Less than 10% petroleum hydrocarbons and additives

Properties
- Comes in wide wax strips and ropes.
- Wax strips are normally 1/16-inch thick, 1½-inch wide, and 12-inch long.

- Wax strips can be purchased in extra thin, which is 0.40-inch thick.
- Withstands heat given off by gypsum products during setting.
- Can be reused.

Precautions   Nonhazardous at room temperature

Processing Wax: Boxing Wax *Continued*

Directions

1. Take one strip and wrap it in a circle to the size of model that is to be poured up.
2. Attach it to itself in a circle pattern.
3. Place it on the counter in an upright position (like a fence around something).
4. The stone or plaster can be placed in this circle and into the model being poured.
5. The circle of wax can be removed easily after the poured model is set. It can be used again on another model if desired.

Processing Wax: Utility Wax

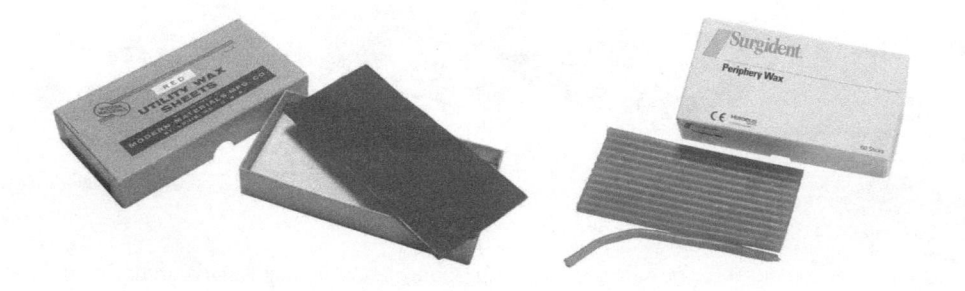

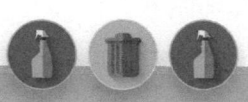

Use Often used on hydrocolloid or alginate trays as beading wax on the periphery of the tray for a cushion or an extension.

Composition
- No hazardous components
- Less than 10% petroleum hydrocarbons and additives

Properties
- Soft wax
- Easily workable and adhesive
- Flame not necessary
- Often called periphery wax
- Comes in long ropes, sheets, or strips and in a number of colors

Precautions Nonhazardous at room temperature

Directions

1. Take one rope of the utility wax and place it onto the impression tray.
2. Form the wax on the border of the tray.
3. Ensure that the wax is not above the height of the base of the tray.
4. Adjust the wax as necessary.

Custom Trays: Coe® Tray Plastic

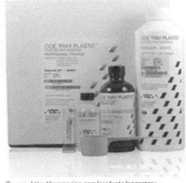

Source: http://gcamerica.com/products/operatory
/Impression_Trays_Accessories/plastic/

Use	To construct accurate fitting, individualized custom impression trays
Composition	• 2-methoxyethanol • Tetraethoxysilane • Ethanol • Dibutyltin dilaurate • Mineral oil
Properties	• Trimming of tray is easy because tray plastic grinds away without clogging burs.

- Will not warp or pull away from the cast during polymerization.
- Powder and liquid mix in seconds and produce smooth dough.
- No additional equipment is needed.
- Tray adhesive available
  - Regular—15 minutes to set
  - Fast set—10 minutes to set

Custom Trays: Coe® Tray Plastic *Continued*

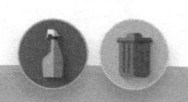

Precautions   Use appropriate PPE and follow all Occupational Safety and Health Administration (OSHA) guidelines.
- Inhalation—May cause nose and throat irritation, nervous system depression, or irritation or burning of mucous membranes. Prolonged exposure may cause brain and nervous system damage.
- Ingestion—May cause abnormal liver and kidney function.
- Skin—May cause irritation or burning of skin. Repeated exposure may cause skin burns and allergic reactions.
- Eyes—May cause irritation or burning of eyes.

Directions

1. Soak the cast in water for 10 minutes prior to making custom tray.
2. Paint a thin film of Coe-Sep™ on cast to prevent sticking.
3. With a pencil, outline the desired periphery of the tray.
4. Adapt a sheet of base plate wax to the cast.
5. Trim the wax to the pencil outline.
6. Cut stops in the wax on areas that are not involved in the impression.
7. Cover the wax spacer with a sheet of polyethylene.
8. Mix 8 ml of liquid with a level scoop of powder.
9. Spatulate together for 30 to 40 seconds.
10. When it is not sticky or tacky, form the mixture into a patty and adapt it to the cast.
11. Trim the excess material from the edges to the pencil outline while it is still soft.
12. Form a handle with the excess material and wet it with the accelerator and adapt it to the custom tray.
13. Remove the custom tray from the model when set, and finish trimming with a bur.

Hydroplastic Beads

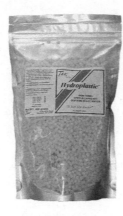

Use To form a custom tray or bleach tray

Composition No hazardous ingredients

Properties
- Nontoxic
- Hypoallergenic
- Softens in hot water
- Comes in 16-oz jar of pellets
- Can be used with Model Bloc to block out undercuts, fill interproximals, and fabricate spacers
- No mixing
- No odor
- No chemical hazard
- Bench set in 5 minutes, or immediately if placed in cold water

Precautions
- Use appropriate PPE and follow all OSHA guidelines
- No evidence of adverse effects from available information

Hydroplastic Beads *Continued*

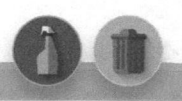

Directions

1. Add a scoop of hydroplastic to hot water (155–180°F).
2. After 1 minute, remove with an instrument and gather together.
3. The material should have turned from a milky color to a clearer color.
4. Knead the material together.
5. Form it to the cast or model (it will not stick to the model).
6. Form a handle out of the material and it will adhere to the material while in a soft stage.
7. Let it bench set for 5 minutes, or place it into cold water for an immediate set.
8. Remove the tray and trim, if necessary, with scissors or make adjustments with a flame.

Triad® True Tray™ Vacuum Forming Machine and Tray Material

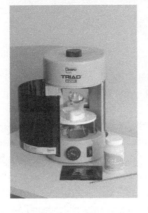

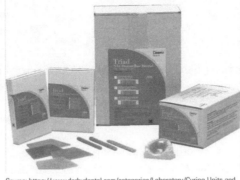

Source: https://www.darbydental.com/categories/Laboratory/Curing-Units-and
-Materials/Triad-Materials/8295020

Use	To fabricate acrylic custom trays
Composition	No hazardous ingredients
Properties	• To be used with Triad 2000™ curing unit • Very low shrinkage • Does not contain methyl methacrylate monomer • Tray made extra-oral only • Store away from direct sunlight • Refrigerate to extend shelf life

Precautions	• Use appropriate PPE and follow all OSHA guidelines. • Nontoxic. • Skin irritation is possible in sensitive individuals.
Curing Time	• On the model initially—2 minutes • Final set off the model—2 minutes

Triad® True Tray™ Vacuum Forming Machine and Tray Material *Continued*

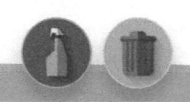

Directions

1. Obtain a properly extended primary cast.
2. Place relief wax and "cutouts" for tray stops, as appropriate for the situation.
3. Coat all surfaces that will contact TruTray custom tray material with a thin layer of Triad Model Release Agent.
4. Remove the rayon film from the TruTray and carefully adapt the material to the cast.
5. Trim the material with a scalpel, knife, or other sharp instrument to the desired outline and remove excess material.
6. Attach a handle by molding excess material into shape and blending edges into the TruTray material on the cast with the Triad modeling tool.
7. Cure the cast with its adapted tray in the Triad curing unit for 2 minutes.
8. Remove the cast from the unit and carefully separate the partially cured tray from the cast. Remove any relief wax from the tray while it is still warm.
9. Cover all surfaces of the custom tray with Triad Air Barrier Coating and return to the Triad curing unit for 2 minutes.
10. Remove the custom tray when the cycle is complete. Scrub gently with warm water and trim if necessary.

Vacuum Former and Materials

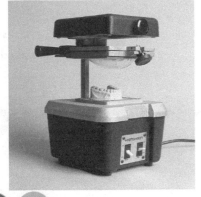

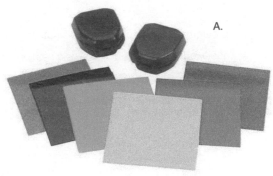

A.

Source: https://dental.keystoneindustries.com/product/mouthguard-resin-sheets-2/

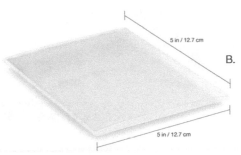

5 in / 12.7 cm

B.

5 in / 12.7 cm

Source: https://dental.keystoneindustries.com/product/soft-eva-2/

Use	• To make custom trays for final impressions • To make whitening trays to be used with whitening materials and techniques • To fabricate mouth guards, night guards, and splints

Composition	• Unit with heating element and vacuum adapter
	• Adjustable arm with heating element and frame to hold sheets under heating unit
	• Vacuum table with holes where model is placed
	• Controls on the base
	• Material:
	  A. Mouth guard tray material
	  B. Whitening tray material

Notes
• Various types of vacuum forming materials are available in different thicknesses.
• Some units have a gasket that needs to be changed to keep a tight seal.
• Once materials are heated, the arm is dropped and the vacuum is turned on to suck the materials tightly to the models.
• Models are wetted to prevent small air bubbles.

Trimming Scissors

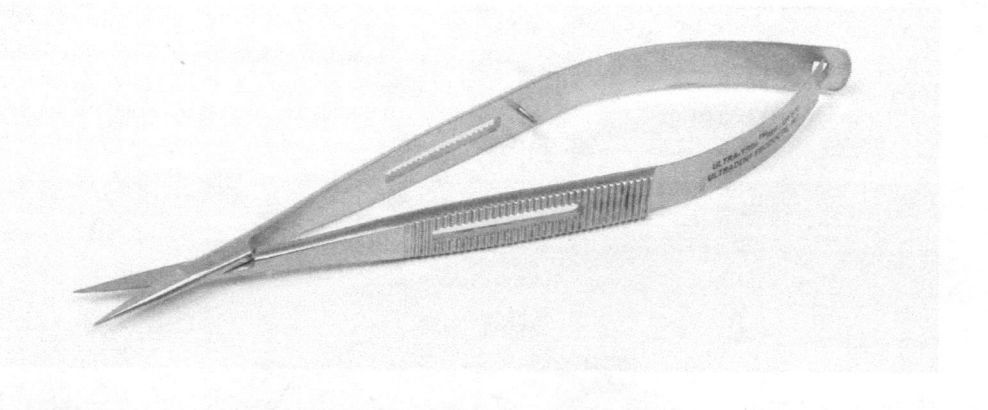

Use	To trim soft tray materials such as whitening trays
Composition	Curved locking handles with sharp pointed blades on working end; lightweight
Notes	• These allow easy manipulation of contours of gingival margin and embrasures. • The cutting tips are sharp.

Soft Tray Trimming Devices

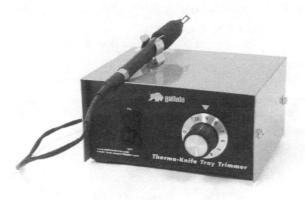

Use
- To trim soft tray materials such as whitening trays
- To trim and contour denture relines, soft night guards, and sports mouth guards

Composition
- Heating unit with adjustable heat settings
- Handpiece-style handle with curved, double-edged tip that is attached by a cord to the unit
- Comes with bracket on the unit to hold the knife handle

Notes
- These are easy to use for cutting and trimming gingival margins.
- They are used with various tray materials.
- They can be used with materials on the models to prevent distortion.
- They can be used interproximally.

Pumice

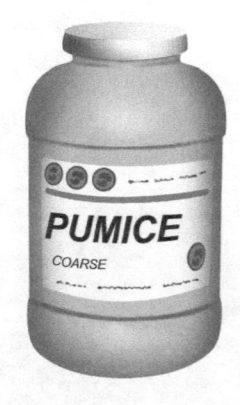

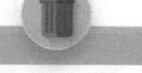

Use	To polish dental appliances such as provisionals, dentures, partials, and bridges
Composition	Volcanic silica manufactured as a loose abrasive. Flour of pumice is extremely fine.
Properties	Available in grades:
	• Pumice, flour
	• Pumice, fine

- Pumice, medium
- Pumice, coarse
- Pumice, extra coarse

Specially ground for fast cutting without scratching or grooving

Mixing and Setting Times	• Used with water and a lathe to smooth the appliance
	• No mixing required

Pumice *Continued*

Directions

1. Remove pumice from canister without contaminating other pumice.
2. Place about 1/3 cup into the slash pan of the lathe.
3. Add water to the pumice to make a putty-like material.
4. Wet the rag wheel and place it on the lathe.
5. If the appliance has not been sterilized, the rag wheel and the splash pan will need to be sterilized/disinfected and the pumice discarded. The EPA issued guidelines for dental issues in 1999 for caring for dental pumice.
6. Place the pumice on the appliance in the area that requires smoothing. Using the rag wheel of the lathe, smooth the area.
7. The pumice needs to be fed into the area that needs polishing during the rotation of the rag wheel.

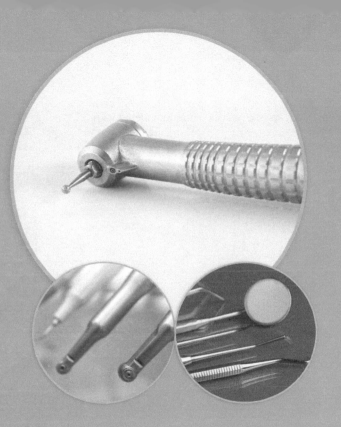

CHAPTER 21

Radiology
Equipment

X-Ray Unit

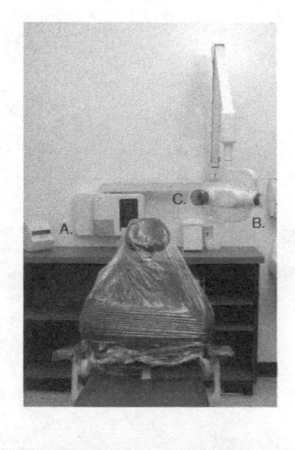

Use To take dental x-rays

Composition A. The control panel has an on/off switch and is where the exposure-time control is located. It may have adjustments for kilovoltage, milliamperage, and radiograph to be taken, and child or adult choices.

B. Tube head where the x-ray tube is located.

C. Cone or position-indicating device (PID) that directs the radiation.

Notes
- Numerous x-ray units are available, each with its own configuration.
- The operating button is located outside the room where the x-ray unit is located.

Handheld X-Ray Machine

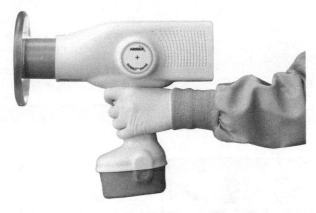

Use	To take/expose x-rays in a variety of dental settings
Composition	Handheld unit includes x-ray tube head, PID or collimator, shielding, handle with digital control panel, and battery
Notes	• This machine is used in dental offices, military bases, teaching facilities, and clinics, as well as to provide global access to dental care in remote areas.

- There are settings for adult or child, anterior or posterior x-rays.
- They can expose dental film, digital sensors, and phosphor plates.
- Units are usually preset at 60 kV and 2 mA.
- The operator is allowed to stay with the patient because the unit is handheld.

Panoramic X-Ray Machine

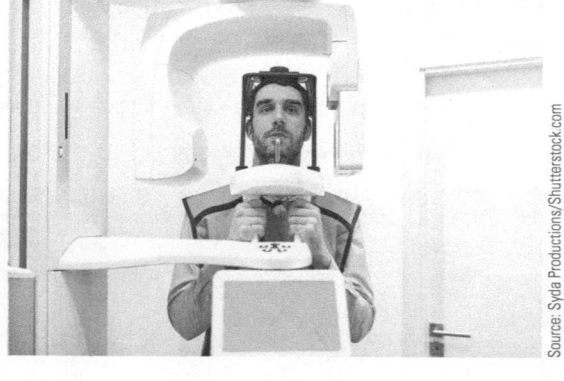

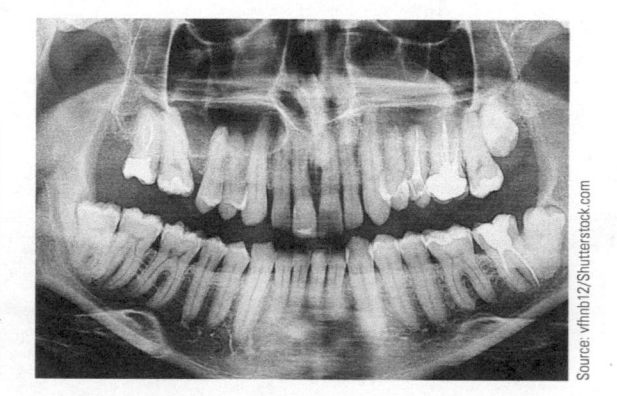

Source: Syda Productions/Shutterstock.com

Source: vhnb12/Shutterstock.com

Use

To expose an x-ray of the entire maxilla and mandible and surrounding tissues in a panoramic view

Composition
- A specialized x-ray machine attached to a column that can be adjusted to the height of the patient
- Rotating attachment with an x-ray tube head on one side, a panoramic sensor holder on the other side, and a head support, bite block, and chin rest in the middle
- Controls for patient height adjustment and a digital touchscreen interface for alignment adjustments

Notes
- Various panoramic machines are available

- The patient wears a double-sided lead apron without a thyroid collar.
- Patients are usually positioned standing up.
- Bite blocks are disposable. Head and chin rests are disinfected after each patient.
- Laser alignment lights are used to ensure correct positioning of the patient's head.
- Some dual-system digital panoramic units will expose temporomandibular joint (TMJ)/sinus nodes and perform tomographic imaging.

Cephalometric X-Ray Machine

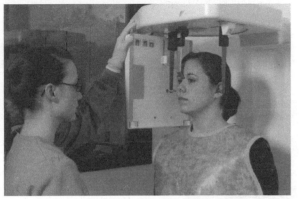

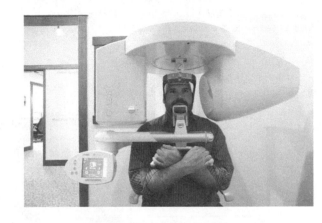

Use
- To expose a radiograph of the patient's skeletal structure and profile
- To aid in orthodontic and oral surgery diagnosis and measurements

Composition
- Specialized x-ray machine attached to a column that is adjustable to the height of the patient
- Rotating attachment with an x-ray tube head on one side, a cephalometric sensor on the other side, and a head-holding device in the middle
- Controls for patient height adjustment and a digital touchscreen interface for alignment adjustments

Notes
- Two views can be taken: lateral and posterior/anterior.
- For lateral views, the side of the patient is positioned parallel with the cassette and earpieces are placed in the patient's ears to align the Frankfort plane.
- For posterior/anterior views, the patient's head is positioned to face the cassette with the earpieces in place. The x-ray beam is then directed at the occipital bone and perpendicular to the cassette.
- Cassettes are specific to the manufacturer of the equipment.
- The patient wears a double-sided lead apron without a thyroid collar.
- Patients are usually positioned standing up.

Cone Beam 3D Imaging System

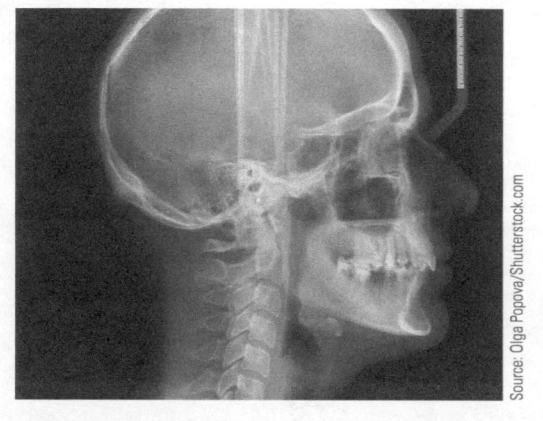

Source: Olga Popova/Shutterstock.com

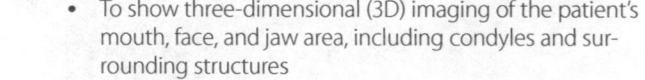

Use
- To show three-dimensional (3D) imaging of the patient's mouth, face, and jaw area, including condyles and surrounding structures
- To produce digital panoramic and cephalometric images, 3D photos, and computed tomography (CT) scans

Composition
- Specialized x-ray machine attached to a column that is adjustable to the height of the patient, with handgrips to stabilize the patient
- Rotating attachment with two sensors to capture 3D images and touchscreen controls for capturing areas of

- Laser lights are used for positioning before scanning.
- 3D software specific to the individual machine and a computer are required.

Notes
- Images are used for diagnosis and treatment planning for caries, endodontic procedures, orthodontics, implants, and other oral surgery procedures and for patient education.
- Images are also used for nerve mapping, accurate measuring, and determining exact tooth location, as they include views from different angles

Cone Beam 3D Imaging System *Continued*

- Several units are designed to take panoramic and cephalometric x-rays and perform 3D options.
- Scans are completed in 8 to 20 seconds.
- Computer software is designed to solve dental problems through perceptive integrations of diagnosis, computer-aided therapy planning, and detailed intraoperative implementation.
- These systems enhance patient understanding of diagnosis and treatment options.

Direct Digital Imaging System

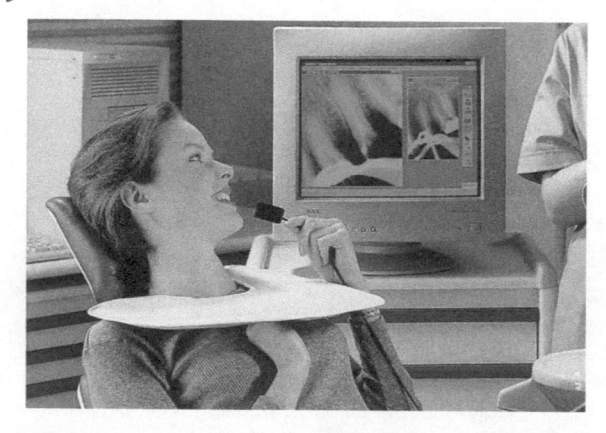

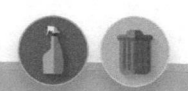

Use	To expose intraoral and extraoral radiographs of the patient and display the images on a computer screen

Composition
- Dental x-ray unit, including control panel, timer, arm assembly, and tube head
- Computer monitor and specific digital imaging software
- Sensors or phosphor plates
- Sensor or phosphor plate holders
- Scanner (with indirect imaging systems)
- Barriers

Notes
- There are several types of digital imaging systems, including

- With the direct imaging systems, the image appears immediately so the dentist can explain findings, diagnoses, and procedures to the patient right at the dental chair.
- With indirect imaging systems, an x-ray is exposed on a phosphor plate, which is then placed on a carousel that is inserted into the scanner to digitize the image to be displayed on the computer screen.
- Both systems have software that allows the digital image to be enhanced, mounted, and stored as part of the patient's records.

Digital Sensor

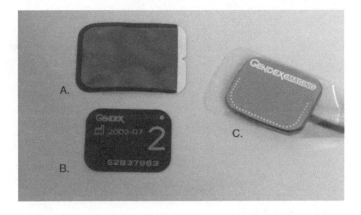

Use	• Electronic or specially coated plate that is positioned in the mouth and then exposed to radiation • Takes the place of traditional x-ray film
Composition	A. Barrier B. Imaging plate C. Direct digital sensor
Notes	• Digital sensors can have a cord that is connected to the computer.

• They can be cordless.
• There are two types of systems:

Direct Digital Imaging
• The sensor is placed in the mouth and the image is produced on the surface of the sensor, digitized, and then transmitted to the computer.
• Sensors come in sizes 0, 1, and 2.

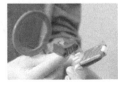

Digital Sensor *Continued*

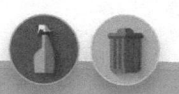

Indirect Digital Imaging

- The plate is placed in the mouth and the image is produced on the surface of the plate. The plate is placed into a scanner that reads the radiographs prior to being transferred to the computer.
- Image plates come in sizes 0, 1, 2, 3, and 4.

Scan X Classic Digital Radiograph System

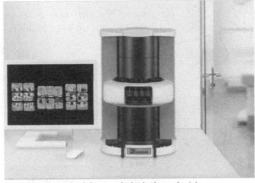

Source: https://www.airtechniques.com/en/product/scanx-classic/

Use	To convert radiographic images taken with digital imaging plates	**Notes**	• With indirect imaging systems, an x-ray is exposed onto a phosphor plate, which is then placed on a carousel that is inserted into the scanner to digitize the image to be displayed on the computer screen.
Composition	• Phosphor plates, barriers, and plate holders • Scanner • Computer system needed		• Systems have software that allows the digital image to be enhanced, mounted, and stored as part of the patient's records. • System consists of thin, flexible reusable plates.

X-Ray XCP (X-Ray Film Holder with One Ring and Arm Positioning System)

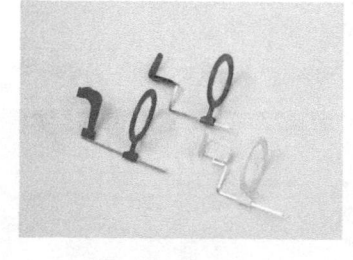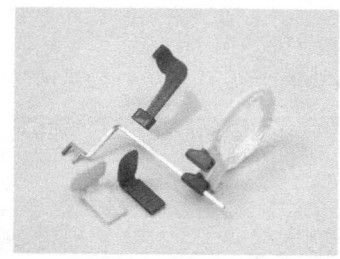

A.

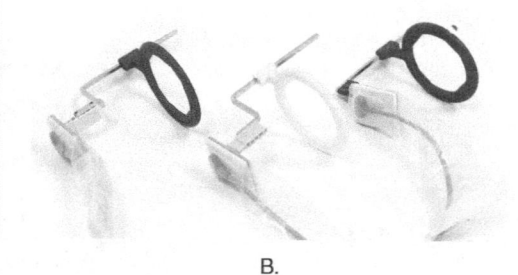

B.

Use	To hold and position x-ray film in patient's mouth and place the PID while exposing a radiograph; available in anterior, posterior, and bite-wing bite blocks
Composition	**A.** Three each of plastic colored rings, metal arms, and color-coordinated plastic bite blocks. One multiring metal arm and three plastic bite blocks
	B. Digital sensors attached to plastic colored rings, metal arms and color-coordinated plastic bite blocks
Notes	• Normally, the red ring and bite block are used for bite-wing images.

- Normally, the blue ring and bite block are used for anterior images.
- Normally, the yellow ring and bite block are used for posterior images.
- The XCP is used with the paralleling exposure technique.
- Digital film holders allow for the cord and have an attachment area.
- They are sterilizable.
- The XCP has brand-specific sensor holders that ensure co-ordination with specific manufacturer's equipment.

X-Ray Film Holder- Snap-A-Ray

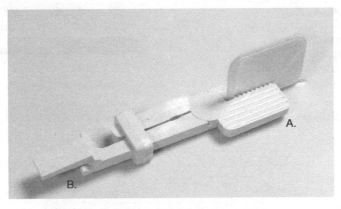

Use To hold and position x-ray film in patient's mouth while exposing a radiograph

Composition Double-ended:
A. The gripping end holds and positions film for posterior teeth and has a biting surface to stabilize the film and holder in the mouth.
B. The end that allows for film to slide in is used on the anterior teeth.

Notes
- Sometimes referred to as an Eezee-Grip holder
- They are sterilizable.
- The anterior or posterior can use either size #1 or size #2.
- They are available for purchase to hold traditional film, sensors, or phosphor plates securely without damaging them.
- The cushioned bite area is good for patient comfort.

Intraoral Film Sizes

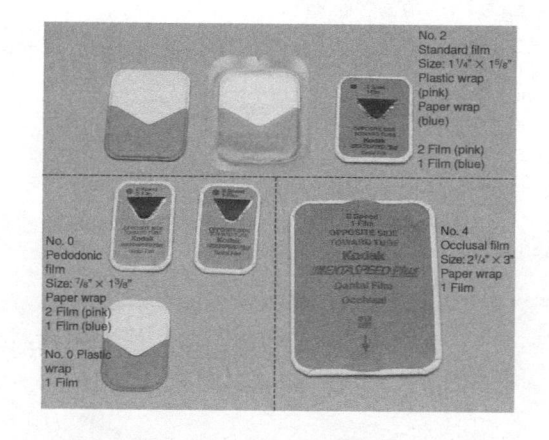

No. 2
Standard film
Size: 1 ¼" × 1⅝"
Plastic wrap
(pink)
Paper wrap
(blue)

2 Film (pink)
1 Film (blue)

No. 0
Pedodonic
film
Size: ⅞" × 1⅜"
Paper wrap
2 Film (pink)
1 Film (blue)

No. 0 Plastic
wrap
1 Film

No. 4
Occlusal film
Size: 2¼" × 3"
Paper wrap
1 Film

Use	Offers different sizes of film needed for the correct radiograph

Composition

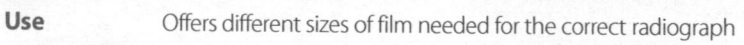

Film Size	Description/Use
No. 0	Child size
No. 1	Narrow anterior film size
No. 2	Adult size
No. 3	Long bite-wing film size
No. 4	Occlusal film size

Notes

- Films packets are available with barriers, or barriers may be purchased separately.
- Films are used to take adult and pedodontic exposures—periapical, occlusal, and bite-wing exposures.
- Packaging color and numbering may differ from manufacturer to manufacturer.

Intraoral Film

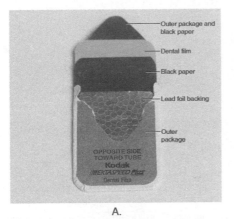

Outer package and black paper
Dental film
Black paper
Lead foil backing
Outer package

OPPOSITE SIDE
TOWARD TUBE
Kodak
EKTASPEED Plus
Dental Film

A.

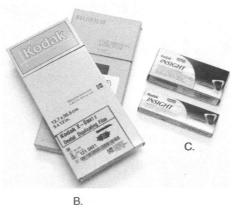

B.

C.

Use	To record intraoral structures such as the teeth and surrounding bone onto the film
Composition	**A.** Film packet

- Outer package and black paper—may be soft plastic or paper
- Dental film—may be a single or double film
- Black paper to protect the film from light
- Lead foil to stop radiation from reaching beyond the film
- Outer package

B. Packaging for x-ray film
C. Comfort strips
- Comfort pads/strips are available to place over the sharp edges of dental packets.

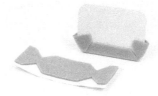

Intraoral Film *Continued*

Notes

- Film packets are waterproof.
- Films are available with barriers.
- Film speeds (A–F) are indicated on the packets. The faster-speed film reduces the amount of radiation exposure for the patient. Currently, F is the most commonly used and results in much less radiation dosing than D or E.
- Available in double-film packets
- Packaging color and numbering may differ from manufacturer to manufacturer.
- Comfort pads come in a variety of sizes and styles and can be used on intraoral film and digital sensors.

Extraoral Film

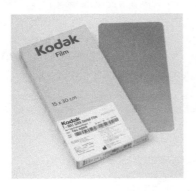
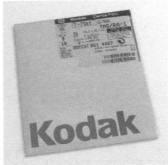
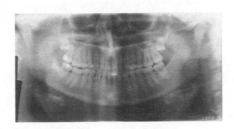
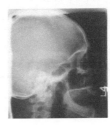

Use	To record extraoral structures such as the teeth and surrounding bone onto the film
Composition	Dental extraoral film held between two screens in a cassette
Notes	• Different extraoral machines require different types of cassettes to hold the film.
	• Extraoral films can be the panoramic type, which shows the maxillary and mandibular and surrounding tissues on one film, or the cephalometric type, which shows a facial profile that includes the bone, teeth, and soft tissue.

• Extraoral films must be loaded and unloaded into the cassette under safelight conditions.
• Some machines have labeling devices to identify patient name and the date the film was exposed.

X-Ray Processing Equipment for Traditional Film

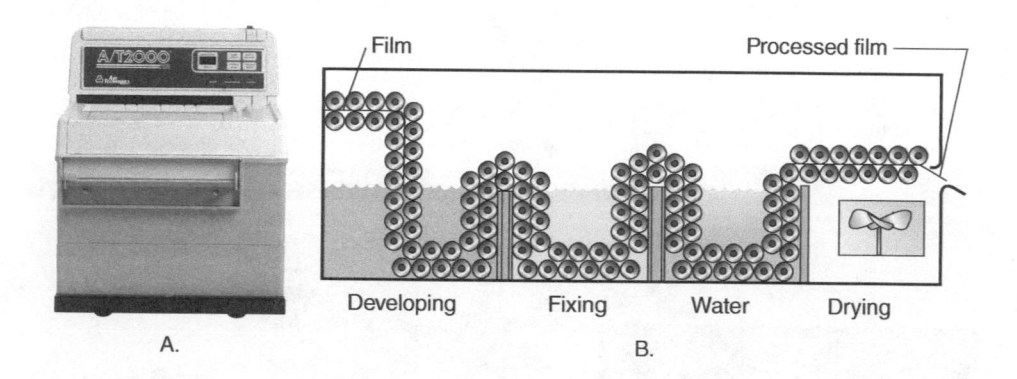

A.

B.

Film

Processed film

Developing Fixing Water Drying

Use	To automatically process exposed radiographs
Composition	**A.** Automatic film processor
	B. Drawing of the inside of a typical automatic film processor

Notes
- These are available with daylight loaders, which allow loading the exposed film in normal light conditions.
- Proper levels of the chemicals must be maintained to ensure correct processing.

- The unit must be turned on prior to processing exposed radiographs to allow the chemicals to be heated to the correct temperatures.
- The film is developed, fixed, washed, dried, and ready to mount within 5 minutes.
- The developing and fixing solutions used with the unit are different from manual developing and fixing solutions.
- The unit must be cleaned and maintained properly.
- Follow the manufacturer's directions.

X-Ray View Box for Traditional Film

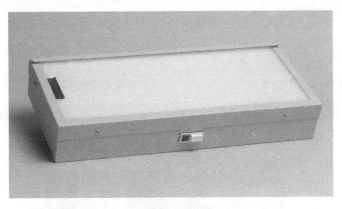

Use	To view/read traditional radiographs
Composition	Small cabinet with bright light covered by a flat frosted surface; has a clip to hold the x-rays and an on/off switch
Notes	• Units may be placed on a counter or mounted on a wall, in a cabinet, or in a dental unit.

- X-rays are placed on the frosted surface with the raised dot in the convex position so they can be read as if the dentist is looking into the patient's mouth.
- There are many styles of view boxes available.
- View boxes are located in each treatment room and also in the x-ray processing area.

Duplicating Machine for Traditional Film

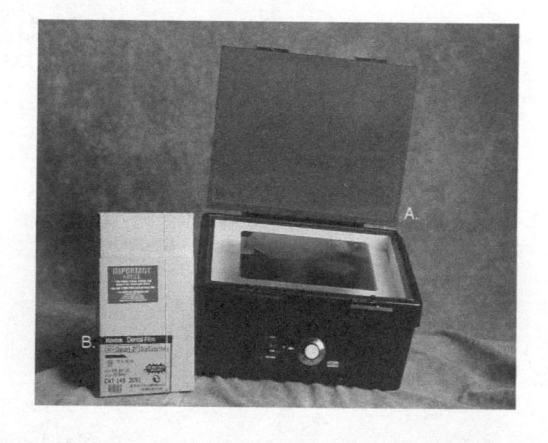

Use   To copy/duplicate x-rays so originals do not have to leave the office

Composition   **A.** Duplicating machine consists of:
- Box with a light
- Glass plate on which to place the original x-rays and then the duplicating film
- Controls for exposure time
- Switch to turn the light on when placing original x-rays and then off to place duplicating film
- Latch to secure the lid during exposure

B. Duplicating dental film
- Available in a variety of sizes
- Can be processed manually or with an automatic processor

Notes
- Duplicating film must be handled under safelight conditions.
- Duplication films are sent with insurance claims and to dental specialty offices when a patient is referred for treatment.
- Duplication films are also used in legal cases, such as malpractice suits or accident cases.

INDEX